Cure and Vaccine, Striking Back at COVID-19

Cure and Vaccine, Striking Back at COVID-19

Lane B. Scheiber II, MD
Lane B. Scheiber, ScD

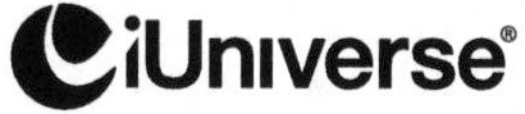

CURE AND VACCINE, STRIKING BACK AT COVID-19

All illustrations were created by Lane B. Scheiber II, MD

iUniverse books may be ordered through booksellers or by contacting:

iUniverse
1663 Liberty Drive
Bloomington, IN 47403
www.iuniverse.com
844-349-9409

ISBN: 978-1-6632-0839-2 (sc)
ISBN: 978-1-6632-0840-8 (e)

Print information available on the last page.

iUniverse rev. date: 09/30/2020

Changing the Global Approach to Medicine, Volume 6

Hunter-Killer Polypeptides to eradicate infectious pathogens.

Intelligent IF-THEN mRNA Directed pharmaceuticals to treat cancers, OA, inflammatory arthritis and modifying genetic disorders. Polyvalent mRNA vaccines.

VIReSOFT Developers of Embedded DNA Vaccines, Molecular Virus Killers, Medically Therapeutic RNA Vector Technologies, Quantum Gene, Executable Gene, Genetic Reference Tables, Prime Genome, Prime Genomic Cube, Genomic Keycode, Essential-Equation-4-Life, Dandelion Rift, the Tritron, the Quadsitron, Quadsitron-Energy Connectivity, the Quadsistor, Fourth Generation Biologics and Molecular Gene Activators, Theory of the Quadsitron Ether, Theory to Unify GLEAM2 (Gravity, Light, Electrons, Atoms, Molecules, Magnetism), Doreen Lightspeed Interstellar Gravity Hypercoil Turbine (DORELIGHT) Engines.

MedStar Labs, Inc.

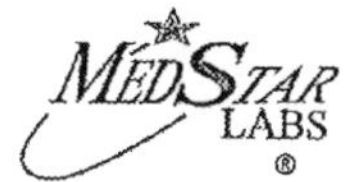

At the time of copyright, the authors believed the novel concepts presented herein to be unique and different from prior art. All figures are meant to be illustrative concepts of otherwise sometimes very complex structures. The novel therapies presented in the text represent medically therapeutic concepts and have not been fully tested. The outcomes of providing such therapies to treat a medical condition is unknown at the time of this writing and requires additional study and testing. This text is intended for educational and entertainment purposes. This text is not intended to take the place of a physician's evaluation or a physician's advice regarding any medical condition. It is recommended the reader consult their physician before starting any medication for any medical condition. All medications have potential side effects. Healthcare providers should be familiar with current prescribing information before prescribing medications; patients should review the latest prescribing information and possible side effects before taking any medication.

The authors apologize for the spelling mistakes and grammatical errors which may be lurking in the pages of this text; the world is in crisis and it was felt the material content was possibly worth more than the missing of a spelling mistake or a grammatical error or just an unglamorous writing style. This is not our daytime job, this is what we pursue in our spare time. Though, I do recall my college freshmen English teacher flat out failing (F) our papers, if we had just three spelling errors (in the days before spell-check software); bless her heart, such an exercise did help drill in the importance of spelling words correctly. I hope your final critique won't be so harsh, in this time of urgency. Thank you for your understanding.

PRIOR ART

DNA VACCINES, Courier Gene Technology
Changing the Global Approach to Medicine Series, Volume 5, 2017
by Lane B. Scheiber II, MD and Lane B. Scheiber, ScD

FOURTH GENERATION BIOLOGICS: Molecular Virus Killers
Changing the Global Approach to Medicine Series, Volume 4, 2014
by Lane B. Scheiber II, MD and Lane B. Scheiber, ScD

CHANGING THE GLOBAL APPROACH TO MEDICINE, Volume 3, 2012
Cellular Command and Control
Also introducing the Prime Genome and the Tritron
by Lane B. Scheiber II, MD and Lane B. Scheiber, ScD

CHANGING THE GLOBAL APPROACH TO MEDICINE, Volume 2, 2011
Medical Vector Therapy
Also introducing the Quantum Gene and the Quadsistor
by Lane B. Scheiber II, MD and Lane B. Scheiber, ScD

CHANGING THE GLOBAL APPROACH TO MEDICINE, Volume 1, 2009
New Perspectives on Treating AIDS, Diabetes, Obesity, Aging, Heart Attacks, Stroke, and Cancer
by Lane B. Scheiber II, MD and Lane B. Scheiber, ScD

THE THEORY OF QUADSITRON-ENERGY CONNECTIVITY,
by Lane B. Scheiber II, MD and Lane B. Scheiber, ScD

IMMORTALITY: QUATERNARY MEDICINE CODE
by Anthony Scheiber

CURSE OF THE SNOW DRAGON
by Anthony Scheiber

THE HUMAN COMPUTER
by Anthony Scheiber

EARTH PRO: The Rings of Sol
by Anthony Scheiber

DEDICATION

Thanks to our wives, Karin and Mary Jane,
for all of their love and support, without which these
efforts could never have been accomplished,...
and we hope to make the world better for Adaline.

ACKNOWLEDGEMENT

The authors would like to honor the dedication and hard work put in by all of the scientists and healthcare providers whom provided the genetic information regarding the coronavirus genome and human genes, which has made access to such data through the NCBI website feasible and accessible. Combating the horrific threat of the coronavirus takes a worldwide effort and collaboration of knowledge from many sources in order to arrive at a practical solution to combat this viral pandemic, which threatens the health and well-being of the entire world. Thank you to all of the researchers who have made the study of human genetics and the analysis of coronavirus and other pathogens possible.

FOREWORD

None of the principle concepts presented in the text

have been proven to date, but when faced

with an unprecedented global crisis, ...

the effort has to start somewhere,

in order to devise and craft,

a novel and decisive solution

to halt such

a catastrophic problem.

Like the saying goes, sometimes you have to
crack some eggs to make an omelette.

INTRODUCTION

The world is on fire. Coronavirus has actively mutated over the past two decades into a virulent form, capable of circumventing the human immune system's security defense systems and threatening the lives of people of every race. COVID-19 has created a pandemic of global proportions. This virus has spread through the population to every corner of the planet. Infection results in approximately a 20% morbidity rate requiring hospitalization and has been leaving in its wake a 2.5-5% kill rate.

To battle this global threat, governments have implemented lockdowns of those communities infected with the virus. Medicine has reacted by attempting to update the 1770's technology of generating a vaccine to combat coronavirus. The coronavirus has effectively evolved into a global humanitarian threat due to the virus's capacity to mutate. Coronavirus carries within the viral genetic code its own replication machinery. The coding for the replication machinery takes up 20,000 bits of information of the virus's approximately 29,900 bits of genetic code. This means the virus does not have to rely on the human cell's reproduction mechanisms to become active, replicate copies of itself and spread. The virus's replication machinery is effective in making copies, but at the same time tends to create errors in those copies, which leads to frequent mutations to the coronavirus's genetic code.

Coronavirus uses the 'S' protein, often referred to as the 'spike' protein, to locate human cells to infect. The 'S' protein is mounted on the surface of the virion, the vessel which carries the virus's genetic code from cell to cell. The 'S' protein is used by the virus's virion to locate the ACE2 receptor on a human cell. Once the spike protein makes contact with an ACE2 receptor, the virion knows it has found a human cell. The virion burrows a hole through the cell membrane and inserts the virus's genetic code into the interior of the human cell. Upon reaching the cytoplasm of a human cell, the virus's genetic code becomes activated and utilizes the resources of energy and materials in the victimized cell to generate copies of itself.

Vaccines developed against viruses tend to react to a particular target, associated with the specific virus, the vaccine is designed to combat. Influenza, a seasonal virus which has an annual lethal rate of 36,000 people in the U.S., mutates frequently. The influenza virus vaccine, provided on an annual basis, requires updating every year in order to try to keep up with the alterations the virus makes to its structure. Unfortunately, the vaccines are generated using the model of the virus from the prior year, so often the vaccine is not fully effective due to the current vaccine does not take into account the changes the virus may have made from one year to the next. The 2018-19 flu shot was 29% effective; the 2019-2020 flu shot reported in February 2020 to be 45% effective per the Center for Disease Control.

If the coronavirus continues to mutate and subsequent copies evolve with substantial alterations to the spike protein, then the current vaccine development may fall short of protecting the population. At the time of this writing, there is at least one variation found in the coronavirus's spike protein which has already developed; variation between the Wuhan and Moscow versions of the spike protein.

There are a whole host of aggressive, harmful viruses found across the world. Some of these viruses which result in severe illnesses in humans include Human Immunodeficiency Virus (HIV), West Nile virus, Dengue Fever virus, Zika virus, Chikungunya virus. There are approximately 219 viral species which are capable of infecting humans.[1] The first discovered was Yellow Fever in 1901. The most well-known and likely the most dreaded is Ebolavirus, given how much this pathogen has been publicized over the years in movies and the media.

The shortcomings revealed by the current coronavirus pandemic point directly to the fact that we need a new means to combat lethal viruses and viral infections in general. Social distancing is effective, but only to a certain point. Though necessary, masks are difficult to wear all of the time, and limit our freedom and individual expression. As we have painfully seen, economies grind to a halt when people are mandated to avoid interactions with others and stay home. Traditional vaccine development is often slow and may not be fully effective as a virus alters its genetic state. In essence, we need to take the fight directly to the virus, deploying a versatile pernicious solution to stop lethal viruses from replicating inside their host cell.

There have been efforts developed over the years to take the fight to infectious viral pathogens. Extensive research has led to a detailed understanding the life-cycle of a number of viruses. Efforts have been contrived to rob certain viruses of their cellular means to complete their life cycle. Agents which inhibit viral replication have been notably developed for HIV and Hepatitis C, which have been very successful. Such viral inhibiting agents have taken significant time to develop, and are often virus specific.

Messenger ribonucleic acid therapy appears to be a promising new approach to not only treating viral infections, but managing many of the difficult medical conditions which currently challenge the medical profession. Here we explore the use of this novel approach, by discussing the topic of crafting mRNA therapies into new medical management tools. First, is to generate a new age of novel hunter-killer proteins specifically designed to be deployed as a cure to combat global pathogens such as COVID-19. Second, is a mRNA based single valent and a revolutionary polyvalent vaccine to protect the population from widespread infection. Both approaches can be easily adapted to thwart future pandemics.

KEY ELEMENTS FOR DISCUSSION

1. **The Threat:** Coronavirus, like computer viruses, is simply bits of information strung together, a little more than 29,900 nucleotides in length, capable of wielding devastating havoc, but instead of hacking computer networks, or laptops or cell phones, COVID-19's target are the ACE2 receptor bearing cells of the human body.

2. **The Vaccine:** Utilize the construct of a CD8 cell surface receptor mRNA, replace the nucleotide coding for the native CD8 cell surface receptor with the nucleotide coding for the COVID-19 'S' probe.

3. **The Cure:** Modify a native human Transcription Factor IIIA polypeptide to seek out, attach and bind to the uracil tail of the negative-sense genome of the coronavirus. Then modify the human Transcription Factor IIIA mRNA to code for this therapeutic Transcription Factor IIIA polypeptide, a protein which is capable of binding to the negative-sense tail of the coronavirus's genome and preventing the virus from replicating, thus neutralizing the infectious nature of COVID-19 and possibly all of the variations of coronavirus.

4. **IF-THEN Intelligent mRNA Pharmaceuticals:** Utilizing the 'AND' codon command of 'UAA', placed strategically in an mRNA to generate versatile mRNA pharmaceuticals, which can generate multiple differing polypeptides and react to differing intracellular environments, delivering a variable, but calculated very effective medical therapeutic response.

THE STRATEGY

To truly, proactively eradicate a viral pandemic, the combined effects of a hunter-killer protein to target and neutralize the virus in infected patients, and a versatile vaccine to prevent healthy people from becoming infected by a pathogen which is continuously modifying itself, need to be brought to bear against such a threat.

STEPS NEEDED TO DEVELOP A CURE TO STOP COVID-19:

1. Determine unique RNA target.
2. Select a molecule to bind to RNA.
3. Develop an algorithm for bonding amino acids to nucleotides.
4. Modification to bonding molecule to create a hunter-killer protein.
5. Package hunter-killer protein.
6. Devise delivery system.

CONTENTS

CHAPTER ONE

VITALS OF RNA AND DNA

BACKGROUND ART

The central dogma of microbiology dictates that inside the nucleus of a cell, genes are transcribed to produce messenger ribonucleic acid (mRNA) molecules, these mRNAs migrate to the cytoplasm where they are translated to produce proteins.

Human genetics is comprised of deoxyribonucleic acid (DNA) separated into 46 chromosomes. The chromosomes are further subdivided into genes. Genes represent units of transcribable DNA. Transcription of the DNA refers to generating one or more forms of ribonucleic acid (RNA) molecules. Transcribable genetic information thus represents the segments of DNA that when transcribed by transcription machinery yield RNA molecules. The nontranscribable genetic information represent segments of DNA that act as either points of attachment for the transcription machinery, or act as commands to direct the transcription machinery, or act as spacers between transcribable segments of genetic information, or have no known function at this time.

When a gene is to be transcribed, approximately forty to seventy proteins (transcription factors) assemble together into what is referred to as a transcription complex, which acts as the transcription machinery. The proteins comprising the transcription complex combine in an area surrounding a segment of DNA either upstream (in the direction of the 5' end of the DNA) from the start of the transcribable genetic information or immediately downstream from the starting point of transcription (transcription start site (TSS)). As a unit, the proteins that comprise the transcription complex attach to the DNA. The transcription complex transcribes the genetic information to produce RNA. It is vital to the cell that the transcription complex is able to locate a specific gene amongst the 3 billion base pairs (bp) comprising the human genome in an orderly and efficient manner to enable the cell to transcribe the proper genes to produce the necessary proteins to perform functions the cell requires to operate, survive, grow and replicate.

For purposes of this text there are several general definitions. A 'ribose' is a five carbon or pentose sugar ($C_5H_{10}O_5$) present in the structural components of ribonucleic acid, riboflavin, and other nucleotides and nucleosides. A 'deoxyribose' is a deoxypentose ($C_5H_{10}O_4$) found in deoxyribonucleic acid. A 'nucleoside' is a compound of a sugar usually ribose or deoxyribose with a nitrogenous base by way of an N-glycosyl link. A 'nucleotide' is a single unit of a nucleic acid, composed of a five-carbon sugar (either a ribose or a deoxyribose), a nitrogenous base and a phosphate group. There are two families of 'nitrogenous bases', which include: pyrimidine and purine. A 'pyrimidine' is a six-member ring made up of carbon and nitrogen atoms; the members of the pyrimidine family include: cytosine (C), thymine (T) and uracil (U). A 'purine' is a five-member ring fused to a pyrimidine type ring; the members of the purine family include: adenine (A) and guanine (G).

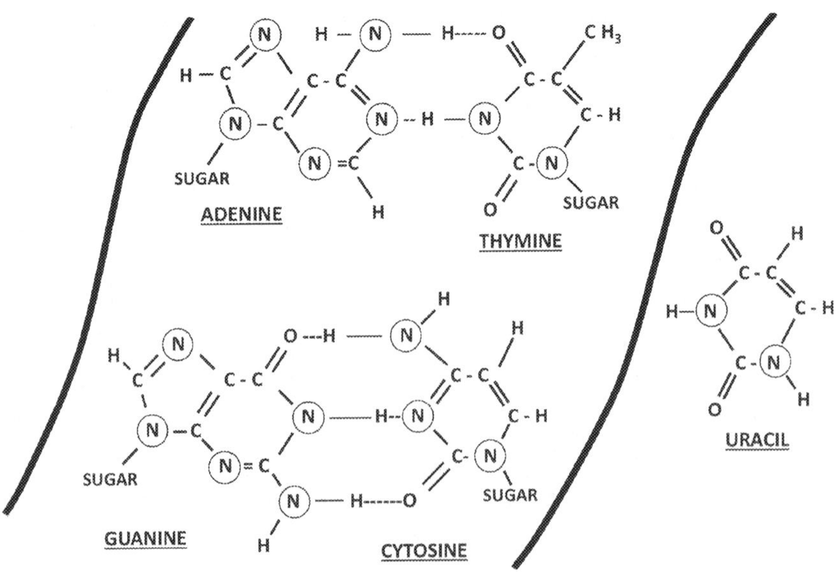

Figure 1

Nucleotides: adenine, cytosine, guanine, thymine, uracil.

The five bases are cytosine (C), thymine (T) and uracil (U), adenine (A) and guanine (G). The differing nucleotides are often referred to by the name of their nitrogenous base. The nucleotide names are technically derived from the base combined with the sugar which are referred to a nucleoside, which when added to a phosphate group is a nucleotide. The five standard nucleosides are cytidine (C), thymidine (T), uridine (U), adenosine (A), and guanosine (G). The nitrogenous base name and nucleoside name for each nucleotide are often used interchangeably with equal authority in the medical literature when referring to a nucleotide.[2,3,4,5,6,7] A 'nucleic acid' refers to a polynucleotide, which is a biologic molecule such as ribonucleic acid or deoxyribonucleic acid, that provides the means for coded genetic information to reproduce organisms. Ribonucleic acid and deoxyribonucleic acid are comprised of chains of nucleotides.[3,6,7,8]

A 'deoxyribose' is a deoxypentose ($C_5H_{10}O_4$) sugar. Deoxyribonucleic acid (DNA) is comprised of molecular subunits comprised of three basic elements: a deoxyribose sugar, a phosphate group and nitrogen containing bases. DNA is a macromolecule made up of two chains of repeating deoxyribose sugars linked by phosphodiester bonds between the 3-hydroxyl group of one and the 5-hydroxyl group of the next; the two chains are held antiparallel to each other by weak hydrogen bonds. DNA strands contain a sequence of nucleotides, these nucleotides are generally referred to by their nitrogenous bases, which include: adenine, cytosine, guanine and thymine. Adenine is always paired with thymine of the opposite strand, and guanine is always paired with cytosine of the opposite strand; one side or strand of a DNA macromolecule is the mirror image, or also referred to as the complement, of the opposing strand. A base pair (bp) refers to a single pair of nucleotides. Nuclear DNA resides in the nucleus of a cell and is regarded as the medium for storing the master plan of hereditary information.

A gene is considered a segment of base pairs of the DNA that represent a unit of inheritance. A gene is transcribed to produce ribonucleic acid (RNA).

A 'ribonucleic acid' (RNA) is a linear polymer of nucleotides formed by repeated riboses linked by phosphodiester bonds between the 3-hydroxyl group of one and the 5-hydroxyl group of the next. RNAs are a single strand macromolecule comprised of a sequence of nucleotides, these nucleotides are generally referred to by their nitrogenous bases, which include: adenine, cytosine, guanine or uracil. Various forms of RNA exist including messenger RNA (mRNA), ribosomal RNA (rRNA), transport RNA (tRNA), and small command RNAs.

It should be noted, by convention the nucleotides are generally written in lower case lettering. In addition, though DNAs are comprised of the four nucleotides adenine, cytosine, guanine, and thymine, and RNAs are comprised of the four nucleotides adenine, cytosine, guanine, and uracil, when writing out the nucleotide code for an RNA the symbolism for DNA is often used in reference sources. Thus, when writing out an RNA sequence, the nucleotides adenine (a), cytosine (c), guanine (g), and thymine (t) are commonly utilized, even though technically the nucleotide uracil (u) should be used instead of thymine. Physically, the mRNA structure as it exists in Nature is comprised of the nucleotides adenine (a), cytosine (c), guanine (g) and uracil (u).

CHAPTER TWO

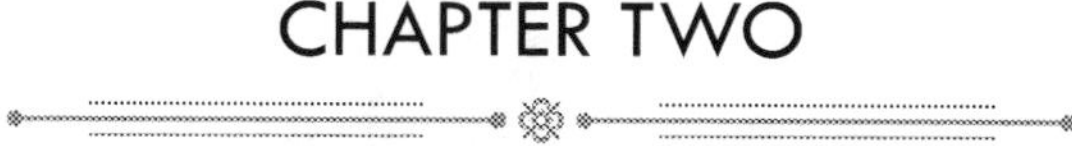

AMINO ACID BASICS

Proteins, also referred to as polypeptides, are comprised of a string of amino acids. There are 20 different amino acids, which are used to generate human proteins. The process of translation creates polypeptides comprised of a specific sequence of amino acids as dictated by the protein generating template carried by mRNA.[5,6]

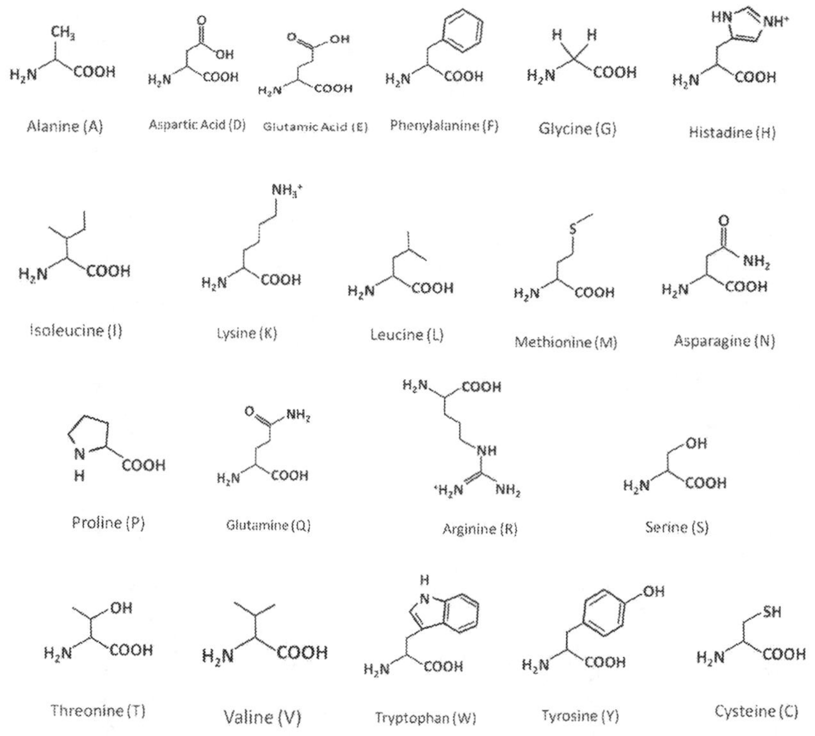

Alanine (A) Aspartic Acid (D) Glutamic Acid (E) Phenylalanine (F) Glycine (G) Histadine (H)

Isoleucine (I) Lysine (K) Leucine (L) Methionine (M) Asparagine (N)

Proline (P) Glutamine (Q) Arginine (R) Serine (S)

Threonine (T) Valine (V) Tryptophan (W) Tyrosine (Y) Cysteine (C)

Figure 2

Structure of the twenty amino acids, the building blocks of life.

Typically, an amino acid is an organic molecule composed of an amine group (-NH_2) attached to a carbon atom which is attached to a carboxyl group (-COOH), which is attached to a side group termed the 'R' group. The 'R' group generally is what is different therefore specific between the amino acids. There are approximately 500 amino acids found in Nature. Twenty different amino acids are coded for in human genetic code and thus can be used to construct protein molecules throughout the human body.

Common amino acid symbol abbreviations as described below in Table 1 are used throughout this discussion:

Inverse table using IUPAC notation.

Amino Acid	Three Letter Abbreviation	One Letter Abbreviation	RNA Nucleotide Codon Codes	DNA Nucleotide Codon Codes
Alanine	Ala	A	GCU, GCC, GCA, GCG	GCT, GCC, GCA, GCG
Arginine	Arg	R	CGU, CGC, CGA, CGG, AGA, AGG	CGT, CGC, CGA, CGG, AGA, AGG
Asparagine	Asn	N	AAU, AAC	AAT, AAC
Aspartic acid	Asp	D	GAU, GAC	GAT, GAC
Cysteine	Cys	C	UGU, UGC	TGT, TGC
Glutamine	Gln	Q	CAA, CAG	CAA, CAG
Glutamic acid	Glu	E	GAA, GAG	GAA, GAG
Glycine	Gly	G	GGU, GGC, GGA, GGG	GGT, GGC, GGA, GGG
Histidine	His	H	CAU, CAC	CAT, CAC
Isoleucine	Ile	I	AUU, AUC, AUA	ATT, ATC, ATA
Leucine	Leu	L	UUA, UUG, CUU, CUC, CUA, CUG	TTA, TTG, CTT, CTC, CTA, CTG
Lysine	Lys	K	AAA, AAG	AAA, AAG
Methionine	Met	M	AUG	ATG
Phenylalanine	Phe	F	UUU, UUC	TTT, TTC
Proline	Pro	P	CCU, CCC, CCA, CCG	CCT, CCC, CCA, CCG
Serine	Ser	S	UCU, UCC, UCA	TCT, TCC, TCA
Threonine	Thr	T	ACU, ACC, ACA, ACG	ACT, ACC, ACA, ACG

Amino Acid	Three Letter Abbreviation	One Letter Abbreviation	RNA Nucleotide Codon Codes	DNA Nucleotide Codon Codes
Tryptophan	Typ	W	UGG	TGG
Tyrosine	Tyr	Y	UAU, UAC	TAT, TAC
Valine	Val	V	GUU, GUC, GUA, GUG	GTT, GTC, GTA, GTG
START	---	---	AUG	ATG
STOP	---	---	UAA, UGA, UAG	TAA, TGA, TAG

Table 1
Amino acid coding.

Notation: IUPAC, International Union of Pure Chemistry and Applied Chemistry at www.IUPAC.org.

Nature uses biologic software code comprised of groupings of three nucleotides, referred to as the 'codon code', to represent amino acids. Proteins, often referred to as polypeptides, are constructed by ribosomes, complexes which string amino acids together. Ribosome protein building machinery is located in the cytoplasm of a cell. Ribosomes translate (decode) mRNAs by deciphering the codon code and stringing amino acids together into linear chains arranged in the order dictated by the consecutive construct of the mRNA nucleotide sequencing.

CHAPTER THREE

KNOWING THE THREAT: THE STRUCTURE OF THE CORONAVIRUS

Coronavirus has been present for at least twenty years.

5′	Location																3′	Virus
Rep 1a		Rep 1b	---	---	S	3a	3b	---	---	---	E	M	---	---	---	---	N	---	HoV-229E
Rep 1a		Rep 1b	2a	HE	S	---	---	4	---	5a	E	M	---	---	---	---	N (I)	---	MHV
Rep 1a		Rep 1b	---	---	S	3a	3b	---	---	---	E	M	5a 5b	6	7a 7b	8a 8b	N (9b)	---	SARS-CoV
Rep 1a		Rep 1b	---	---	S	3	--	4a	4b	5	E	M	---	---	---	---	N (8b)	---	MERS-CoV
Rep 1a		Rep 1b	---	---	S	3a	3b	---	---	---	E	M	5a 5b	---	---	---	N	---	IBV
Orflab nsp1 leader protein nsp2 nsp3 proteinase nsp4 (TM2) nsp5 3C proteinase nsp6 transmembrn nsp7 nsp8 nsp9 ssRNA bind pr nsp10 growth-factor nsp12 RdRp nsp13 helicase nsp14 exonuclease nsp15 endoRNAse nsp16 2'-O-MT nsp16	1-265 266-805 806-2719 2720-8554 8555-10054 10055-10972 10973-11842 11843-12091 12092-12685 12686-13024 13025-13441 13442-13468 13468-16236 16237-18039 18040-19620 19621-20658 20659-21552	---	---	---	S	Orf 3a	---	---	---	---	E	M	---	Orf 6	Orf 7a 7b	Orf 8	N (9)	Orf 10	**2019-nCoVid 1-29,903 Wuhan-Hu-1 ncbi.nlm** NC: 045512.2 28Jan20

Table 2
Comparison of various coronavirus genomes.

There have been a number of versions of coronavirus genome identified in the last twenty years.[8,9] Table 2 demonstrates six versions of coronavirus and compares the subsegments comprising their genomes. The six versions of coronavirus listed in Table 2 include: Human Coronavirus 229E (HoV 229E), Mouse Hepatitis Virus Coronavirus (MHV), Severe Acute Respiratory Syndrome Coronavirus (SARS-CoV), Middle East Respiratory syndrome related coronavirus (MERS-CoV), Avian coronavirus (IBV), 2019-nCoVid. Each of the coronavirus entities has had a slightly different composition to the viral genome. The latest version, Severe Acute Respiratory Syndrome Coronavirus-2 (SARS-CoV-2), also previously called 2019-nCoVid, most recently referred to as COVID-19, is comprised of nonstructural proteins 1-16, S, 3a, E, M, 6, 7a, 7b, 8, N, 10. The front end of the COVID-19 genome positive sense from 5' to 3' starting at nucleotide 266 through 21552, assist the virus in replicating. From nucleotides 21563 to 29674 are considered structural proteins and effector instructions. The 'S' protein is coded between 21563-25384.

5' END	1-265
nonstructural protein 1 (nsp1) leader protein	266-805
nsp2	806-2719
nsp3 proteinase	2720-8554
nsp4 transmembrane 2 (TM2)	8555-10054
nsp5 3C proteinase	10055-10972
nsp6 transmembrane	10973-11842
nsp7	11843-12091
nsp8	12092-12685
nsp9 ssRNA binding protein	12686-13024
nsp10 growth-factor	13025-13441
nsp12 RNA dependent RNA polymerase (RdRp)	13442-13468
	13468-16236
nsp13 helicase	16237-18039
nsp14 exonuclease	18040-19620
nsp15 endoRNAse	19621-20658
nsp16 2'-O-MT (methyltransferase function)	20659-21552
nsp16	
(+11)	
S (spike protein)	21563-25384
(+9)	
3a	25393-26220
(+25)	

E	26245-26472
(+51)	
M	26523-27191
(+196)	
6	27202-27387
7a + 7b	27394-27759
8	27756-27887
(+15)	
N (9)	28274-29533
(+25)	
10	29558-29674
3' END (+229)	29675-29903

Table 3
Breakdown of the COVID-19 viral genome.

COVID-19's genome is broken down in Table 3. This is based off the Wuhan-Hu-1 version of coronavirus. The genome of Wuhan-Hu-1 is found at the NCBI website.[10]

COVID-19 genome is carried inside a transport vehicle referred to as a virion. See Figure 3. The transport vehicle is comprised of a protein shell to protect the viral genome concealed inside the inner chamber of the virion. The transport vehicle has the 'S' or spike protein mounted on the surface of the virion. This 'S' protein is used as a probe to seek out an appropriate host cell, which will facilitate replication of copies of the virus. The 'S' protein probe seeks an angiotensin-converting-enzyme 2 (ACE2) receptor on a human cell as the target it is searching for in the human body. Once the 'S' protein probe bind to and ACE2 receptor, the virion injects the viral genome cargo it carries into the target host cell.

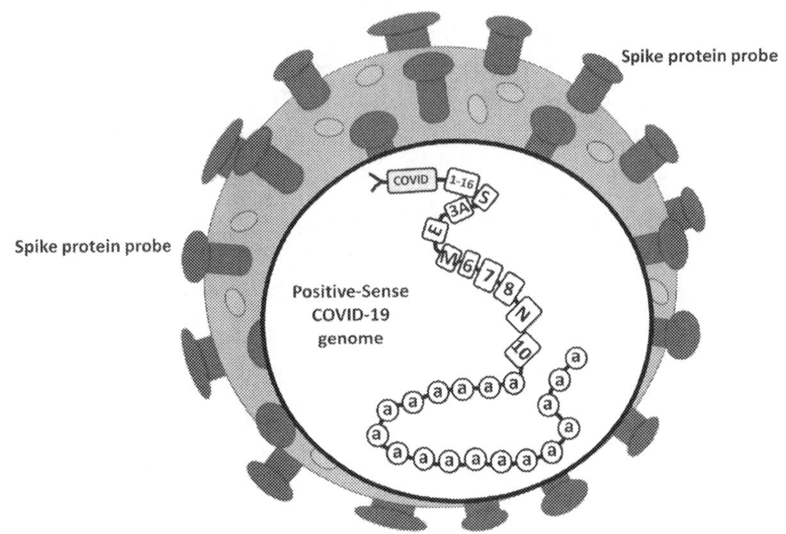

Figure 3
Coronavirus virion with positive-sense genome.

The life-cycle of the coronavirus involves intercepting a human cell with an ACE2 cell surface receptor, entering the cell, replicating the genetics and virion, then being released by the victimized cell to venture off and infect another cell to repeat the process.[11,12] See Figure 4. The coronavirus's genetic code is injected into the cell as a positive-sense RNA. The COVID-19 genetic code is translated as a positive-sense mRNA genome. The positive-sense genome is then converted to a negative-sense genome to facilitate making copies of the genome in order to replicate the virus. The negative-sense genome is the complement of the positive-sense genome. The structural proteins are generated using the host cell's bio-machinery. The structural proteins are combined into a virion and the replicated copies of the positive-sense single stranded viral genome are inserted into the replica virions. The completed copies of the virus are inserted into a vacuole. The viral virions are then released from the storage vacuole into the extracellular environment to seek out and infect other host cells in order to continue the life-cycle process of coronavirus.

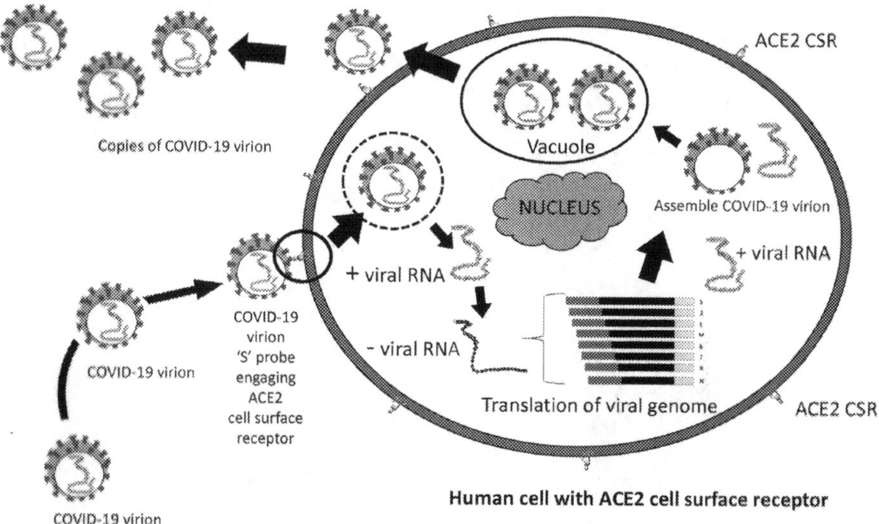

Figure 4
Life-cycle of the COVID-19

Coronavirus is a positive-sense RNA virus. Inside the virion, the viral genome is carried as the positive-sense of the viral genome to be transported from host cell to host cell. A positive-sense single stranded RNA can serve directly as a messenger ribonucleic acid (mRNA), be read by the host cell's ribosomes, and be translated to produce proteins. Positive RNA viruses make up a large number of known human viruses including hepatitis C, West Nile virus, Dengue Fever virus, SARS, MERS, and COVID-19. Rhinovirus which is responsible for the common cold is also a positive-sense virus.

As with most mRNAs, coronavirus possesses an adenine tail. The adenine tail at the 3' terminal end of an mRNA dictates to the ribosomes reading and decoding the codon code of the mRNA, the number of times to repeat the translation process. If there are 15 adenines at the 3' end of an mRNA, the strip of RNA genetic code will be translated 15 times. The COVID-19 viral positive-sense genetic code has 33 adenine nucleotides positioned at the 3' terminal end. See Figure 5.

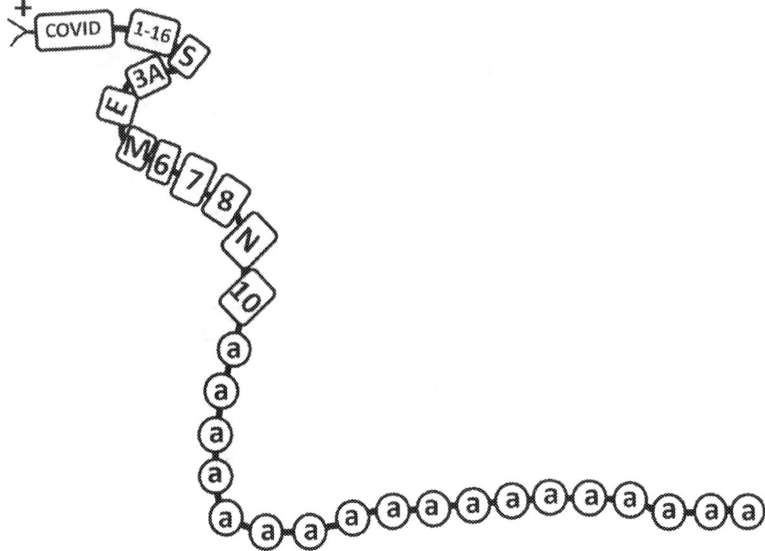

Figure 5

Positive Sense version of the COVID-19 virus.

In the life-cycle of COVID-19 the viral genome changes from the positive-sense RNA, which is the original form delivered to the host cell, to a negative-sense version of the viral genome. When a viral genome transforms from positive-sense to negative-sense, the adenine (a) nucleotides each are converted to thymine (t), cytosines (c) are converted to guanines (g), then guanines (g) are converted to cytosines (c) and thymines (t) are converted to adenines (a). Since in DNA, adenine always binds to thymine, and cytosine always binds to guanine, the negative-sense version of a positive-sense single stranded RNA virus is like the mirror image of the viral genome.

The interesting phenomenon which occurs with respect to COVID-19 genome, is that where the tail of the positive-sense version of the genome possesses a tail of 33 adenine nucleotides, the mirror image negative-sense version would then possess a tail of 33 thymine nucleotides. See Figure 6. Since native mRNAs all have an adenine tail, a lengthy string of thymine nucleotides seen in the negative-sense coronavirus genome is an unusual finding in the cytoplasm of the host cell.

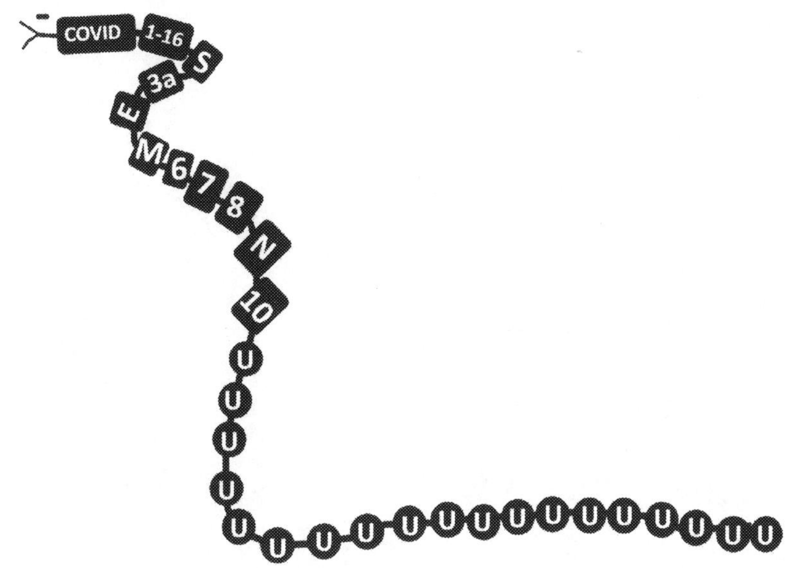

Figure 6
Covid-19 negative-sense genome.

Within the DNA, there may exist long stretches of thymine nucleotides. In the cytoplasm, there will be segments of continuous thymine nucleotides, but generally not nearly to the length of what would be seen in the tail of the negative-sense COVID-19 genome. Given the uniqueness of a long uracil tail in the cytoplasm, this phenomena in the life-cycle of the coronavirus is possibly a high-value target specific to COVID-19 and could be capitalized upon as a therapeutic target to neutralize COVID-19 in an infected host cell.

CHAPTER FOUR

TAKING THE FIGHT DIRECTLY TO COVID-19 WITH A MODIFIED TFIIIA POLYPEPTIDE

Knowing your threat is half the battle when waging war against an adversary whom is comprising your life-style, freedom and very existence. The other half the battle is deriving a scheme by which one can neutralize the hazard imposed by an adversary. Determining a means to neutralize the COVID-19 pandemic requires detailed analysis of the virus's genome and life-cycle in order to arrive at a strategy to subdue the danger posed by such a complicated threat.

The chilling realization is that to defeat coronavirus, one has to take the fight directly to the virus. One has to develop a solution which engages the virus directly in the environment where the virus replicates and stop the viral genome from making copies of itself. This strategy has been employed with a few viruses, such as Hepatis C, by blocking virus specific proteins, required by the virus to replicate. Often though, viruses use the same machinery as the human cell and therefore there may not be a specific viral protein which can be targeted without causing widespread interference in native cell's metabolism. In the process of deriving an anti-viral therapy, the obvious objective is to create a means to fight an infection with minimum side effects to patients.

Broadening the perspective of defense against viral infections, one could employ a native protein to engage and neutralize a specific part of the virus's genome. Wuhan-Hu-1 coronavirus has a genome consisting of 29,903 nucleotides; the number of nucleotides varies depending upon the version of the virus being studied. Locating a segment of the coronavirus's genome which is specific to the coronavirus and not otherwise seen in other native RNAs in a host cell, would be key to deriving a means of neutralizing the virus, without causing side effects to the patient.

Transcription factors generally either regulate decoding of the genetic information stored in DNA or combine together and form complexes which transcribe the DNA to produce messenger RNAs (mRNAs). In some instances, it takes the combination of 72 different transcription factor proteins to assemble together into a transcription complex, in order for a segment of DNA to be read and an mRNA to be generated. Of the 72 proteins which assemble to form a transcription complex, a few of the transcription factor proteins will interact directly with the DNA, while most of the transcription factors will simply interact with each other to build the transcription machinery.

Transcription Factor IIIA (TFIIIA) is one of the transcription factor proteins which interacts with the DNA. Certain amino acids comprising the TFIIIA protein temporarily bind to specific nucleotides found in certain gene segments of the DNA. Since TFIIIA is a protein derived from an mRNA in the cytoplasm of the cell, it would seem reasonable that modification of the design of the native TFIIIA protein, by recoding the amino acids which bind to the DNA to a specific code to target coronavirus would offer a means to engage COVID-19 directly, inside infected human cells. A modified TFIIIA would allow humans to constructively and proactively take the battle directly to the virus inside the cells which have been infected.

CHAPTER FIVE

STRUCTURE OF THE NATIVE TFIIIA POLYPEPTIDE

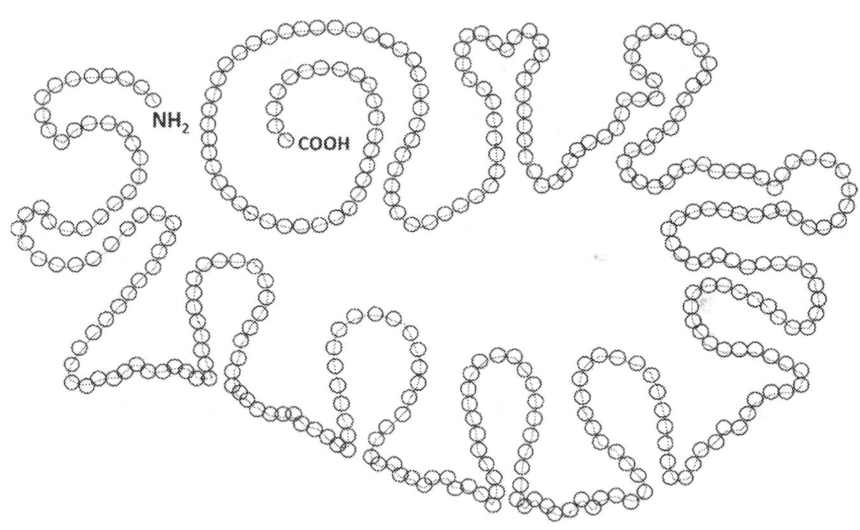

Figure 7

Illustration of 365 amino acids comprising Transcription Factor IIIA.

The following three hundred sixty-five amino acid sequence comprises the Transcription Factor III A molecule, Taxonomic identifier 9606 [NCBI]:

```
1          10         20         30         40         50         60
MDPPAVVAES VSSLTIADAF IAAGESSAPT PPRPALPRRF ICSFPDCSAN YSKAWKLDAH
        70         80         90        100        110        120
LCKHTGERPF VCDYEGCGKA FIRDYHLSRH ILTHTGEKPF VCAANGCDQK FNTKSNLKKH
       130        140        150        160        170        180
```

```
FERKHENQQK QYICSFEDCK KTFKKHQQLK IHQCQHTNEP LFKCTQEGCG KHFASPSKLK
       190        200        210        220        230        240
RHAKAHEGYV CQKGCSFVAK TWTELLKHVR ETHKEEILCE VCRKTFKRKD YLKQHMKTHA
       250        260        270        280        290        300
PERDVCRCPR EGCGRTYTTV FNLQSHILSF HEESRPFVCE HAGCGKTFAM KQSLTRHAVV
       310        320        330        340        350        360
HDPDKKKMKL KVKKSREKRS LASHLSGYIP PKRKQGQGLS LCQNGESPNC VEDKMLSTVA
  365
VLTLG
```

The TFIIIA 9606 is utilized naturally by a human cell to assist in the transcription of 5S RNA molecules.

The TFIIIA protein is comprised of nine zinc fingers. All nine zinc fingers may attach to the DNA in some situation. The fourth, fifth, sixth and seventh finger from 5- to the 3' end of the molecule may attach to an RNA molecule. The eighth zinc finger may attach at times to a TFIIIC molecule. The ninth zinc finger may attach at times to TFIIID molecule.

The TFIIIA 9606 is utilized naturally by a human cell to assist in the transcription of 5S RNA molecules. The TFIIIA molecule also assists in transcribing some viral DNA genomes

The following is taken from the NCBI website and represents how the gene which is responsible for the construct of the Transcription Factor III A molecule (Taxonomic identifier 9606 [NCBI])[13,14,15] is described:

```
FEATURES             Location/Qualifiers
     source          1..11166
                     /organism="Homo sapiens"
                     /mol _type="genomic DNA"
                     /db _xref="taxon:9606"
                     /chromosome="13"
     gene            1..11166
                     /gene="GTF3A"
                     /gene _synonym="AP2; TFIIIA"
                     /note="general transcription factor IIIA;
                     Derived by automated computational analysis
                     using gene prediction method: BestRefSeq."
                     /db _xref="GeneID:2971"
                     /db _xref="HGNC:HGNC:4662"
                     /db _xref="MIM:600860"
```

```
mRNA            join(1..395,2549..2649,5327..5423,5990..6078,8188
                ..8261, 9596..9676,10262..10491,10590..10649,1089
                0..11166)
                /gene="GTF3A"
                /gene _synonym="AP2; TFIIIA"
                /product="general transcription factor IIIA"
                /note="Derived by automated computational
                analysis using gene prediction method:
                BestRefSeq."
                /transcript _id="NM  002097.2"
                /db _xref="GI:166063994"
                /db _xref="GeneID:2971"
                /db _xref="HGNC:HGNC:4662"
                /db _xref="MIM:600860"
CDS             join(195..395,2549..2649,5327..5423,5990..6078,
                8188..8261,9596..9676,10262..10491,10590..10649,
                10890..11054)
                /gene="GTF3A"
                /gene _synonym="AP2; TFIIIA"
                /note="non-AUG (CUG) translation initiation
                codon; Derived by automated computational
                analysis using gene prediction
                method: BestRefSeq."
                /codon _start=1
                /product="transcription factor IIIA"
                /protein _id="NP  002088.2"
                /db _xref="GI:166063995"
                /db _xref="CCDS:CCDS45019.1"
                /db _xref="GeneID:2971"
                /db _xref="HGNC:HGNC:4662"
                /db _xref="MIM:600860"
```

CDS: 'Coding DNA Sequence'

The amino acid sequence for general TFIIIA molecule. The TFIIIIA molecule is comprised of 365 amino acid molecules. The amino acid sequence for the TFIIIA molecule is as follows:

/translation="MDPPAVVAESVSSLTIADAFIAAGESSAPTPPRPALPRRFICSF

PDCSANYSKAWKLDAHLCKHTGERPFVCDYEGCGKAFIRDYHLSRHILTHTGEKPFVC

AANGCDQKFNTKSNLKKHFERKHENQQKQYICSFEDCKKTFKKHQQLKIHQCQHTNEP

LFKCTQEGCGKHFASPSKLKRHAKAHEGYVCQKGCSFVAKTWTELLKHVRETHKEEIL

CEVCRKTFKRKDYLKQHMKTHAPERDVCRCPREGCGRTYTTVFNLQSHILSFHEESRP

FVCEHAGCGKTFAMKQSLTRHAVVHDPDKKKMKLKVKKSREKRSLASHLSGYIPPKRK

QGQGLSLCQNGESPNCVEDKMLSTVAVLTLG"

The gene that when transcribed generates the mRNA to produce the general TFIIIA molecule. Gene comprised of 11,166 nucleotides. The underlined segments are the nucleotide strings that represent bonding sites of the TFIIIA molecule's zinc fingers. Note the bonding sites are twelve amino acids in length. Thirty-six nucleotides are required to code for twelve amino acids (using the codon code methodology). The nucleotides comprising the DNA, when being used to code for an amino acid, function by three consecutive nucleotides coding for a single amino acid. There are sixty-four three-nucleotide combinations. Sixty-one of the three-nucleotide combinations code for the twenty amino acids. Three nucleotide combinations (taa, tag, tga) code specifically as stop codes. One three amino acid combination 'atg' codes for the amino acid methionine and also, in the proper setting, is recognized as a start code.

```
ORIGIN
        1 atgcgcgatc tcccggagca tgcgcagcag cggcgccgac gcggggcggt gcctggtgac
       61 cgcgcgcgct cccggaagtg tgccggcgtc gcgcgaaggt tcagcaggga gccgtgggcc
      121 gggcgcgccg gttcccggca cgtgtctcgg cacgtggcag cgcgcctggc cctgggcttg
      181 gaggcgccgg cgccctggat ccgccggccg tggtcgccga gtcggtgtcg tccttgacca
      241 tcgccgacgc gttcattgca gccggcgaga gctcagctcc gaccccgccg cgccccgcgc
      301 ttcccaggag gttcatctgc tccttccctg actgcagcgc caattacagc aaagcctgga
      361 agcttgacgc gcacctgtgc aagcacacgg gggaggtgag gggggcgagg ctgccaaccc
```

421 tgggcctagg gatggcgcgt ggccccgggg tagccactgc agtcgtggcc agggccgcag
481 gccccgctgt gcagcgcgtt cagctttgac atccaggact tggggaagga gctgaggaag
541 tagacaggaa gttgtaggac cttcgttctg cgaccttgat atccatggca ggggctcggg
601 atttactaag cagtcattga tcgtgagtct cggccagcca agtgcctccc gtaatctgca
661 aataagtgtg aggtttgagg gggcccaccg ctactagaca cctgccaaac actggcccct
721 ggagctggta cagaagatgg gttacatgta ccaggggtcg tgaaagcagc atgtgctcat
781 ttcttcgtaa ctccacactg gagagagcag tgagcaaaac aggcaaaccc aaggtttctg
841 ctgccatgga cctttgttcc tgggtcgagc cgaccacagg ataggtggga atgacatgca
901 gtgttgtggt caggaaaggc ctctctgtgt gagccgtgta agaaggaagg atctagccat
961 gcagacattt gtgctaggta gagagaacac aaagggagcc tgtgaccctt ggggtgggag
1021 gcaggtgggt gtgtttgggt gcggagatca ccatatgagg tctgagaagt aggcccatta
1081 ggagtttgga ttttattttg agggcaggag aatgtcagat accatgatat gacgtggcag
1141 cccatgtcac acacaagtga ggaaaacgag ggtcatggag gtcaaggaat ctgcccagct
1201 tcccagtttt tggcagagct aggcttcaca ctgcctcagc ttaaagccct taatttctta
1261 aaccactggg ctgcagtcca tacctttgcc ccttgcacct cctctaattt atgggccacc
1321 ttctccaggt gtcctccggg gcctcattcc ttaacctctc cagcactgga aggccgaccg
1381 cttcttcctt gagaccttct ctggttcttt tcctcttcct cgtctgccct tttcgttgga
1441 tcctcttctg ccctctgcat gttccacccc gcccagctcc ctcttgcggt cttacatagc
1501 caccggcatg actcataaca tcctttatgc tttgcccctc tgcccttcct cttgcccgtt
1561 ctagcctcta aattctgggc tctgtattac cagtagatcc acgtaagagc ttgcctttcc
1621 ttttagaccg gtgtgctgta ttttggatac tggcgctacc agtttcctta atacaggttg
1681 aaaaacttgg agtcatcttt gttgtcccag atctctcatg cagattaatt tgacaaatgt
1741 ttattgagcc tactccacgc ctgccgctgt gcaaggttct gtggctccgc ccctggtggt
1801 atgtagctca ctgtgttcct gtttgcttgt tttgctccta gtactctcat ggaggcctcg
1861 gtgcctccct cctggacgcc ttggtagtat gcttttcata gtttgatgca ccaaactggt
1921 tatttggtta tttggggtgt gtgtttggct tttactatag gttcaaaatg agtcaccccc
1981 tcccaactcc tgggttacaa aaggtggttg catttagggt gttgagctgt tttctttgct
2041 tcgccctggc acctgtgagc tttttcaggt gtgacacact ttcctatagc tgtgcttggc
2101 attatcctag cacagaccct gggcttgtct gggatgagac aggcctccct cgttcctctg
2161 ccctaggctt gctttttac atgttaaatc atgcggtggt ggggatccat gcagacaagc
2221 catgctaaca gccagggcgt ctttaagagg gggttgctgt gaaagcctgc tgccgggttg
2281 ggagcaggtt aaaaatgcta tgcctgctta ttttaaatgc tgttcatgga acaaaaatct
2341 gtgtagtgac tttgtgagaa gttgtgatgt ttatgttgtg taactttgtg caggaacact
2401 gcgtcttgca gtgggtgcac agctctgagt agaaaccacc tcttcatagg aagcctgtgg
2461 ccttaacact aggcagttta agcttttaaa taataccaga gttactaact agtgcagaag
2521 tgacatgctt tttcttttt cctgctag**ag accatttgtt tgtgactatg aagggtgtgg**
2581 **caaggccttc atcagggact accatctgag ccgccacatt ctgactcaca caggagaaaa**
2641 **gccgtttgt**g taagtagaga cctgttttta ggcttttgaa gtgggttgtg ttgggcatat
2701 agacccagta agaagattga tgttaactca cgagatcagg aatgtgaagc ctggcagggc
2761 tcggtggctc atgcctgtaa tcccagcact ttgggaggcg gagatgggca gatcacttga
2821 acccaggagt ttgagacaaa cctgggcaac atggtgaaac cccgtatgta caaaaataca

2881 aaaattagtc agggatggtg gtttgtgcct gtaatcctag ctacccagga ggctgagcta
2941 acataaaatg ctcatgggtg gggacaagct aaagtatatc aacacaatgg gataccctac
3001 agccaggaaa atgaatgcag atgctctctg caaagccatg agaaaatcac cagggcactt
3061 taattgaaaa accaaggtgc agaagagtcc tctttaggct acttttatgt gtgtaaaaaa
3121 gctagggggt agggggaggg gtgagtagtg ggtgttgggt aggcaggaag caactatatt
3181 tgtatttgtt cctatttgta aagaagtctt aaaagttaca taacaaaact aaaaatgtca
3241 tctgttttgg gagcagtggg ggatcctggc caagtagggg gtggggatgg taggaaatgc
3301 catgcaacca ggaactactg gacatgactc ttccagctca tgatctaacc cagaccctgc
3361 ccctctttag ctgtagttcc ccgtttccca ctgctcgctg gacagtgcta cttggctatc
3421 tctgtgtctt cttaaattcc atgtggtagg ctgggtgtgg tggctcatgc ctgtaatccc
3481 agcactttga gaggctgagg tgggaggatt gctttgaggc caggagttca ggctgggcaa
3541 gatggtcagg tccatctcta ttaaagaaat aaataaataa aaaattccac atggcccaaa
3601 tttgtcacag tcaaactgag ctcacttttc tgtttgatct tctctcatgt tcttgtctgg
3661 agaggtggcc tcgctgtctg tccagtgacc catagcaaag ataaggcagc tccctggact
3721 ctccattctt tctcccatcc cttgcaacag gtgggttgcc agatcctgta actgacccat
3781 cagatccagc agccactgtc ttatctcggt cccttcctct ggctggaatg acagtttgca
3841 ggccagccct ctcccccagt gccctcccgt gtgcttccct taaagctgtg cagtgctttc
3901 aagcacggcc tacatgtgaa atccaggttt caagtgtgtc ctacaatgac ctgcgtgatt
3961 tagccctttt ctgcttatct tgccccattt gcttgacttg caggcatgaa gctgtggtcc
4021 agctgtgcta actaaccagc cccctctcca agtgtgccgg ggtctctcac gcccacttgg
4081 gtcttgtcag gactcttcct ggcctgtcct cctatcccat acccggttgg gttagatgcc
4141 tgtgtcaggt ttagagtgaa gaatggcagg aaccccagca caagagatgc ttaaacaaga
4201 tgggctcttt gtcttgtgcg actgaaatac agaaatacag aggcaggagc tctggagcct
4261 cttctgactg gtctctgcca tcctcatctt gggctttaac ctcactgtga tgcctgtttg
4321 ggcccatctg tcacataagc atgccactgg caggaaggag gaaagggcat aagaggcatg
4381 ccccctatt tagagacttt gtgggggttg agcaggatgg gctggactca gccatgagcc
4441 gccctaattg caggggaggc cggagagtgc actttctgtc ggccacctgc ccagctaaca
4501 ctcagcattc tgtccctgca gttagggggg cttctagggt ctctgccaca gcgcccctcc
4561 catttgtggg cctctgtgct gtgcctccca tggtcactgc tggcttgttt gtctctgctt
4621 ggccctagga atgggacagt gcctgcctca gggttatcag tgagtgatgg ctaagattga
4681 gcctgggaaa ggaagtcctg cttcatccct caagcttacg aaggctcatc acaagaggca
4741 caaattttct tttgggaaaa aaaaaaaaaa aaaaggaaaa ggctttgcag aggatttaga
4801 tcattcaaag ccaagatgcc aagataaggg gaaccagaat ggcttggtaa gccagagaac
4861 ataatggtta tggttctgct ctaagtatct gttttacctc taatgataag ccaagacaag
4921 ttttatggag gcctttctgg aaatccagtt cataatgaca tctcaagcag cattaaggtt
4981 gtcagattct aagctgagaa taatttgtct taagcatgat ttaggcctag tgtaggcttt
5041 tgggactagt gtatttcacc ttcccatctg cccagtgtgt ataaaagatg actgatgtag
5101 tgtgtataat ttcagaagcc taatatgaaa aagcattttg ttacatgata gtcatcaggt
5161 tgagagtcta tgtggtatgg cttaacactc tggaattcgc taagactatt ttatagtatt
5221 actattcttt ggaagaatta gcttctataa agtaggaaga tatatgtgtc ttaaaacttc
5281 ttctcccttg gtttattaat attttggttt atataacttc ttacagt**tgt gcagccaatg**

5341 **gctgtgatca aaaattcaac acaaaatcaa acttgaagaa acattttgaa cgcaaacatg**

5401 **aaaatcaaca aaaacaatat ata**gtaagta tgattttata tgcttaaatt ttttgagtat

5461 ttttacactt actgcctatg tttctgacat tttcagccag gtgcggtggc tcaagcctat

5521 aatcgtagct tgaggccagg aatttgagac cagcctggga aacatagtga aatgctgtct

5581 ctgaaaaaaa aaaacaaaaa cagaaaacaa aacaaaaaat tttggggtaa cagagaccct

5641 gtctctaaaa aataaaagtg aaaaataaag ttttcgtcaa ccaaattttg tctgccaaat

5701 gtctgaattt acttaatgcc atcataatga taaaggtttt aatttggaag cagacattgt

5761 gcaaattagt gtattgggag actattccaa ctgaaacagt tttgcttttt caaatgttat

5821 atgattcttc aaaccttttt gagataaagc agaattttac agtaacaaaa tgggtgaaag

5881 cagaaatttt atacagtctc caaaattgtt ttatcttgag gattctgtta cgaactgttc

5941 attttgtttt gactttccat aagactaacg agcctttaca atttaacag**t gcagttttga**

6001 **agactgtaag aagaccttta agaaacatca gcagctgaaa atccatcagt gccagcatac**

6061 **caatgaacct ctattcaag**t aggtacttca tgtggctgaa aatgcctgga ttctaggtgt

6121 gaataagatt ggaaatgcaa gggtggtgtt gagcattgtt tcatgttttt tggccatttg

6181 tatatcttct gagaaatgtc tgttcatatc ctttgcccac ttttcgatgg attgtttttt

6241 tcttgctgat ctgagttccc tgtagatcct ggatatacat tctttattgg atgcataatg

6301 tgccagtatt ttctcccact ctctgggttg tctgtttact ctgctgatta tttcttttgc

6361 tgtgcagaag ctttttagtt taattaggtc ccatttattt atttctattt ttgttgcatt

6421 tgctttcagg gccttagtaa gaattctttg cctaggctga tgtccagaag tttttccaat

6481 gttttcattt tgaattttta gtttcaggtc ataaacttaa tttgagttga tttttgtata

6541 aggtgagaga tagggatcca gtttttccag caccatttat tgaataggga gtcctttccc

6601 cagtttacgt ttttatatgc tttgttgaag atcgggtggc tgtaagtatt tggctttatt

6661 tctgttttgt tccattggtc taagtgccta tttttaaacc agtgccaccc tgttttggta

6721 actgtagcct cgtagtataa tctgaagtct ggtcaaagga aaagaagtca ctatatgaaa

6781 aagacacatg cacacacgtt tacagcagca cagttcacaa ttgcaaatac atggagccaa

6841 tttaagtgcc catcgaccaa tgagtagata aagaaaacgt gatgtatata caccatggaa

6901 tactacacag ccataaaagg gaacaaaatg atgtcttttg cagcagcttg gatggagctg

6961 gaggccatta ttctcagtga agtaactcag gaatggaaaa ccaaatacca tagttttcac

7021 taagtgggca ctaaactatg aggacaaaaa gacacagtga tttcataaac tttggggact

7081 tggggtgggg agtttgggga gggggtgag ggatgaaaga ctacatattg ggtacagtgt

7141 atgctgcttg agtgatggtg cgctaaaatc tcagcaccac tataggattc atccacgtaa

7201 cgaaaaaaca cttgcaaccc caaaagccat tgaaatttaa agcaacggtg ggacaaatct

7261 tctgaaagct tcctaatcaa catttttctg ttaaaatgta ctgcatatgc acatttatat

7321 attgggagca ttttaaaggt ttactttgct ctgaaagaaa tatttaatgt gtttcaaaat

7381 aatttttgag attattctag ttgtggttaa gcttaaaggc tgagaaatta cttaactatt

7441 caaatagagc ctgtgcaact atatgaaatg tcattatgga gacactcatt atgcttttcc

7501 tgtagaacaa aacaagtagt tgggtttatc tgcaattagg gtttttgag gaacgtgagg

7561 gtggctggac aagttgggta gacctgcaaa agggccagcg gctctctgca tggctctggc

7621 catccggcac tttcccttga cttgcacagg ctgccctgtg ccttggagtt gctgcagtga

7681 ccttgcctgt ccttgcttgt gggtctgctg ctgctgcttt gctgctgatg gctttagcac

7741 agagggggcc cgtgcttttt attgctcacc agaggcagat gcatctactg ctgtgctgtc

7801 tcgcacaccc cctatgcagc atcattagga aagctagaca caagtgattc agaatggctt

7861 aggggtttat ctaagccaag tcagataacc tcttgaacta tctttttgta gccatgaaag

7921 cagagtatat ttccagaggt ataaagatga aaactgttta aatgggtcaa aaaaagtaac

7981 gtgacttttt tctccaacag tttgttttgt cctaaagctg gtcaagtaac ttgaatctca

8041 cctgtgatga gagctacatt ttaacatggg tttggttatg ggaagaggca agactttggt

8101 gggagaaaca ggacaaagtg ccattgacct tgagcggagt tctctgtgaa aatggattgg

8161 ctaatacctc atgtgttgcc aatgcagg**tg** **tacccaggaa** **ggatgtggga** **aacactttgc**

8221 **atcacccagc** **aagctgaaac** **gacatgccaa** **ggcccacgag** **g**gtgtgtacg gatagcctgg

8281 gtgtgctccg agggggatgc caaatcctgg gcgcctttga atctgttctg tgatcacgct

8341 gaaaagatgg gaaccctgtg aacaggggac accatcctgc ttatttgggt cttacactct

8401 tgtccaaaga ggcactgtat atgtctgttt ttccactacc gtatcattgc tgttcacatg

8461 taatgtgttg tttgttcaca acaagcgcct ggttacacat tacactgacg aatgtgctga

8521 tgctccagcc atggctttga tgcttctgtc atttttaacc tcttctatta atatttactg

8581 cctgtgccat tcttttcctt gttggccatt cacaaggctt ggataatcgt gtgacatttt

8641 gagagccatc agatgttacg tttctcaaaa aaaaaaaaaa aagacttgat tatattaact

8701 atttgaatct atgatctgtt tccttgaggg atttttgcta atctgtattt caatttccca

8761 ggtcctagaa tttatgattt tttttttttt aagaggttag tagctaacag tgagaggcag

8821 cctcattgtt tttagtttct agttgggtgg aactcagccc tagtgttgta tacttattaa

8881 tcccatttta gtgctttgca catatccatt gttattcagt gtttttctct gggtccttcc

8941 agtttatttt cttccttagc tgtactcttt taaaaaaaaa aaacaaaaaa aaactttttt

9001 tttttttttt gtgataaagt taaaatataa tgtaccctac tttttttgtg cagtatgaca

9061 cttacaagat ggccagacta gaggaagcca gaggtgggca tggtaacact actgaaaagt

9121 tggtggtgtg ccatggacaa gggaccgact gcagagtatg tttgctgagg aaaatagagg

9181 cgaggataga gcaggcaggg gaagggaaat aagacatgga gataggaggt taaagcagtt

9241 gggagtccat acacagccta cccaacttcc tgagaactct tagagaggaa aaggcatcct

9301 taggcatcct tcctgtgaag tttgcctatt ccgtgatcac gctgagaaga tgggaactct

9361 gaagtttgct tcacaggaag gtaaaatcct taaagggagg caccttgctg tgccactgtt

9421 cagttttact ataacatcaa tcttttttta gtttttattc ccacctcaag aggctgagtt

9481 gaatactatt aggcggggaa tggaaaatta tataggcacc taagtttcct ttctagttat

9541 ggtcagtgtt tacactgagt attcatgaca gacaatgcac caattttttt aatag**gctat**

9601 **gtatgtcaaa** **aaggatgttc** **ctttgtggca** **aaaacatgga** **cggaacttct** **gaaacatgtg**

9661 **agagaaaccc** **ataaag**gtaa ggcaggcatg aatggcaggc atggtgtaaa tgtttgtccc

9721 cacagaactg atttagtgct tttcaagagt gaaatgctgt gtgctttaaa gtaaaagggt

9781 ttctctatga tattttgtga agtgctgggt atgatgttgt tggaaaggtg agcagagctg

9841 tgccaggtct ctgagccacc ccaccatgca caattagcat gctgaaggcg gtggcaggtc

9901 tgtagtgaag aatttcggga ggcactgctg ttctgtggga ccgcctggga aacagtaccc

9961 tgcatactgg gggacaagga aggacactgg tctgcttcat tttctgtacc tccccacagt

10021 caccttcctg agagccctgc ctcttggcaa gtgaacaatg actgtgtggc atttaagaac

10081 ttcagagaat tgagacaaac ttcctaggtg ataaaaactg gggttgtttc cttgggaatt

10141 tctgatttgt atatagtgat caggtttcag gcactgaatg ttacttatat attaggtatt

10201 aatttttct aaatggtaat atctggggaa atttgtgaaa tttgtctgtc tgtcccacca

10261 g**aggaaatac tatgtgaagt atgccggaaa acatttaaac gcaaagatta ccttaagcaa**
10321 **cacatgaaaa ctcatgcccc agaaagggat gtatgtcgct gtccaagaga aggctgtgga**
10381 **agaacctata caactgtgtt taatctccaa agccatatcc tctccttcca tgaggaaagc**
10441 **cgcccttttg tgtgtgaaca tgctggctgt ggcaaaacat ttgcaatgaa a**gtaagcact
10501 caccctcata ctcatggtcc tatagtctat gctttcacaa catggttttc atattaatat
10561 ttcattaata actttctctt tcattgtag**c aaagtctcac taggcatgct gttgtacatg**
10621 **atcctgacaa gaagaaaatg aagctcaaa**g taagttgaaa ctacttaggc aagcttagtt
10681 ttcaagtgga aattgtttaa ggccagaagg agtctgtttg gaattctttt cacctgcttt
10741 actgtttgag tctgcactac tgttgaagac tttacttcct cataaagcaa tgttgtacac
10801 tatatctgct ggtacatatg actatcgtaa aattaactca gacagttttg attttgaatt
10861 ctaatcgtgt gtcttcctta ttcccaaag**g tcaaaaaatc tcgtgaaaaa cggagtttgg**
10921 **cctctcatct cagtggatat atccctccca aaaggaaaca agggcaaggc ttatctttgt**
10981 **gtcaaaacgg agagtcaccc aactgtgtgg aagacaagat gctctcgaca gttgcagtac**
11041 **ttacccttgg ctaagaactg cactgctttg tttaaaggac tgcagaccaa ggagcgagct**
11101 **ttctctcaga gcatgctttt ctttattaaa attactgatg cagaacattt gattccttat**
11161 **catttc**

Details of how the general TFIIIA molecule is constructed per coding instructions from the genetic code:[14,15,16,17]

CDS join(195..395,2549..2649,5327..5423,5990..6078,8188..8261,
9596..9676,10262..10491,10590..10649,10890..11054)

ORIGIN

TFIIIA GENE EXON ONE:

TFIIIA mRNA 5′ UPSTREAM UNTRANSLATABLE SEGMENT:

1 **atg**cgcgatc tcccggagca tgcgcagcag cggcgccgac gcggggcggt gcctggtgac
61 cgcgcgcgct cccggaagtg tgccggcgtc gcgcgaaggt tcagcaggga gccgtgggcc
121 gggcgcgccg gttcccggca cgtgtctcgg cacgtggcag cgcgcctggc cctgggcttg
181 gaggcgccgg cgcc

***LOOP ALPHA BINDING TO DNA**

TFIIIA MOLECULE AMINO ACIDS 1-47:

```
     L   D   P   P   A   V   V   A   E   S   V   S   S   L   T
195 ctg gat ccg ccg gcc gtg gtc gcc gag tcg gtg tcg tcc ttg acc

     I   A   D   A   F   I   A   A   G   E   S   S   A   P   T
240 atc gcc gac gcg ttc att gca gcc ggc gag agc tca gct ccg acc
```

```
     P   P   R   P   A   L   P   R   R   F   I   C   S   F   P
286 ccg ccg cgc ccc gcg ctt ccc agg agg ttc atc tgc tcc ttc cct

     D   C
330 gac tgc
```

TFIIIA MOLECULE ZINC FINGER 'ONE' DNA BONDING SITES, AMINO ACIDS 48-59:

```
     S    A    N    Y    S    K    A    W    K    L    D    A
336 agc  gcc  aat  tac  agc  aaa  gcc  tgg  aag  ctt  gac  gcg
```

TFIIIA MOLECULE AMINO ACIDS 60-67:

```
     H   L   C   K   H   T   G   E
372 cac ctg tgc aag cac acg ggg gag
```

TFIIIA GENE INTRON ONE:

```
 396 gtgag gggggcgagg ctgccaaccc
 421 tgggcctagg gatggcgcgt ggccccgggg tagccactgc agtcgtggcc agggccgcag
 481 gccccgctgt gcagcgcgtt cagctttgac atccaggact tggggaagga gctgaggaag
 541 tagacaggaa gttgtaggac cttcgttctg cgaccttgat atccatggca ggggctcggg
 601 atttactaag cagtcattga tcgtgagtct cggccagcca agtgcctccc gtaatctgca
 661 aataagtgtg aggtttgagg gggcccaccg ctactagaca cctgccaaac actggcccct
 721 ggagctggta cagaagatgg gttacatgta ccaggggtcg tgaaagcagc atgtgctcat
 781 ttcttcgtaa ctccacactg gagagagcag tgagcaaaac aggcaaaccc aaggtttctg
 841 ctgccatgga cctttgttcc tgggtcgagc cgaccacagg ataggtggga atgacatgca
 901 gtgttgtggt caggaaaggc ctctctgtgt gagccgtgta agaaggaagg atctagccat
 961 gcagacattt gtgctaggta gagagaacac aaagggagcc tgtgaccctt ggggtgggag
1021 gcaggtgggt gtgtttgggt gcggagatca ccatatgagg tctgagaagt aggcccatta
1081 ggagtttgga ttttattttg agggcaggag aatgtcagat accatgatat gacgtggcag
1141 cccatgtcac acacaagtga ggaaaacgag ggtcatggag gtcaaggaat ctgcccagct
1201 tcccagtttt tggcagagct aggcttcaca ctgcctcagc ttaaagccct taatttctta
1261 aaccactggg ctgcagtcca tacctttgcc ccttgcacct cctctaattt atgggccacc
1321 ttctccaggt gtcctccggg gcctcattcc ttaacctctc cagcactgga aggccgaccg
1381 cttcttcctt gagaccttct ctggttcttt tcctcttcct cgtctgccct tttcgttgga
1441 tcctcttctg ccctctgcat gttccacccc gcccagctcc ctcttgcggt cttacatagc
1501 caccggcatg actcataaca tcctttatgc tttgcccctc tgcccttcct cttgcccgtt
1561 ctagcctcta aattctgggc tctgtattac cagtagatcc acgtaagagc ttgcctttcc
1621 ttttagaccg gtgtgctgta ttttggatac tggcgctacc agtttcctta atacaggttg
1681 aaaaacttgg agtcatcttt gttgtcccag atctctcatg cagattaatt tgacaaatgt
1741 ttattgagcc tactccacgc ctgccgctgt gcaaggttct gtggctccgc ccctggtggt
1801 atgtagctca ctgtgttcct gtttgcttgt tttgctccta gtactctcat ggaggcctcg
1861 gtgcctccct cctggacgcc ttggtagtat gcttttcata gtttgatgca ccaaactggt
1921 tatttggtta tttggggtgt gtgtttggct tttactatag gttcaaaatg agtcaccccc
1981 tcccaactcc tgggttacaa aaggtggttg catttagggt gttgagctgt tttctttgct
2041 tcgccctggc acctgtgagc tttttcaggt gtgacacact ttcctatagc tgtgcttggc
2101 attatcctag cacagaccct gggcttgtct gggatgagac aggcctccct cgttcctctg
2161 ccctaggctt gctttttac atgttaaatc atgcggtggt ggggatccat gcagacaagc
2221 catgctaaca gccagggcgt ctttaagagg gggttgctgt gaaagcctgc tgccgggttg
2281 ggagcaggtt aaaaatgcta tgcctgctta ttttaaatgc tgttcatgga acaaaaatct
2341 gtgtagtgac tttgtgagaa gttgtgatgt ttatgttgtg taactttgtg caggaacact
2401 gcgtcttgca gtgggtgcac agctctgagt agaaaccacc tcttcatagg aagcctgtgg
2461 ccttaacact aggcagttta agcttttaaa taataccaga gttactaact agtgcagaag
2521 tgacatgctt tttcttttt cctgctag
```

TFIIIA GENE EXON TWO:

***LOOP BETA BINDING TO DNA**

TFIIIA MOLECULE AMINO ACIDS 68-77:

```
      R   P   F   V   C   D   Y   E   G   C
2549 aga cca ttt gtt tgt gac tat gaa ggg tgt
```

TFIIIA MOLECULE ZINC FINGER 'TWO' DNA BONDING SITES, AMINO ACIDS 78-89

```
      G   K   A   F   I   R   D   Y   H   L   S   R
2579 ggc aag gcc ttc atc agg gac tac cat ctg agc cgc
```

TFIIIA MOLECULE AMINO ACIDS 90-101:

```
      H   I   L   T   H   T   G   E   K   P   F   V
2615 cac att ctg act cac aca gga gaa aag ccg ttt gtg
```

TFIIIA GENE INTRON TWO:

2651 **taa (STOP)**

```
2654 gtagaga cctgtttta ggcttttgaa gtgggttgtg ttgggcatat
2701 agacccagta agaagattga tgttaactca cgagatcagg aatgtgaagc ctggcagggc
2761 tcggtggctc atgcctgtaa tcccagcact ttgggaggcg gagatgggca gatcacttga
2821 acccaggagt ttgagacaaa cctgggcaac atggtgaaac cccgtatgta caaaaataca
2881 aaaattagtc agggatggtg gtttgtgcct gtaatcctag ctacccagga ggctgagcta
2941 acataaaatg ctcatgggtg gggacaagct aaagtatatc aacacaatgg gataccctac
3001 agccaggaaa atgaatgcag atgctctctg caaagccatg agaaaatcac cagggcactt
3061 taattgaaaa accaaggtgc agaagagtcc tctttaggct acttttatgt gtgtaaaaaa
3121 gctagggggt agggggaggg gtgagtagtg ggtgttgggt aggcaggaag caactatatt
3181 tgtatttgtt cctatttgta aagaagtctt aaaagttaca taacaaaact aaaaatgtca
3241 tctgttttgg gagcagtggg ggatcctggc caagtagggg gtggggatgg taggaaatgc
3301 catgcaacca ggaactactg gacatgactc ttccagctca tgatctaacc cagaccctgc
3361 ccctctttag ctgtagttcc ccgtttccca ctgctcgctg gacagtgcta cttggctatc
3421 tctgtgtctt cttaaattcc atgtggtagg ctgggtgtgg tggctcatgc ctgtaatccc
3481 agcactttga gaggctgagg tgggaggatt gctttgaggc caggagttca ggctgggcaa
3541 gatggtcagg tccatctcta ttaaagaaat aaataaataa aaaattccac atggcccaaa
3601 tttgtcacag tcaaactgag ctcacttttc tgtttgatct tctctcatgt tcttgtctgg
3661 agaggtggcc tcgctgtctg tccagtgacc catagcaaag ataaggcagc tccctggact
3721 ctccattctt tctcccatcc cttgcaacag gtgggttgcc agatcctgta actgacccat
3781 cagatccagc agccactgtc ttatctcggt cccttcctct ggctggaatg acagtttgca
3841 ggccagccct ctcccccagt gccctcccgt gtgcttccct taaagctgtg cagtgctttc
3901 aagcacggcc tacatgtgaa atccaggttt caagtgtgtc ctacaatgac ctgcgtgatt
3961 tagccctttt ctgcttatct tgccccattt gcttgacttg caggcatgaa gctgtggtcc
4021 agctgtgcta actaaccagc cccctctcca agtgtgccgg ggtctctcac gcccacttgg
4081 gtcttgtcag gactcttcct ggcctgtcct cctatcccat acccggttgg gttagatgcc
4141 tgtgtcaggt ttagagtgaa gaatggcagg aaccccagca caagagatgc ttaaacaaga
4201 tgggctcttt gtcttgtgcg actgaaatac agaaatacag aggcaggagc tctggagcct
4261 cttctgactg gtctctgcca tcctcatctt gggctttaac ctcactgtga tgcctgtttg
4321 ggcccatctg tcacataagc atgccactgg caggaaggag gaaagggcat aagaggcatg
4381 ccccttatt tagagacttt gtgggggttg agcaggatgg gctggactca gccatgagcc
4441 gccctaattg caggggaggc cggagagtgc actttctgtc ggccacctgc ccagctaaca
4501 ctcagcattc tgtccctgca gttagggggg cttctagggt ctctgccaca gcgcccctcc
```

4561 catttgtggg cctctgtgct gtgcctccca tggtcactgc tggcttgttt gtctctgctt
4621 ggccctagga atgggacagt gcctgcctca gggttatcag tgagtgatgg ctaagattga
4681 gcctgggaaa ggaagtcctg cttcatccct caagcttacg aaggctcatc acaagaggca
4741 caaattttct tttgggaaaa aaaaaaaaaa aaaaggaaaa ggctttgcag aggatttaga
4801 tcattcaaag ccaagatgcc aagataaggg gaaccagaat ggcttggtaa gccagagaac
4861 ataatggtta tggttctgct ctaagtatct gttttacctc taatgataag ccaagacaag
4921 ttttatggag gcctttctgg aaatccagtt cataatgaca tctcaagcag cattaaggtt
4981 gtcagattct aagctgagaa taatttgtct taagcatgat ttaggcctag tgtaggcttt
5041 tgggactagt gtatttcacc ttcccatctg cccagtgtgt ataaaagatg actgatgtag
5101 tgtgtataat ttcagaagcc taatatgaaa aagcattttg ttacatgata gtcatcaggt
5161 tgagagtcta tgtggtatgg cttaacactc tggaattcgc taagactatt ttatagtatt
5221 actattcttt ggaagaatta gcttctataa agtaggaaga tatatgtgtc ttaaaacttc
5281 ttctcccttg gtttattaat attttggttt atataacttc ttacagt

TFIIIA GENE EXON THREE:

***LOOP GAMMA BINDING TO DNA**

TFIIIA MOLECULE AMINO ACIDS 102-107:

C A A N G C
5328 tgt gca gcc aat ggc tgt

TFIIIA MOLECULE ZINC FINGER 'THREE' DNA BONDING SITES, AMINO ACIDS 108-119

D Q K F N T K S N L K K
5349 gat caa aaa ttc aac aca aaa tca aac ttg aag aaa

TFIIIA MOLECULE AMINO ACIDS 120-133:

H F E R K H E N Q Q K Q Y I
5381 cat ttt gaa cgc aaa cat gaa aat caa caa aaa caa tat ata

TFIIIA GENE INTRON THREE:

5424 gtaagta tgattttata tgcttaaatt ttttgagtat
5461 ttttacactt actgcctatg tttctgacat tttcagccag gtgcggtggc tcaagcctat
5521 aatcgtagct tgaggccagg aatttgagac cagcctggga aacatagtga aatgctgtct
5581 ctgaaaaaaa aaaacaaaaa cagaaaacaa aacaaaaaat tttggggtaa cagagaccct
5641 gtctctaaaa aataaaagtg aaaaataaag ttttcgtcaa ccaaattttg tctgccaaat
5701 gtctgaattt acttaatgcc atcataatga taaaggtttt aatttggaag cagacattgt
5761 gcaaattagt gtattgggag actattccaa ctgaaacagt tttgcttttt caaatgttat
5821 atgattcttc aaaccttttt gagataaagc agaattttac agtaacaaaa tgggtgaaag
5881 cagaaatttt atacagtctc caaaattgtt ttatcttgag gattctgtta cgaactgttc
5941 atttgtttt gactttccat aagactaacg agcctttaca atttaacag

TFIIIA GENE EXON FOUR:

***LOOP DELTA BINDING TO DNA**

TFIIIA MOLECULE AMINO ACIDS 134-139:

```
        C    S    F    E    D    C
  5990 tgc  agt  ttt  gaa  gac  tgt
```

TFIIIA MOLECULE ZINC FINGER 'FOUR' DNA BONDING SITES, AMINO ACIDS 140-151

```
        K    K    T    F    K    K    H    Q    Q    L    K    I
  6008 aag  aag  acc  ttt  aag  aaa  cat  cag  cag  ctg  aaa  atc
```

TFIIIA MOLECULE AMINO ACIDS 152-164:

```
        H    Q    C    Q    H    T    N    E    P    L    F    K
  6044 cat  cag  tgc  cag  cat  acc  aat  gaa  cct  cta  ttc  aag
```

TFIIIA GENE INTRON FOUR:

6080 tag (STOP)

```
6083 gtacttca tgtggctgaa aatgcctgga ttctaggtgt
6121 gaataagatt ggaaatgcaa gggtggtgtt gagcattgtt tcatgttttt tggccatttg
6181 tatatcttct gagaaatgtc tgttcatatc ctttgcccac ttttcgatgg attgtttttt
6241 tcttgctgat ctgagttccc tgtagatcct ggatatacat tctttattgg atgcataatg
6301 tgccagtatt ttctcccact ctctgggttg tctgtttact ctgctgatta tttcttttgc
6361 tgtgcagaag cttttagtt taattaggtc ccatttattt atttctattt ttgttgcatt
6421 tgctttcagg gccttagtaa gaattctttg cctaggctga tgtccagaag tttttccaat
6481 gttttcattt tgaattttta gtttcaggtc ataaacttaa tttgagttga tttttgtata
6541 aggtgagaga tagggatcca gtttttccag caccatttat tgaataggga gtcctttccc
6601 cagtttacgt ttttatatgc tttgttgaag atcgggtggc tgtaagtatt tggctttatt
6661 tctgttttgt tccattggtc taagtgccta tttttaaacc agtgccaccc tgttttggta
6721 actgtagcct cgtagtataa tctgaagtct ggtcaaagga aaagaagtca ctatatgaaa
6781 aagacacatg cacacacgtt tacagcagca cagttcacaa ttgcaaatac atggagccaa
6841 tttaagtgcc catcgaccaa tgagtagata aagaaaacgt gatgtatata caccatggaa
6901 tactacacag ccataaaagg gaacaaaatg atgtcttttg cagcagcttg gatggagctg
6961 gaggccatta ttctcagtga agtaactcag gaatggaaaa ccaaatacca tagttttcac
7021 taagtgggca ctaaactatg aggacaaaaa gacacagtga tttcataaac tttggggact
7081 tggggtgggg agtttgggga gggggtgag ggatgaaaga ctacatattg ggtacagtgt
7141 atgctgcttg agtgatggtg cgctaaaatc tcagcaccac tataggattc atccacgtaa
7201 cgaaaaaaca cttgcaaccc caaaagccat tgaaatttaa agcaacggtg ggacaaatct
7261 tctgaaagct tcctaatcaa cattttctg ttaaaatgta ctgcatatgc acatttatat
7321 attgggagca ttttaaaggt ttactttgct ctgaaagaaa tatttaatgt gtttcaaaat
7381 aattttgag attattctag ttgtggttaa gcttaaaggc tgagaaatta cttaactatt
7441 caaatagagc ctgtgcaact atatgaaatg tcattatgga gacactcatt atgcttttcc
7501 tgtagaacaa aacaagtagt tgggtttatc tgcaattagg gtttttttgag gaacgtgagg
7561 gtggctggac aagttgggta gacctgcaaa agggccagcg gctctctgca tggctctggc
7621 catccggcac tttcccttga cttgcacagg ctgccctgtg ccttggagtt gctgcagtga
7681 ccttgcctgt ccttgcttgt gggtctgctg ctgctgcttt gctgctgatg gctttagcac
7741 agagggggcc cgtgcttttt attgctcacc agaggcagat gcatctactg ctgtgctgtc
7801 tcgcacaccc cctatgcagc atcattagga aagctagaca caagtgattc agaatggctt
7861 aggggtttat ctaagccaag tcagataacc tcttgaacta tctttttgta gccatgaaag
7921 cagagtatat ttccagaggt ataaagatga aaactgttta aatgggtcaa aaaaagtaac
7981 gtgacttttt tctccaacag tttgttttgt cctaaagctg gtcaagtaac ttgaatctca
8041 cctgtgatga gagctacatt ttaacatggg tttggttatg ggaagaggca agactttggt
8101 gggagaaaca ggacaaagtg ccattgacct tgagcggagt tctctgtgaa aatggattgg
8161 ctaatacctc atgtgttgcc aatgcagg
```

TFIIIA GENE EXON FIVE:

***LOOP EPSILON BINDING TO DNA**

TFIIIA MOLECULE AMINO ACIDS 164-169:

```
      C   T   Q   E   G   C
8189 tgt acc cag gaa gga tgt
```

TFIIIA MOLECULE BONDING TO DNA AMINO ACIDS 170-181:

```
      G   K   H   F   A   S   P   S   K   L   K   R
8207 ggg aaa cac ttt gca tca ccc agc aag ctg aaa cga
```

TFIIIA MOLECULE AMINO ACIDS 182-187:

```
      H   A   K   A   H   E
8243 cat gcc aag gcc cac gag
```

TFIIIA GENE EXON FIVE:

```
      G
8261 ggt
```

```
8264 gtgtacg gatagcctgg
8281 gtgtgctccg aggggatgc caaatcctgg gcgcctttga atctgttctg tgatcacgct
8341 gaaaagatgg gaaccctgtg aacaggggac accatcctgc ttatttgggt cttacactct
8401 tgtccaaaga ggcactgtat atgtctgttt ttccactacc gtatcattgc tgttcacatg
8461 taatgtgttg tttgttcaca acaagcgcct ggttacacat tacactgacg aatgtgctga
8521 tgctccagcc atggctttga tgcttctgtc atttttaacc tcttctatta atatttactg
8581 cctgtgccat tcttttcctt gttggccatt cacaaggctt ggataatcgt gtgacatttt
8641 gagagccatc agatgttacg tttctcaaaa aaaaaaaaaa aagacttgat tatattaact
8701 atttgaatct atgatctgtt tccttgaggg atttttgcta atctgtattt caatttccca
8761 ggtcctagaa tttatgattt tttttttttt aagaggttag tagctaacag tgagaggcag
8821 cctcattgtt tttagtttct agttgggtgg aactcagccc tagtgttgta tacttattaa
8881 tcccatttta gtgctttgca catatccatt gttattcagt gtttttctct gggtccttcc
8941 agtttatttt cttccttagc tgtactcttt taaaaaaaaa aaacaaaaaa aaactttttt
9001 tttttttttt gtgataaagt taaaatataa tgtaccctac tttttttgtg cagtatgaca
9061 cttacaagat ggccagacta gaggaagcca gaggtgggca tggtaacact actgaaaagt
9121 tggtggtgtg ccatggacaa gggaccgact gcagagtatg tttgctgagg aaaatagagg
9181 cgaggataga gcaggcaggg gaagggaaat aagacatgga gataggaggt taaagcagtt
9241 gggagtccat acacagccta cccaacttcc tgagaactct tagagaggaa aaggcatcct
9301 taggcatcct tcctgtgaag tttgcctatt ccgtgatcac gctgagaaga tgggaactct
9361 gaagtttgct tcacaggaag gtaaaatcct taaagggagg caccttgctg tgccactgtt
9421 cagttttact ataacatcaa tcttttttta gtttttattc ccacctcaag aggctgagtt
9481 gaatactatt aggcggggaa tggaaaatta tataggcacc taagtttcct ttctagttat
9541 ggtcagtgtt tacactgagt attcatgaca gacaatgcac caattttttt aata
```

TFIIIA GENE EXON SIX:

***LOOP ZETA BINDING TO TRANSCRIPTION FACTORS**

TFIIIA MOLECULE AMINO ACIDS 188-195:

```
     G   Y
9595 ggc tat

     V   C   Q   K   G   C
9601 gta tgt caa aaa gga tgt
```

TFIIIA MOLECULE BIND TO TRANSCRIPTION FACTOR AMINO ACIDS 196-207:

```
     S   F   V   A   K   T   W   T   E   L   L   K
9619 tcc ttt gtg gca aaa aca tgg acg gaa ctt ctg aaa
```

TFIIIA MOLECULE AMINO ACIDS 208-214:

```
     H   V   R   E   T   H   K
9655 cat gtg aga gaa acc cat aaa
```

GENE INTRON SIX

```
 9676 ggtaa ggcaggcatg aatggcaggc atggtgtaaa tgtttgtccc
 9721 cacagaactg atttagtgct tttcaagagt gaaatgctgt gtgctttaaa gtaaaagggt
 9781 ttctctatga tattttgtga agtgctgggt atgatgttgt tggaaaggtg agcagagctg
 9841 tgccaggtct ctgagccacc ccaccatgca caattagcat gctgaaggcg gtggcaggtc
 9901 tgtagtgaag aatttcggga ggcactgctg ttctgtggga ccgcctggga aacagtaccc
 9961 tgcatactgg gggacaagga aggacactgg tctgcttcat tttctgtacc tccccacagt
10021 caccttcctg agagccctgc ctcttggcaa gtgaacaatg actgtgtggc atttaagaac
10081 ttcagagaat tgagacaaac ttcctaggtg ataaaaactg ggttgtttc cttgggaatt
10141 tctgatttgt atatagtgat caggtttcag gcactgaatg ttacttatat attaggtatt
10201 aattttttct aaatggtaat atctggggaa atttgtgaaa tttgtctgtc tgtcccacca
```

TFIIIA GENE EXON SEVEN:

***LOOP ETA BINDING TO TRANSCRIPTION FACTORS**

TFIIIA MOLECULE AMINO ACIDS 215-222:

```
      E   E   I   L   C   E   Y   C
10261 gag gaa ata cta tgt gaa gta tgc
```

TFIIIA MOLECULE AMINO ACIDS 223-234:

```
      R   K   T   F   K   R   K   D   Y   L   K   Q
10285 cgg aaa aca ttt aaa cgc aaa gat tac ctt aag caa
```

TFIIIA MOLECULE AMINO ACIDS 235-253:

```
      H   M   K   T   H   A   P   E   R   D   V   C   R   C
10321 cac atg aaa act cat gcc cca gaa agg gat gta tgt cgc tgt
```

```
       p   R   E   G   C
10363 cca aga gaa ggc tgt
```

*LOOP THETA BINDING TO TRANSCRIPTION FACTORS

TFIIIA MOLECULE AMINO ACIDS 254-265:

```
       G   R   T   Y   T   T   V   F   N   L   Q   S
10378 gga aga acc tat aca act gtg ttt aat ctc caa agc
```

TFIIIA MOLECULE AMINO ACIDS 266-284:

```
       H   I   L   S   F   H   E   E   S   R   P   F
10414 cat atc ctc tcc ttc cat gag gaa agc cgc cct ttt

       V   C   E   H   A   G   C
10450 gtg tgt gaa cat gct ggc tgt
```

*LOOP IOTA BINDING TO TRANSCRIPTION FACTORS

TFIIIA MOLECULE AMINO ACIDS 285-291:

```
       G   K   T   F   A   M   K
10471 ggc aaa aca ttt gca atg aaa
```

GENE INTRON SEVEN

```
10492 gtaagcact
10501 caccctcata ctcatggtcc tatagtctat gctttcacaa catggttttc atattaatat
10561 ttcattaata actttctctt tcattgtag
```

*LOOP IOTA (CONTINUED) BINDING TO TRANSCRIPTION FACTORS

TFIIIA MOLECULE AMINO ACIDS 292-296:

```
       Q   S   L   T   R
10590 caa agt ctc act agg
```

TFIIIA MOLECULE AMINO ACIDS 297-311:

```
       H   A   V   V   H   D   P   D   K   K   K   M   K
10605 cat gct gtt gta cat gat cct gac aag aag aaa atg aag

       L   K
10644 ctc aaa
```

GENE INTRON EIGHT

```
10650 gtaagttgaa actacttagg caagcttagt t
10681 ttcaagtgga aattgtttaa ggccagaagg agtctgtttg gaattctttt cacctgcttt
```

```
10741 actgtttgag tctgcactac tgttgaagac tttacttcct cataaagcaa tgttgtacac
10801 tatatctgct ggtacatatg actatcgtaa aattaactca gacagttttg attttgaatt
10861 ctaatcgtgt gtcttcctta ttcccaaag
```

3′ END OF THE TFIIIA MOLECULE

TFIIIA MOLECULE AMINO ACIDS 312-365:

```
       V   K   K   S   R   E   K   R   S   L   A   S   H
10890 gtc aaa aaa tct cgt gaa aaa cgg agt ttg gcc tct cat

       L   S   G   Y   I   P   P   K   R   K   Q   G   Q
10929 ctc agt gga tat atc cct ccc aaa agg aaa caa ggg caa

       G   L   S   L   C   Q   N   G   E   S   P   N   C
10968 ggc tta tct ttg tgt caa aac gga gag tca ccc aac tgt

       V   E   D   K   M   L   S   T   V   A   V   L   T
11007 gtg gaa gac aag atg ctc tcg aca gtt gca gta ctt acc


11046  L   G
      ctt ggc

11052 taa  (STOP)
```

TFIIIA GENE 3′ DOWNSTREAM REGION

```
11055 gaactg cactgctttg tttaaaggac tgcagaccaa ggagcgagct
11101 ttctctcaga gcatgctttt ctttattaaa attactgatg cagaacattt gattccttat
11161 catttc
```

CHAPTER SIX

STUDY OF OPTIMAL BONDING RELATIONSHIPS BETWEEN AMINO ACIDS AND NUCLEOTIDES

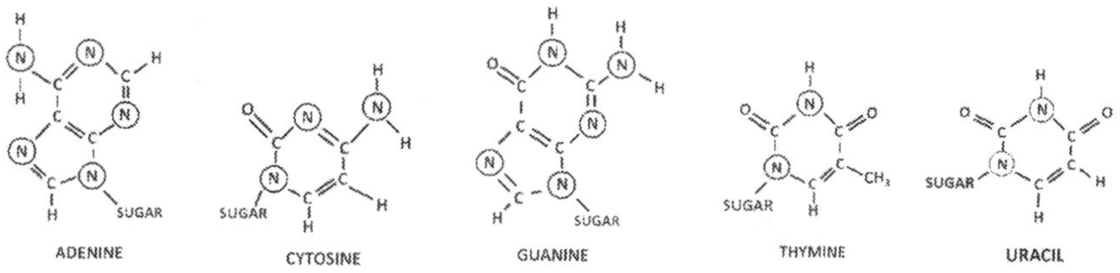

Figure 8

The five nucleotides comprising DNA and RNA.

There are five nucleotides which make up the bits of biologic information found in deoxyribonucleic acid (DNA) and ribonucleic acid (RNA). The five nucleotides include adenine, cytosine, guanine, thymine and uracil. DNA is a double stranded sequence of nucleotides, composed of adenine, cytosine, guanine, and thymine. RNA is a single stranded sequence of nucleotides composed of adenine, cytosine, guanine, and uracil. DNA is located in the nucleus and mitochondria of a cell. RNA is generated by transcribing the DNA, so messenger RNAs (mRNA), ribosomal RNAs (rRNAs) and transport RNAs (tRNAs) travel from the nucleus to the cytoplasm, and are active in the cytoplasm of the cell in which they were generated.

In the DNA, where two nucleotide strands comprise the double helix architecture of the deoxyribonucleic acid, the two genetic strands are opposite of one another. In the nucleotide coding, adenine always pairs with thymine and cytosine always pairs with guanine. The pairing is dictated by the chemical construct of the nucleotides. See Figure 9.

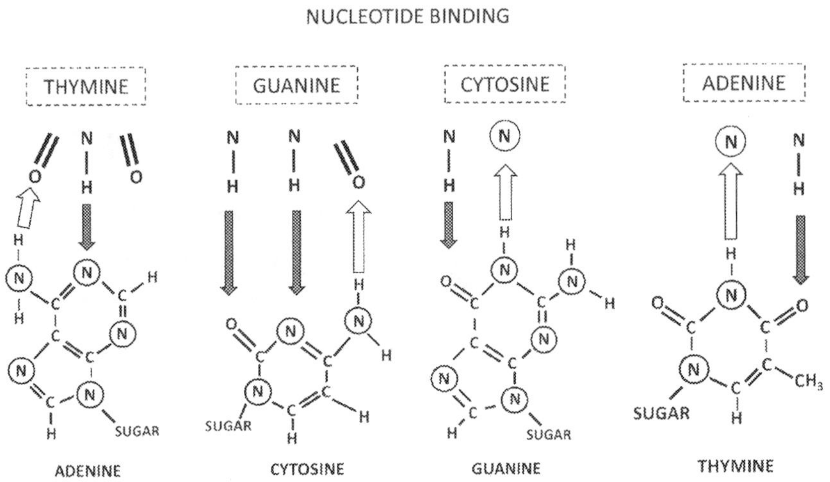

NUCLEOTIDE BINDING

THYMINE GUANINE CYTOSINE ADENINE

ADENINE CYTOSINE GUANINE THYMINE

Figure 9
Nucleotide to nucleotide bonding.

Detailed in Appendix I at the end of this text, is the analysis which describes how the optimal semi-permanent amino acid to nucleotide bonding characteristics were determined. Shown in Figure 10 is an illustration of the proposed chemical binding sites between the amino acids and the four DNA nucleotides. It turns out the binding of lysine to thymine is similar to lysine to uracil. For all four amino acids which bind semi-permanently to a DNA nucleotide, the length and construct of the R side chain of the amino acid is what facilitates the bonding characteristic of amino acid to nucleotide.

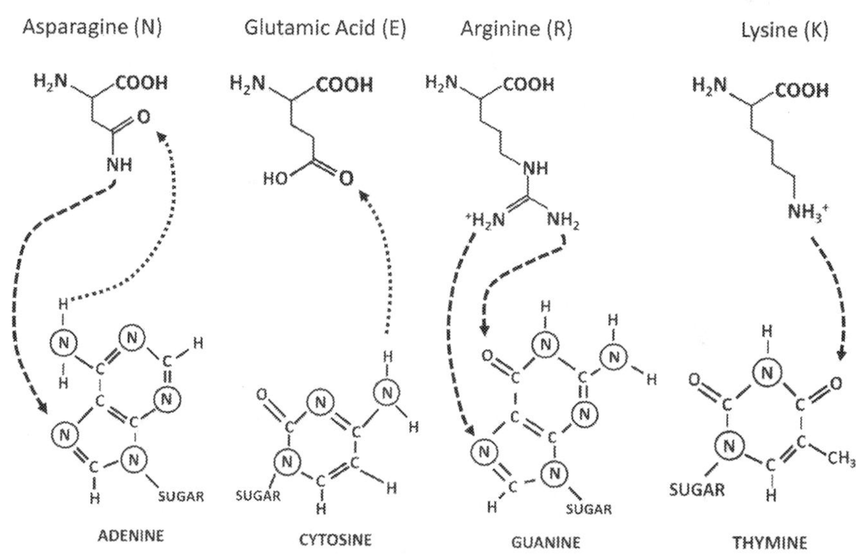

Figure 10
Optimal amino acid to nucleotide bonding.

Utilizing these key amino acids to nucleotide bonding characteristics, one can construct polypeptides which bond to segments of the DNA or the RNA. Such a concept of amino acid to nucleotide bonding could be utilized in the modification of a transcription factor IIIA (TFIIIA) polypeptide or other transcription factor, to seek out and bind to a specific portion of the DNA or to a specific portion of a messenger RNA. Furthering this concept, if the preferential binding scheme of amino acid binding to nucleotide is as illustrated above, asparagine (N) binds to adenine (a), glutamic acid (E) binds to cytosine, arginine (R) binds to guanine and lysine (K) binds to thymine, then given a segment of nucleotide coding, the binding segment of amino acids can be easily determined. The sizes of amino acids are smaller than nucleotides, so when constructing a sequence of amino acids to bind to a segment of nucleic acids, spacer amino acids need to be added in order to match the binding amino acids properly to the target nucleotides.

The amino acids which bind to nucleotides in the construct of the native TFIIIA polypeptide are known and have been mapped out. The amino acids which act as spacers has also been identified. To target a particular known segment of nucleotides present in the DNA or RNA, the sequence of nucleotides simply needs to be identified and the corresponding amino acids built into the construct of a transcription factor polypeptide such as TFIIIA. A virus like coronavirus has a vulnerable target nucleotide sequence consisting of a string of thymine (uracil) nucleotides. The TFIIIA polypeptide need only be modified such that the binding amino acids of the relevant zinc fingers of the protein are all coded to attach to thymine (uracil) nucleotides.

CHAPTER SEVEN

MODIFYING TFIIIA POLYPEPTIDE TO SEEK OUT AND NEUTRALIZE DNA VIRUSES

Ideally, a molecule could be developed to silence the HIV genome by modifying assets already in routine use by normal cells. Hormones direct cellular function and in some cases, such as the thyroid hormone, nuclear transcription. Nuclear signaling proteins generated in a cell's cytoplasm regulate nuclear function. These are examples of extranuclear proteins regulating nuclear function by engaging the DNA and either activating or blocking gene transcription.

Several nuclear and extranuclear ligands exist. These include hormones produced remotely outside the cell, intrinsic nuclear signaling proteins originating in the cytoplasm or smooth endoplasmic reticulum, and possibly control RNA molecules originating in the nucleus. Some hormones interact with nuclear receptors either combining with a nuclear receptor in the cytoplasm then migrating to the nucleus or combining with the nuclear receptor in the nucleus. Each of these modalities target a specific gene or grouping of genes once the molecule or molecular complex is in the nucleus. Some form of genetic identification must exist for the nuclear signaling protein complexes to activate or deactivate the proper genes as required. See Figure 11. Genes have unique identifiers.[15]

HIV GENOME

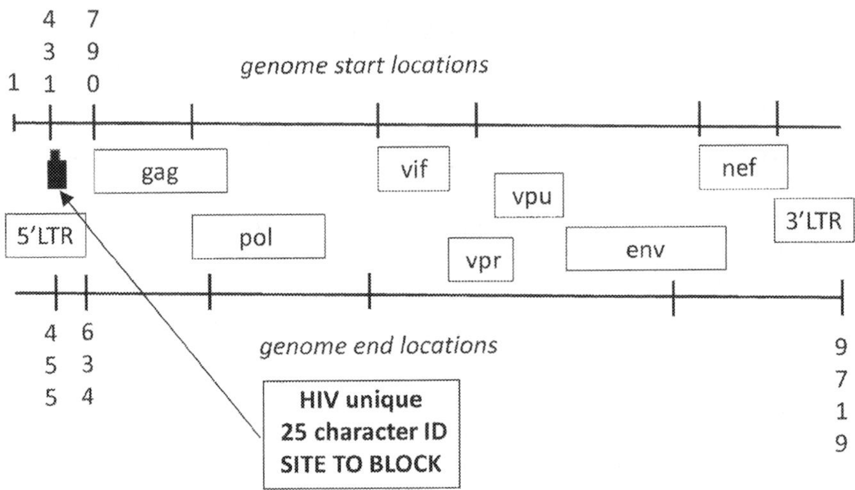

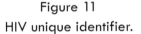

Figure 11
HIV unique identifier.

Taking advantage of the presence of a unique identifier associated with DNA embedded viruses, a nuclear binding protein could be fashioned to seek out the viral unique identifier. Therapeutic nuclear binding proteins would adhere to the DNA only in locations of the virus's unique identifier.

A unique identifier is a subsegment of DNA or RNA, which is exclusive to that sequence of genetic code. Such a unique subsegment may be 12 or more linear nucleotides; though some complex unique identifiers may be two or more linear segments of nucleotides, separated by segment(s) of uninvolved nucleotides. The unique identifier can be utilized by the cell to locate the particular segment of DNA or RNA for purposes of transcription and translation respectfully. Due to the fact the unique identifier is exclusive to a sequence of DNA or RNA, the unique identifier can be used as a target sequence to intercept the segment of DNA or RNA inside the cell. A protein can be crafted to seek out and interact with a particular sequence of DNA or RNA by targeting the sequence's unique identifier to perform a medically therapeutic function.

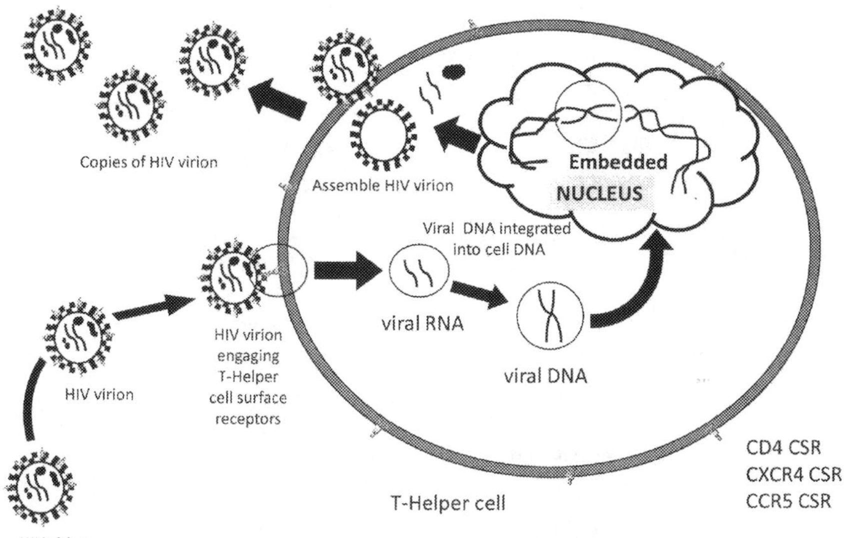

Figure 12
Life cycle of HIV.

Several choices exist for therapeutic nuclear binding proteins. The Transcription Factor III A (TFIIIA) molecule has been shown to be generated in the cytoplasm of a cell and migrate to the nucleus of a cell. The TFIIIA molecule has been implicated in viral transcription. See Figure 13. In the construct of a transcription complex, TFIIIA attaches to the DNA upstream from the transcription start site (TSS).

Modifying the TFIIIA molecule to seek out HIV's unique identifier would cause the modified TFIIIA molecule to attach to the HIV genome when embedded in the human genome. The modified TFIIIA redesigned such that once it attaches to the embedded HIV genome, the configuration of the TFIIIA molecule prevents the formation of a transcription complex that would otherwise transcribe the HIV genome. Once TFIIIA and other transcription factors have bound to the DNA, additional transcription factors and polymerase III assemble to generate the transcription complex. The transcription complex transcribes the gene targeted by TFIIIA.

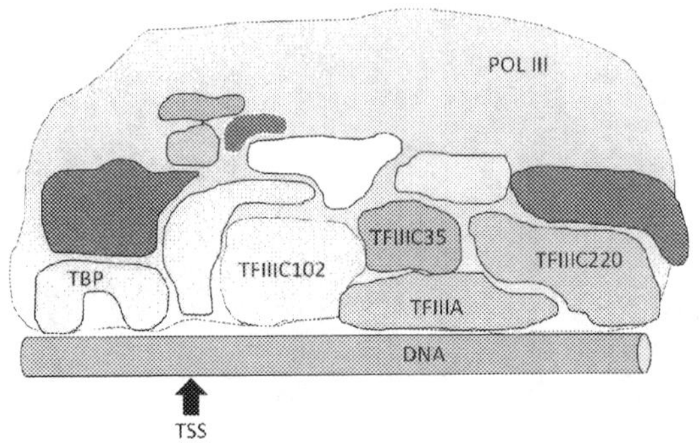

Figure 13
TFIIIA binds to DNA to assist initiation of assembly of a transcription complex.

The TFIIIA molecule is comprised of 365 amino acids. The generic TFIIIA molecule is presented in Figure 14 in a concept drawing.

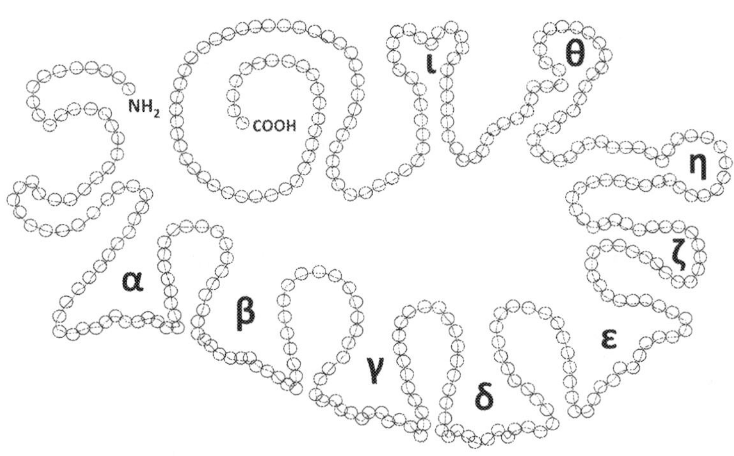

Figure 14
Concept drawing of the TFIIIA molecule.

Combining the concept that HIV has a unique identifier and nuclear binding proteins travel from the cytoplasm to the nucleus, a transcription factor molecule can be modified to seek out and target HIV's unique identifier. Human immunodeficiency virus 1 (HXB2), complete genome; HIV1/HTLV-III/LAV reference genome, GenBank K03455.1. (Accessed

October 20, 2013 at http://www.ncbi.nlm.nih.gov/nuccore/1906382.) The human immunodeficiency virus (HIV) type 1 HXB2 DNA genome at position 431 to 455 has the twenty-five nucleotide sequence 5'-agcagctgctttttgcctgtactgg-3' as a unique sequence located between HIV's TATA box and the TSS and is referred to as the unique identifier of HIV. The zinc fingers designated alpha, beta, gamma, delta and epsilon are the amino acid loops that bind to nuclear DNA. The zinc fingers designated zeta, eta, theta and iota are loops that bind with other transcription factors as the transcription complex becomes assembled.

Proper modification of zinc fingers: alpha, beta, gamma, delta, and epsilon cause the TFIIIA molecule to target the unique identifier of the HIV genome. Artful modification of the fingers designated zeta, eta, theta, and iota could prevent binding of transcription factors to the TFIIIA molecule when the TFIIIA molecule is bound to the DNA.

The alpha zinc finger's original native nucleotide sequence is SANYSKAWKLDA. As shown in Figure 15, the alpha zinc finger amino acid sequence of the TFIIIA polypeptide is converted to NSSRESSNSSRE in order to modify the TFIIIA protein to target HIV.

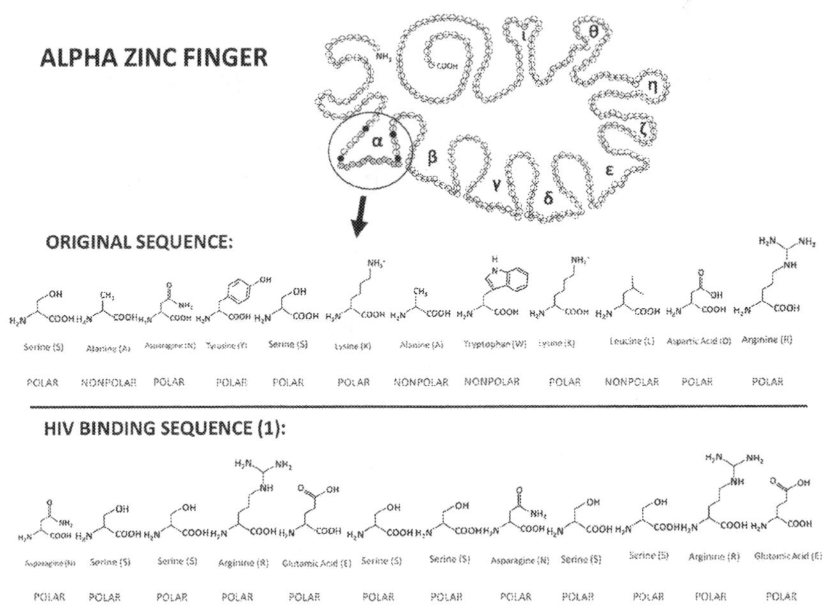

Figure 15

Alteration of the alpha zinc finger coding to neutralize HIV.

The beta zinc finger's original native nucleotide sequence is GKAFIRDYHLSR. As shown in Figure 16, the beta zinc finger amino acid sequence of the TFIIIA polypeptide is converted to KSSRESSKSSKK in order to modify the TFIIIA protein to target HIV.

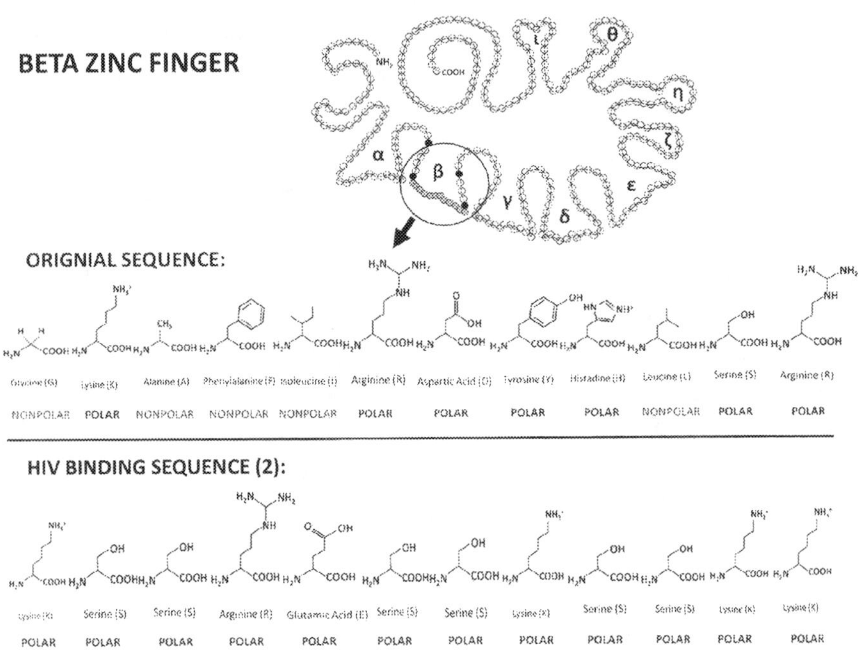

Figure 16
Alteration of the TFIIIA beta zinc finger coding to neutralize HIV.

The gamma zinc finger's original native nucleotide sequence is DQKFNTKSNLKK. As shown in Figure 17, the gamma zinc finger amino acid sequence of the TFIIIA polypeptide is converted to KSSKRSSESSEK in order to modify the TFIIIA protein to target HIV.

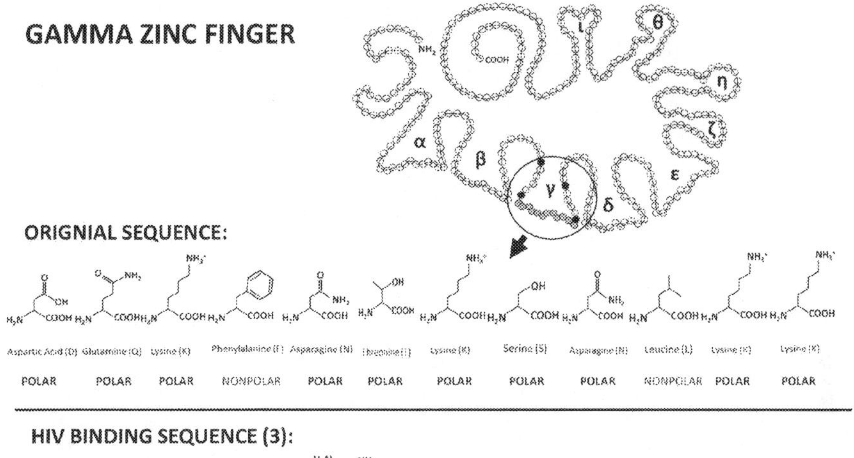

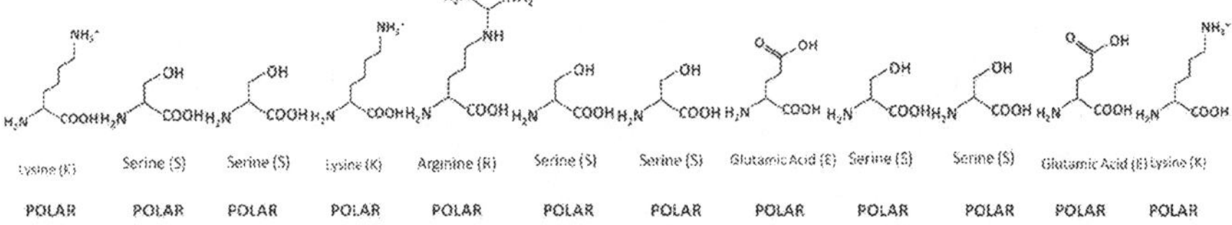

Figure 17

Alteration of the TFIIIA gamma zinc finger coding to neutralize HIV.

The delta zinc finger's original native nucleotide sequence is KKTFKKHQQLKI. As shown in Figure 18, the delta zinc finger amino acid sequence of the TFIIIA polypeptide is converted to RSSKNSSESSKR in order to modify the TFIIIA protein to target HIV.

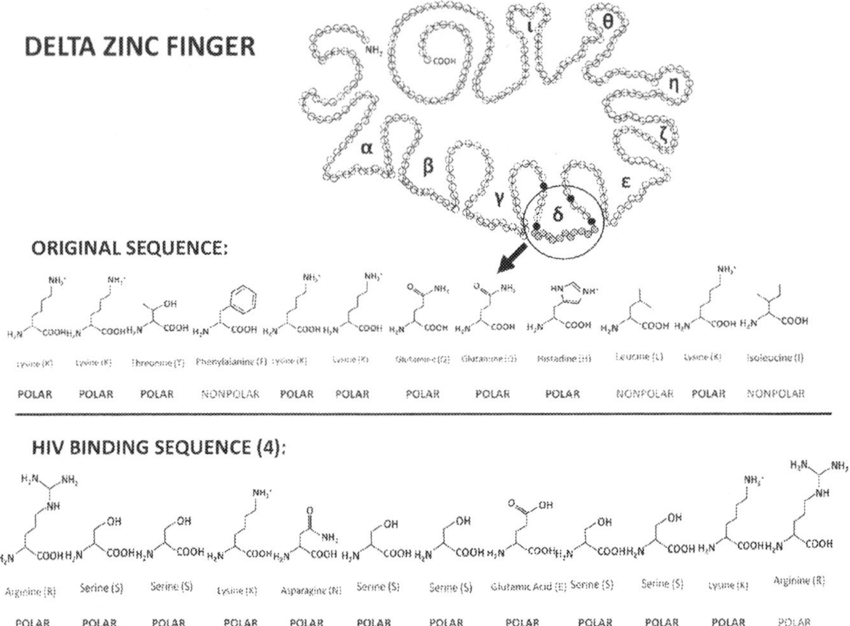

Figure 18
Alteration of the TFIIIA delta zinc finger coding to neutralize HIV.

The epsilon zinc finger's original native nucleotide sequence is GKHFASPSKLKR. As shown in Figure 19, the epsilon zinc finger amino acid sequence of the TFIIIA polypeptide is converted to RSSRKSSESSKE in order to complete the targeting sequence of the modified TFIIIA protein to facilitate the polypeptides binding to the HIV double stranded gene when embedded in human DNA.

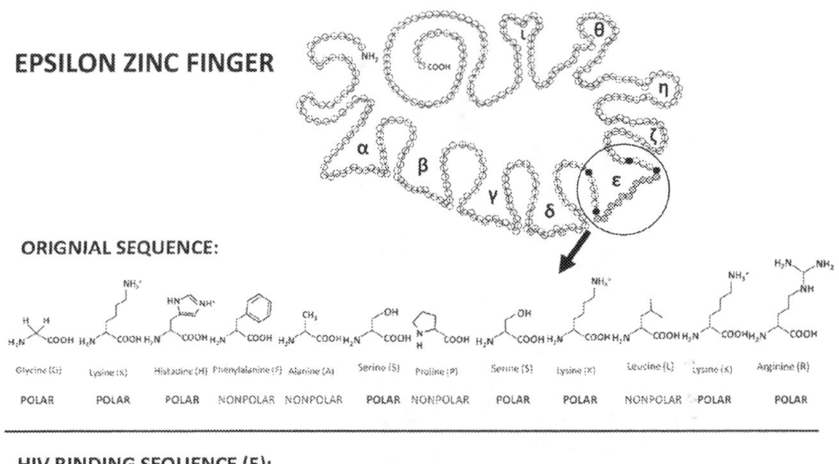

HIV BINDING SEQUENCE (5):

Arginine (R) Serine (S) Serine (S) Arginine (R) Lysine (K) Serine (S) Serine (S) Glutamic Acid (E) Serine (S) Serine (S) Lysine (K) Glutamic Acid (E)

POLAR POLAR POLAR POLAR POLAR POLAR POLAR POLAR POLAR POLAR POLAR POLAR

Figure 19

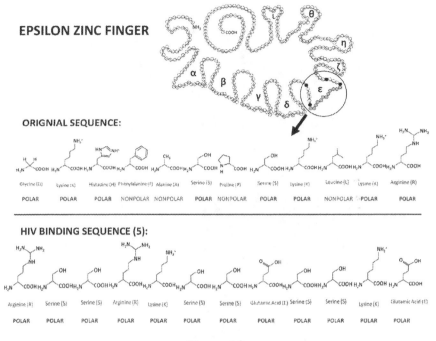

Alteration of the TFIIIA epsilon zinc finger coding to neutralize HIV.

Compiling the reconstruction of the TFIIIA polypeptide as illustrated in above Figures 15-19, results in a final modified TFIIIA polypeptide. This final modified polypeptide is designed to seek out and bind to the thirty nucleotides comprising the unique identifier of the HIV DNA genome.

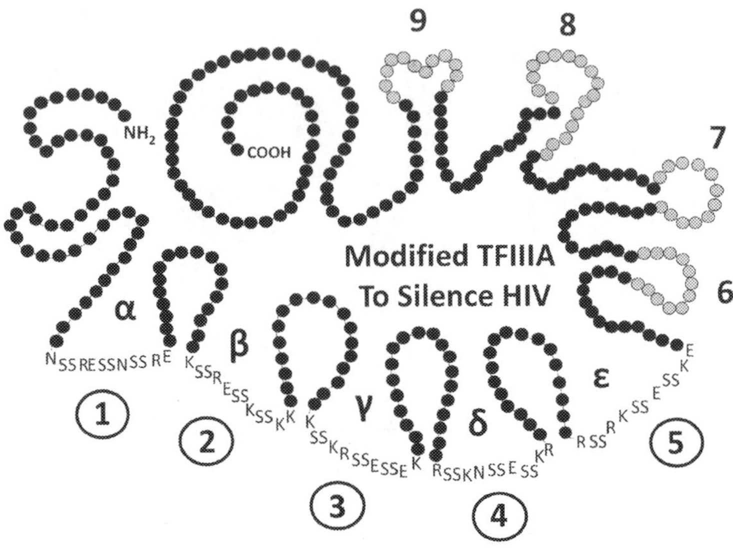

Figure 20
TFIIIA molecule to bind to HIV unique identifier.

Figure 20 represents the generic molecule that may be termed a Molecular Virus Killer due to the concept whereby if a TFIIIA molecule is modified to target a specific virus, such a TFIIIA molecule would be capable of semi-permanently binding to a viral genome and preventing transcription of the virus's genetic material. If a virus's genome is prevented from being transcribed, then the virus is unable to generate copies of its virion and in effect the viral infection has been halted.

MOLECULAR VIRUS KILLER TO SILENCE HIV GENOME

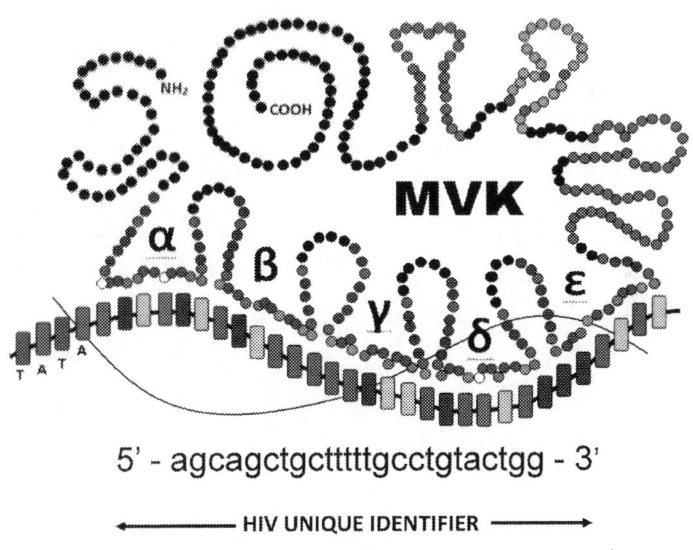

Figure 21
TFIIIA binding to HIV unique identifier post TATA box
to neutralize HIV DNA genome from replicating.

This example was an exercise to modify the TFIIIA polypeptide to neutralize HIV which is a DNA virus. A similar design strategy could be employed to alter the construct of the TFIIIA polypeptide to seek out and attach to RNA viruses, such as coronavirus.

CHAPTER EIGHT

STEPPING UP THE DESIGN EFFORT TO ACCOUNT FOR THE DIFFERENT CHALLENGES REQUIRED TO COMBAT RNA VIRUSES

Designing a means to neutralize an RNA virus, like coronavirus, enlists similar strategies as to what is necessary to create a polypeptide to bind to a segment of DNA, such as described for the HIV DNA virus. There is are several distinct differences when designing a therapeutic molecule to target a viral messenger RNA genome.

First, there may not be a signature segment in the viral mRNA which would be a unique target for which to design a modified TFIIIA molecule. That is, where most genes likely have some subsegment or segments, which acts as a unique identifier so that the cell transcription machinery can locate the gene when needed, mRNAs may not need employ any form of unique code in order for the ribosome to find and translate the mRNA. In fact, it may be more efficient for the cell for all mRNAs to have a universal appearance such that ribosomal complexes simply translate any mRNA the decoders encounters, rather than having the ribosomal complex try to decide if it should or shouldn't translate a segment of mRNA.

Second, transcription factors once generated, are meant to migrate from the cytoplasm to inside the nucleus of the cell. Coronavirus spends its intracellular life in the cytoplasm. Therefore, the structure of the modified medically therapeutic transcription factor needs to be further altered to prevent our RNA virus seeking TFIIIA, from leaving the cytoplasm and entering the nucleus.

Third, binding to a segment of DNA entails accounting for the curving physical nature of the deoxyribonucleic acid structure. The DNA is somewhat of a predicable physical target given that two strands of nucleotide sequences bond together and support each other. Coronavirus on the other hand is represented as a single strand of nucleotides. There may be unforeseen challenges presented by trying to bind to a portion of the single strand of nucleotides as the molecule floats in the 3D dynamic fluid environment of the cell's cytoplasm. Thus, targeting the virus's negative-sense thymine (uracil) tail, may offer the simplest, most efficient and successful means of neutralizing coronavirus.

CHAPTER NINE

RECONFIGURING TRANSCRIPTION FACTOR IIIA INTO A HUNTER-KILLER POLYPEPTIDE TO ENGAGE AND BIND TO THE URACIL TAIL OF THE COVID-19 NEGATIVE-SENSE RNA VIRAL GENOME

Abstract

A modified version of the human TFIIIA polypeptide is designed to seek out the poly uracil tail of a negative-sense version of the coronavirus's genome with the intention to act as a practical means to neutralize the global pandemic. Altering zinc fingers 1-6 of the native TFIIIA polypeptide causes the protein to seek out and bind to the 33 amino acid uracil tail of the negative-sense coronavirus genome. See Figure 22. Attaching a 365 amino acid polypeptide to the coronavirus genome will interfere with the replication of the virus and halt the infectious nature of the virus.

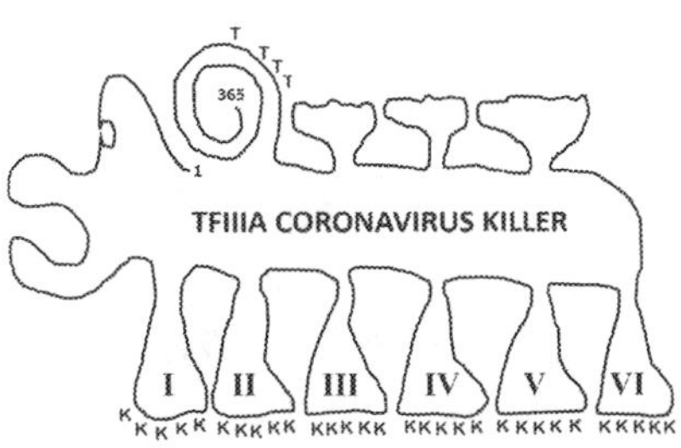

Figure 22
Artistic illustration of the Transcription Factor IIIA to seek out and neutralize COVID-19.

FIELD OF THE INVENTION

This invention relates to any medical device intended to intercept, engage and bind to a segment of nucleotides in a target messenger ribonucleic acid or viral genome.

BACKGROUND ART

Transcription Factor IIIA is often referred to as TFIIIA or AP2. Transcription factor IIIA is the product of the gene referred to as GTF3A NC_ 000013.11. GTF3A is a human DNA gene 11,205 base pairs in length.

Transcription Factor IIIA (TFIIIA) (TI9606) is a human polypeptide fashioned to seek out and attach to the DNA and RNA. Zinc fingers 1-3 and 5, are interactive projections of the 365 amino acid TFIIIA molecule, which inherently are meant to bind to nucleotides in the DNA, with zinc fingers 4 and 6 acting as spacers. Zinc fingers 7-9 bind to other transcription factors resulting in the assembly of a larger transcription complex.

OBJECTIVE

To redesign the native human Transcription Factor IIIA (TFIIIA) polypeptide, recoding the DNA binding sites, in order to modify the protein into a hunter-killer molecule programmed specifically to seek out and neutralize the coronavirus genome inside infected host cells.

NATIVE TRANSCRIPTION FACTOR IIIA

The following three hundred sixty-five amino acid sequence comprises the Transcription Factor III A molecule, Taxonomic identifier 9606 [NCBI]:

```
1         10         20         30         40         50         60
MDPPAVVAES VSSLTIADAF IAAGESSAPT PPRPALPRRF ICSFPDCSAN YSKAWKLDAH
```

```
        70          80          90         100         110         120
LCKHTGERPF  VCDYEGCGKA  FIRDYHLSRH  ILTHTGEKPF  VCAANGCDQK  FNTKSNLKKH
       130         140         150         160         170         180
FERKHENQQK  QYICSFEDCK  KTFKKHQQLK  IHQCQHTNEP  LFKCTQEGCG  KHFASPSKLK
       190         200         210         220         230         240
RHAKAHEGYV  CQKGCSFVAK  TWTELLKHVR  ETHKEEILCE  VCRKTFKRKD  YLKQHMKTHA
       250         260         270         280         290         300
PERDVCRCPR  EGCGRTYTTV  FNLQSHILSF  HEESRPFVCE  HAGCGKTFAM  KQSLTRHAVV
       310         320         330         340         350         360
HDPDKKKMKL  KVKKSREKRS  LASHLSGYIP  PKRKQGQGLS  LCQNGESPNC  VEDKMLSTVA
  365
VLTLG
```

The TFIIIA TI9606 is utilized naturally by a human cell to assist in the transcription of 5S RNA molecules. The TFIIIA molecule also assists in transcribing some viral DNA genomes. The amino acid sequence of TFIIIA's zinc fingers can auspiciously be recoded to bind to an alternative segment of DNA or bind to an RNA.

Studies indicate a preferential tight bonding relationship of amino acid-to-nucleobases is accomplished with the amino acid 'asparagine' binding to 'adenine', 'arginine' binding to 'guanine', 'glutamic acid' binding to 'cytosine' and 'lysine' binding to 'thymine' or 'uracil'. With such a bonding strategy, the amino acid sequence of the native TFIIIA molecule can be restructured to seek out and hunt down a signature nucleotide sequence in the native DNA or native RNA or a viral genome.

COVID-19 is a positive-sense single-stranded RNA virus when delivered to a host cell by the virus's virion. Once in the cytoplasm of a host cell, the positive-sense COVID-19 genome is converted to the complement of the genome's original self, which is referred to as a negative-sense genome. The complementary negative-sense RNA would exist such that each adenine in the original RNA would be replaced by uracil, each uracil replaced by adenine, each cytosine replaced by guanine and each guanine replaced by cytosine. At the terminal aspect of the 3' end of the positive-sense coronavirus genome there is a tail comprised of as many as thirty-three adenine nucleotides. In the negative-sense version of the COVID-19 genome, 'adenine' is represented as its complement nucleobase 'uracil'. The tail of the negative-sense version of the COVID-19 viral genome is therefore comprised of a sequence of as many as thirty-three uracil nucleotides.

Human messenger RNAs use adenine tails for regulation of translation. Typically, mRNAs possess a number of adenine nucleotides at the 3' end of the sequence of nucleotides which is often used by the ribosomes decoding the mRNA template to determine the number of times to translate proteins from the mRNA template. A long sequence of native thymine nucleotides would be found in the nucleus of the cell coded into the human genome, but not in the cytoplasm of the cell. Messenger RNA would typically have long 3' tails consisting of adenine nucleotides. Messenger RNAs would not typically have extensive sequences of uracil nucleotides comprising their coding. When the coronavirus exists in the complementary negative-sense genome state, the 3' tail consisting of more than thirty uracil nucleotides becomes an inviting target to attach polypeptide. Binding a large polypeptide to the coronavirus genome will prevent the virus from replicating and thus halt the infectious nature of coronavirus.

The structure of the native human TFIIIA polypeptide can be modified so as to change the binding sites of amino acid-to-nucleobases in zinc fingers 1-6 so that all represent lysine (K) to institute binding to uracil. Floating free in the cytoplasm of a host cell, lysine rich zinc fingers 1-6 would target the uracil tail of the negative-sense coronavirus genome. Once attached to the coronavirus genome, the modified TFIIIA polypeptide would prevent replication of the virus's genome.

The nucleotide sequence PDKKKMKLK present in the 3' tail of the native TFIIIA polypeptide is proposed to act as the nuclear location sequence (NLS), giving the molecule access to the cell's nucleus.[18] It is desirable to maintain the modified TFIIIA in the cytoplasm and prevent the polypeptide from entering into the nucleus. In order to trap the modified TFIIIA polypeptide in the cytoplasm the lysine amino acids of the native NSL can be changes to threonine.

SUMMARY DESCRIPTION

The amino acid sequence of the human TFIIIA TI 9606 polypeptide can be modified to cause the TFIIIA polypeptide to seek out and bind to a specific sequence of amino acids present in the genome of a mRNA or RNA viral genome.

The amino acid sequence comprising the TFIIIA polypeptide can be modified such that the amino acid-nucleotide binding sites present in zinc fingers 1-6 can be altered such that the modified TFIIIA polypeptide seeks out the poly uracil tail of a negative-sense RNA version of the coronavirus genome. The TFIIIA's zinc fingers 7-9 can be modified such that the molecule does not interact with other transcription factors. The segment of the TFIIIA polypeptide that allows the molecule to gain access to the nucleus of the host cell can be altered such that the modified TFIIIA molecule is restricted to the cytoplasm of the cell.

The modified form of the TFIIIA molecule is as follows, with the original amino acid sequence comprising the molecule modified as mentioned above and the new amino acid sequences appearing in their defined position and underlined for clarity.

1 10	20	30	40	50	60
MDPPAVVAES	VSSLTIADAF	IAAGESSAPT	PPRPALPRRF	ICSFPDCKSS	KKSSKSSKKH
70	80	90	100	110	120
LCKHTGERPF	VCDYEGCKSS	KKSSKSSKKH	ILTHTGEKPF	VCAANGCKSS	KKSSKSSKKH
130	140	150	160	170	180
FERKHENQQK	QYICSFEDCK	SSKKSSKSSK	KHQCQHTNEP	LFKCTQEGCK	SSKKSSKSSK
190	200	210	220	230	240
KHAKAHEGYV	CQKGCSFVKK	KWKKLLKHVR	ETHKEEILCE	VCATTFTATD	YLTQHMKTHA
250	260	270	280	290	300
PERDVCRCPA	AGCGATYTTV	FALQAHILSF	HEESRPFVCE	HAGCGTTFAM	TQALTAHAVV
310	320	330	340	350	360
HDPDTTTMTL	TVKKSREKRS	LASHLSGYIP	PKRKQGQGLS	LCQNGESPNC	VEDKMLSTVA
365					
VLTLG					

DETAILED DESCRIPTION

The three hundred sixty-five amino acid sequence of the native TFIIIA polypeptide:

1 10	20	30	40	50	60
MDPPAVVAES	VSSLTIADAF	IAAGESSAPT	PPRPALPRRF	ICSFPDCSAN	YSKAWKLDAH

```
        70         80         90        100        110        120
LCKHTGERPF VCDYEGCGKA FIRDYHLSRH ILTHTGEKPF VCAANGCDQK FNTKSNLKKH
       130        140        150        160        170        180
FERKHENQQK QYICSFEDCK KTFKKHQQLK IHQCQHTNEP LFKCTQEGCG KHFASPSKLK
       190        200        210        220        230        240
RHAKAHEGYV CQKGCSFVAK TWTELLKHVR ETHKEEILCE VCRKTFKRKD YLKQHMKTHA
       250        260        270        280        290        300
PERDVCRCPR EGCGRTYTTV FNLQSHILSF HEESRPFVCE HAGCGKTFAM KQSLTRHAVV
       310        320        330        340        350        360
HDPDKKKMKL KVKKSREKRS LASHLSGYIP PKRKQGQGLS LCQNGESPNC VEDKMLSTVA
  365
VLTLG
```

Represents the naturally occurring Transcription Factor IIIA molecule, Taxonomic identifier 9606 [NCBI] (TFIIIA9606) found at http://www.uniprot.org/uniprot/Q92664. The TFIIIA TI9606 protein is 365 amino acids in length.

The human TFIIIA (TI 9606) polypeptide is 365 amino acids in length. There are nine zinc fingers in the structure moving from the 5' (NH2) to 3' (COOH) end of the molecule designated as zinc finger 1, zinc finger 2, zinc finger 3, zinc finger 4, zinc finger 5, zinc finger 6, zinc finger 7, zinc finger 8, and zinc finger 9. There is a nucleus locating sequence near the terminal portion of the molecule at the 3' end. To create a modified TFIIIA polypeptide to seek out the poly uracil tail of a negative-sense viral genome the native human TFIIIA amino acid sequence would be recoded as follows:

Zinc finger 1 is considered to include amino acids 40 to 64.
Within zinc finger 1, the amino acids 48 to 59 'SANYSKAWKLDA' are changed to the amino acid sequence 'KSSKKSSKSSKK'.

Zinc finger 2 is considered to include amino acids 70 to 94.
Within zinc finger 2, amino acids 78 to 89 'GKAFIRDYHLSR' are changed to the amino acid sequence 'KSSKKSSKSSKK'.

Zinc finer 3 is considered to include amino acids 100 to 125.
Within zinc finger 3, amino acids 108 to 119 'DQKFNTKSNLKK' are changed to the amino acid sequence 'KSSKKSSKSSKK'.

Zinc finger 4 is considered to include amino acids 132 to 154. Within zinc finger 4, amino acids 140 to 151 'KKTFKKHQQLKI' are changed to the amino acid sequence 'KSSKKSSKSSKK'.

Zinc finger 5 is considered to include amino acids 162 to 186. Within zinc finger 5, amino acids 170 to 181 'GKHFASPSKLKR' are changed to the amino acid sequence 'KSSKKSSKSSKK'.

Zinc finger 6 is considered to include amino acids 189 to 213. Zinc finger 6, amino acids 196 to 207 'SFVAKTWTELLK' are changed to the amino acid sequence 'SFVKKKWKKLLK'.

Zinc finger 7 is considered to include amino acids 217 to 239. Within zinc finger 7, amino acids 223 TO 234 'RKTFKRKDYLKQ' are changed to the amino acid sequence 'ATTFTATDYLTQ'.

Zinc finger 8 is considered to include amino acids 246 to 271. Within zinc finger 8, amino acids 249 to 265 'PREGCGRTYTTVFNLQS' are changed to the amino acid sequence 'PAAGCGATYTTVFALQA'.

Zinc finger 9 is considered to include the amino acids 277 to 301. Within zinc finger 9, amino acids 285 TO 296 'GKTFAMKQSLTR' are changed to the amino acid sequence 'GTTFAMTQALTA'.

The cell restricts flow of molecules which enter into the nucleus from the cytoplasm. In the cycle of protein production, messenger RNAs are generated in the nucleus as a result of transcription complexes decoding the DNA. The mRNAs travel from the nucleus to the cytoplasm, where the mRNAs are translated by ribosomes and polypeptides are created. A portion of the polypeptides generated in the translation process are required to enter the nucleus to perform duties required by cell metabolism and to satisfy the structural requirements of the cell's nuclear architecture. Polypeptides destined to enter the nucleus are labeled with a particular sequence of amino acids termed the nuclear location sequence (NLS). The gateways through the nuclear membrane separating the cytoplasm from the inner chamber of the nucleus recognize the NLS coded into the structure of the polypeptide and grant access to polypeptides which possess the proper NLS.

The amino acid sequence 'PDKKKMKLK' present in the 3' tail of the native TFIIIA polypeptide (TI9606) from amino acid 303 to 311 acts as the nuclear location sequence, giving the molecule access to the translocate from the cell's cytoplasm to the nucleus of the cell.[18] It is desirable to maintain the modified TFIIIA in the cytoplasm and prevent the polypeptide from entering into the nucleus. In order to trap the modified TFIIIA polypeptide in the cytoplasm of a cell to optimize the molecule's effectiveness, the lysine amino acids of the native NSL are changed to threonine. The modified TFIIIA polypeptide is to possess the modified amino acid sequence of amino acids 303 to 311 as described as 'PDTTTMTLT'.

The modified form of the TFIIIA molecule is as follows with the original amino acid sequence comprising the molecule modified as mentioned above and the new amino acid sequences appearing in their defined position and underlined for clarity.

```
1          10          20          30          40          50          60
   MDPPAVVAES  VSSLTIADAF  IAAGESSAPT  PPRPALPRRF  ICSFPDCKSS  KKSSKSSKKH
           70          80          90         100         110         120
   LCKHTGERPF  VCDYEGCKSS  KKSSKSSKKH  ILTHTGEKPF  VCAANGCKSS  KKSSKSSKKH
          130         140         150         160         170         180
   FERKHENQQK  QYICSFEDCK  SSKKSSKSSK  KHQCQHTNEP  LFKCTQEGCK  SSKKSSKSSK
          190         200         210         220         230         240
   KHAKAHEGYV  CQKGCSFVKK  KWKKLLKHVR  ETHKEEILCE  VCATTFTATD  YLTQHMKTHA
          250         260         270         280         290         300
   PERDVCRCPA  AGCGATYTTV  FALQAHILSF  HEESRPFVCE  HAGCGTTFAM  TQALTAHAVV
          310         320         330         340         350         360
   HDPDTTTMTL  TVKKSREKRS  LASHLSGYIP  PKRKQGQGLS  LCQNGESPNC  VEDKMLSTVA
   365
VLTLG
```

Coronavirus replicates its RNA genome in the cytoplasm of the host cell and passes a copy of the genetic code onto the next generation of virus virions. Once constructed with a copy of the viral code, the coronavirus virion exits the host cell and travels to other potential host cells to repeat the replication process. The TFIIIA polypeptide reconstructed in the above manner will transform this modified TFIIIA polypeptide into a medically therapeutic agent that will seek out and bind to the poly uracil tail of the negative-sense coronavirus genome or other similar negative-sense RNA viral genome. Once the modified TFIIIA polypeptide has attached itself to the poly uracil tail of the negative-sense coronavirus genome or other similar negative-sense RNA viral genome, the presence of the modified TFIIIA polypeptide attached to the viral genome will interfere with the replication process meant to copy the virus's genome.

If the viral genome is prevented from being replicated by the physical attachment of TFIIIA to the virus's genome, there will be no copies of the viral genome to pass on to the next generation and the infectious nature of the virus is neutralized. The impotent viral genome will be broken down and destroyed cellular enzymes.

Targeting the unique poly uracil tail of the negative-sense coronavirus genome with a modified TFIIIA polypeptide as described should not affect other native mRNAs, nor the translation of native mRNAs.

Likely other specific segments of viral RNA, in addition to the poly uracil tail, can be determined to be unique target sequences, which modified TNFIIIA polypeptides can be constructed to seek out and bind to in order to neutralize coronavirus or other RNA viruses.

Introducing modified TFIIIA therapeutic polypeptides into host cells infected by the coronavirus may be accomplished by a number of practical means. Once infused into the body, the modified TFIIIA molecule might diffuse across the cell membrane or become invaginated by the cell. A carrier protein or vacuole might be enlisted to transport TFIIIA into cells.

To introduce the therapeutic modified TFIIIA polypeptide into a cell, an interesting approach would be editing COVID-19's own genome, extruding unnecessary viral elements, while embedding programming code sufficient to construct the modified TFIIIA molecule. Coronavirus virion's spike probe seeks out and binds to the ACE2 cell surface receptor present on a number of different human cells. Paradoxically, the bio-programming comprising the coronavirus's genome could be rewritten to generate COVID-19 virions which would deliver therapeutic TFIIIA molecules to the same human cells the virus targets.

DISCUSSION

The human race cannot allow a misguided scrap of malignant bio-programming code to ravage the world's population without being heatedly contested by our best efforts at innovation. We must capitalize on the advancements in the knowledge of how the DNA is decoded, the construct of transcription factors and how mRNAs are translated. A modified TFIIIA polypeptide designed to seek out the poly uracil tail of a negative-sense version of the coronavirus is a practical means to neutralize the COVID-19 viral global pandemic threat.

CHAPTER TEN

SEARCH FOR THE IDEAL THERAPEUTIC TARGET IN COVID-19 NUCLEOTIDE SEQUENCING

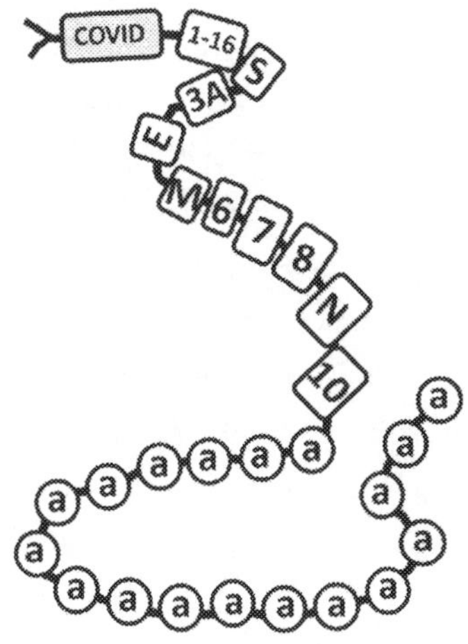

Figure 23
Searching for the optimal target amongst COVID-19's 29,900 amino acids.

The topic reviewed and discussed in the previous chapter was to target the negative sense tail of the coronavirus in order to neutralize the virus and prevent the virus from replicating. There may be numerous nucleotide segments in the coronavirus's genome unique to the virus, which could be used as possibly an even more effective target signature with which to construct a transcription factor to neutralize COVID-19. A 20-30 nucleotide sequence unique to coronavirus could be used worldwide to neutralize all existing generations of coronavirus and all future variations of the virus. A nucleotide sequence unique to coronavirus may offer a more specific and better treatment target than the thymine tail of the negative sense version of the virus's genome.

To discover such a unique 20-30 nucleotide sequence, if it exists, likely requires taking the coronavirus genome and matching all of the 20-30 nucleotide segments to the mRNA data base for humans. This can be done with a simple computer program, but requires interfacing with NCBI more intimately than can be done as a private home investigator. There was an attempt by the authors to search out a unique segment of the coronavirus by hand and it was quickly realized that the amount of time it would take to complete such as task by hand was beyond the scope of time we had available to solve the problem.

Additionally, as mentioned earlier, there may be unforeseen challenges presented by trying to bind a therapeutic molecule to a portion of a single strand of nucleotides comprising mRNA as the molecule floats in the 3D dynamic fluid environment of the cell's cytoplasm. A single strand of nucleotides may whip violently around in the dynamic flow of the complex fluid environment of the cytoplasm. Erratic and sporadic movement of mRNA may make it difficult for a therapeutic molecule to bond to a target segment located internal to the overall structure of the molecule. Thus, targeting the virus's negative-sense thymine tail, may in the end offer the most efficient and successful means of neutralizing coronavirus.

The designer of such an intervention must be leery that the 3D orientation of one or more zinc fingers of the TFIIIA polypeptide may be reversed in relation to how the nucleotides are physically linearly written. Thus, re-coding a TFIIIA molecule to seek out a unique identifier present in the coronavirus genome may be a little tricky. On the other hand, re-coding a TFIIIA polypeptide to seek out a long sequence of consecutive uracil nucleotides mitigates the targeting problems related to the 3D orientation of trying to bond to a pliant RNA molecule.

CHAPTER ELEVEN

MESSENGER RIBONUCLEIC ACID TO PRODUCE A MODIFIED TRANSCRIPTION FACTOR IIIA POLYPEPTIDE TO ENGAGE AND BIND TO THE URACIL TAIL OF COVID-19 RNA VIRAL GENOME

Abstract

A modified version of the human TFIIIA polypeptide messenger ribonucleic acid molecule is designed so that when translated will produce a modified TFIIIA polypeptide to seek out the poly uracil tail of a negative-sense version of the coronavirus's genome with the intention to act as a practical means to neutralize the global pandemic. Altering zinc fingers 1-6 of the native TFIIIA polypeptide causes the protein to seek out and bind to the 33 amino acid uracil tail of the negative-sense coronavirus genome. Attaching a 365 amino acid polypeptide to the coronavirus genome will interfere with the replication of the virus and halt the infectious nature of the virus. New advances in inhaled mRNA therapies make this modified mRNA strategy a practical therapeutic management option.

Messenger Ribonucleic Acid to Produce a Modified Transcription Factor IIIA Polypeptide to Engage and Bind to the Uracil Tail of COVID-19 RNA Viral Genome

FIELD OF THE INVENTION

This invention relates to any medical device intended to generate a protein which will intercept, engage and bind to a segment of nucleotides in a target messenger ribonucleic acid or viral genome.

DESCRIPTION

Transcription Factor IIIA is often referred to as TFIIIA or AP2. Transcription factor IIIA is the product of the gene referred to as GTF3A NC_ 000013.11. GTF3A is a human DNA gene 11,205 base pairs in length.

Transcription Factor IIIA (TFIIIA) (TI9606) is a human polypeptide fashioned to seek out and attach to the DNA and RNA. Zinc fingers 1-3 and 5, are interactive projections of the 365 amino acid TFIIIA molecule, which inherently are meant to bind to nucleotides in the DNA, with zinc fingers 4 and 6 acting as spacers. Zinc fingers 7-9 bind to other transcription factors resulting in the assembly of a larger transcription complex.

The following three hundred sixty-five amino acid sequence comprises the Transcription Factor III A molecule, Taxonomic identifier 9606 [NCBI]:

```
1         10          20          30          40          50          60
 MDPPAVVAES  VSSLTIADAF  IAAGESSAPT  PPRPALPRRF  ICSFPDCSAN  YSKAWKLDAH
         70          80          90         100         110         120
 LCKHTGERPF  VCDYEGCGKA  FIRDYHLSRH  ILTHTGEKPF  VCAANGCDQK  FNTKSNLKKH
        130         140         150         160         170         180
 FERKHENQQK  QYICSFEDCK  KTFKKHQQLK  IHQCQHTNEP  LFKCTQEGCG  KHFASPSKLK
        190         200         210         220         230         240
 RHAKAHEGYV  CQKGCSFVAK  TWTELLKHVR  ETHKEEILCE  VCRKTFKRKD  YLKQHMKTHA
        250         260         270         280         290         300
 PERDVCRCPR  EGCGRTYTTV  FNLQSHILSF  HEESRPFVCE  HAGCGKTFAM  KQSLTRHAVV
        310         320         330         340         350         360
 HDPDKKKMKL  KVKKSREKRS  LASHLSGYIP  PKRKQGQGLS  LCQNGESPNC  VEDKMLSTVA
        365
 VLTLG
```

The TFIIIA TI9606 is utilized naturally by a human cell to assist in the transcription of 5S RNA molecules. The TFIIIA molecule also assists in transcribing some viral DNA genomes. The amino acid sequence of TFIIIA's zinc fingers can auspiciously be recoded to bind to an alternative segment of DNA or bind to an RNA.

Studies indicate a preferential tight bonding relationship of amino acid-to-nucleobases is accomplished with the amino acid 'asparagine' binding to 'adenine', 'arginine' binding to 'guanine', 'glutamic acid' binding to 'cytosine' and 'lysine' binding to 'thymine' or 'uracil'.[1,2] With such a bonding strategy, the amino acid sequence of the native TFIIIA molecule can be restructured to seek out and hunt down a signature nucleotide sequence in the native DNA or native RNA or a viral genome.

COVID-19 is a positive-sense single-stranded RNA virus when delivered to a host cell by the virus's virion. Once in the cytoplasm of a host cell, the positive-sense COVID-19 genome is converted to the complement of the genome's original self, which is referred to as a negative-sense genome. The complementary negative-sense RNA would exist such that each adenine in the original RNA would be replaced by uracil, each uracil replaced by adenine, each cytosine replaced by guanine and each guanine replaced by cytosine. At the terminal aspect of the 3' end of the positive-sense coronavirus genome there is a tail comprised of as many as thirty-three adenine nucleotides. In the negative-sense version of the COVID-19 genome, 'adenine' is represented as its complement nucleobase 'uracil'. The tail of the negative-sense version of the COVID-19 viral genome is therefore comprised of a sequence of as many as thirty-three uracil nucleotides.

Human messenger RNAs use adenine tails for regulation of translation. Typically, mRNAs possess a number of adenine nucleotides at the 3' end of the sequence of nucleotides which is often used by the ribosomes decoding the mRNA template to determine the number of times to translate proteins from the mRNA template. A long sequence of native thymine nucleotides would be found in the nucleus of the cell coded into the human genome, but not in the cytoplasm of the cell. Messenger RNA would typically have long 3' tails consisting of adenine nucleotides. Messenger RNAs would not typically have extensive sequences of uracil nucleotides comprising their coding. When the coronavirus exists in the complementary negative-sense genome state, the 3' tail consisting of more than thirty uracil nucleotides becomes an inviting target to attach polypeptide. Binding a large polypeptide to the coronavirus genome will prevent the virus from replicating and thus halt the infectious nature of coronavirus.

The structure of the native human TFIIIA polypeptide can be modified so as to change the binding sites of amino acid-to-nucleobases in zinc fingers 1-6 so that all represent lysine (K) to institute binding to uracil. Floating free in the cytoplasm of a host cell, lysine rich zinc fingers 1-6 would target the uracil tail of the negative-sense coronavirus genome. Once attached to the coronavirus genome, the modified TFIIIA polypeptide would prevent replication of the virus's genome.

The nucleotide sequence PDKKKMKLK present in the 3' tail of the native TFIIIA polypeptide is proposed to act as the nuclear location sequence (NLS), giving the molecule access to the cell's nucleus. It is desirable to maintain the modified TFIIIA in the cytoplasm and prevent the polypeptide from entering into the nucleus. In order to trap the modified TFIIIA polypeptide in the cytoplasm the lysine amino acids of the native NSL can be changes to threonine.[18]

SUMMARY OF THE 'CURE' DESCRIPTION

The amino acid sequence of the human TFIIIA TI 9606 polypeptide can be modified to cause the TFIIIA polypeptide to seek out and bind to a specific sequence of amino acids present in the genome of a mRNA or RNA viral genome.

The amino acid sequence comprising the TFIIIA polypeptide can be modified such that the amino acid-nucleotide binding sites present in zinc fingers 1-6 can be altered such that the modified TFIIIA polypeptide seeks out the poly uracil tail of a negative-sense RNA version of the coronavirus genome. The TFIIIA's zinc fingers 7-9 can be modified such that the molecule does not interact with other transcription factors. The segment of the TFIIIA polypeptide that allows the molecule to gain access to the nucleus of the host cell, the nuclear location sequence, can be altered such that the modified TFIIIA molecule is restricted to the cytoplasm of the cell.

The modified TFIIIA molecule is constructed to seek out the uracil tail of the negative-sense COVID-19 genome. Bonding the medically therapeutic TFIIIA to the uracil tail of the intracellular negative-sense COVID-19 genome would prevent coronavirus from being able to replicate. See Figure 24.

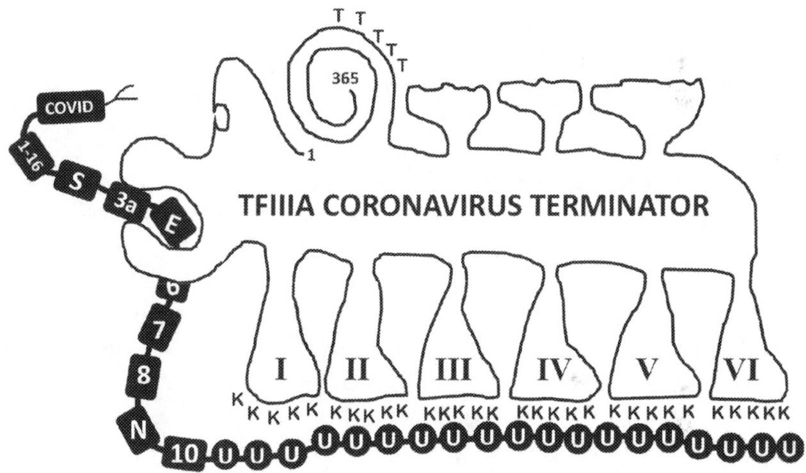

Figure 24
Transcription Factor IIIA designed to engage and bond to the uracil tail of COVID-19.

The modified form of the mRNA which when translated generates the said modified TFIIIA molecule is as follows, with the original nucleotide sequence comprising the molecule modified as mentioned above and the new nucleotide sequences appearing in their defined position and underlined for clarity. Note, this is an mRNA, but by convention, t's are used to represent the uracil (u) nucleotides.

Sequence for the modified mRNA to generate the said modified TFIIIA protein:

5' end

1 aagtgtgccg gcgtcgcgcg aaggttcagc agggagccgt gggccgggcg cgccggttcc 60
61 cggcacgtgt ctcggcacgt ggcagcgcgc ctggccctgg gcttggaggc gccggcgcc 119

Messenger Ribonucleic Acid to Produce a Modified Transcription Factor IIIA Polypeptide to Engage and Bind to the Uracil Tail of COVID-19 RNA Viral Genome

(*Note the first amino acid is coded as an L (ctg) rather than the expected M (atg).)

120/1 (nucleotide # / amino acid #) 179/20
L D P P A V V A E S V S S L T I A D A F
ctg gat ccg ccg gcc gtg gtc gcc gag tcg gtg tcg tcc ttg acc atc gcc gac gcg ttc

180/21 239/40
I A A G E S S A P T P P R P A L P R R F
att gca gcc ggc gag agc tca gct ccg acc ccg ccg cgc ccc gcg ctt ccc agg agg ttc

240/41 299/60
I C S F P D C S S S K S K S K K S K K H
atc tgc tcc ttc cct gac tgc agc tcc tct aag agc aaa tcc aag aag tct aag aag cac

300/61 359/80
L C K H T G E R P F V C D Y E G C K K S
ctg tgc aag cac acg ggg gag aga cca ttt gtt tgt gac tat gaa ggg tgt aag aag tcc

360/81 419/100
K K S S K S S S K H I L T H T G E K P F
aag aag tcg tcc aag tct tcg acg aag cac att ctg act cac aca gga gaa aag ccg ttt

420/101 479/120
V C A A N G C K S K K K S K S S S K K H
gtt tgt gca gcc aat ggc tgt aaa tca aaa aag aag tca aaa tca tcc tcg aag aaa cat

480/121 539/140
F E R K H E N Q Q K Q Y I C S F E D C K
ttt gaa cgc aaa cat gaa aat caa caa aaa caa tat ata tgc agt ttt gaa gac tgt aag

540/141 599/160
K S K K K S K S S K K H Q C Q H T N E P
aag tcc aaa aag aaa tct aag tcg tcg aaa aag cat cag tgc cag cat acc aat gaa cct

600/161 659/180
L F K C T Q E G C K K S K K S S S K S K
cta ttc aag tgt acc cag gaa gga tgt aag aaa tcc aaa aaa tca tcc agc aag tcg aaa

660/181 719/200
K H A K A H E G Y V C Q K G C S S S K K
aag cat gcc aag gcc cac gag ggc tat gta tgt caa aaa gga tgt tcc tct tcg aaa aaa

720/201 779/220
S S K S S K K H V R E T H K E E I L C E
tca tcg aag tca tct aag aaa cat gtg aga gaa acc cat aaa gag gaa ata cta tgt gaa

780/221 839/240

Y C A T T F T A T D Y L T Q H M K T H A

gta tgc gcg aca aca ttt aca gcc aca gat tac ctt acg caa cac atg aaa act cat gcc

840/241 899/260

P E R D V C R C P A A G C G A T Y T T V

cca gaa agg gat gta tgt cgc tgt cca gca gca ggc tgt gga gca acc tat aca act gtg

900/261 959/280

F A L Q A H I L S F H E E S R P F V C E

ttt gct ctc caa gcc cat atc ctc tcc ttc cat gag gaa agc cgc cct ttt gtg tgt gaa

960/281 1019/300

H A G C G T T F A M T Q A L T A H A V V

cat gct ggc tgt ggc aca aca ttt gca atg aca caa gct ctc act gcg cat gct gtt gta

1020/301 1079/320

H D P D T T T M T L T V K K S R E K R S

cat gat cct gac acg acg aca atg acg ctc aca gtc aaa aaa tct cgt gaa aaa cgg agt

1080/321 1139/340

L A S H L S G Y I P P K R K Q G Q G L S

ttg gcc tct cat ctc agt gga tat atc cct ccc aaa agg aaa caa ggg caa ggc tta tct

1140/341 1199/360

L C Q N G E S P N C V E D K M L S T V A

ttg tgt caa aac gga gag tca ccc aac tgt gtg gaa gac aag atg ctc tcg aca gtt gca

1214/365 STOP

V L T L G ◎

gta ctt acc ctt ggc taa

3' end

1218 gaactgcact gctttgttta aaggactgca gaccaaggag cgagctttct ctcagagcat 1277

1278 gcttttcttt attaaaatta ctgatgcaga acatttgatt ccttatcatt tccatggtct 1337

1338 ttgttcaaag tgtctctttc ctgggtctct tgagtttctt tatatgcctt ctcctcattt 1397

1398 ttgctgaaag cacgaagaac acacattaaa gcttttcctc cttgaa 1443

The modified mRNA is 1443 nucleotides long, though the final length depends upon the number of adenosine nucleotides comprising the 3' tail of the mRNA.

DETAILED DESCRIPTION

The three hundred sixty-five amino acid sequence of the native TFIIIA polypeptide:

```
1         10         20         30         40         50         60
MDPPAVVAES VSSLTIADAF IAAGESSAPT PPRPALPRRF ICSFPDCSAN YSKAWKLDAH
          70         80         90        100        110        120
LCKHTGERPF VCDYEGCGKA FIRDYHLSRH ILTHTGEKPF VCAANGCDQK FNTKSNLKKH
         130        140        150        160        170        180
FERKHENQQK QYICSFEDCK KTFKKHQQLK IHQCQHTNEP LFKCTQEGCG KHFASPSKLK
         190        200        210        220        230        240
RHAKAHEGYV CQKGCSFVAK TWTELLKHVR ETHKEEILCE VCRKTFKRKD YLKQHMKTHA
         250        260        270        280        290        300
PERDVCRCPR EGCGRTYTTV FNLQSHILSF HEESRPFVCE HAGCGKTFAM KQSLTRHAVV
         310        320        330        340        350        360
HDPDKKKMKL KVKKSREKRS LASHLSGYIP PKRKQGQGLS LCQNGESPNC VEDKMLSTVA
  365
VLTLG
```

Represents the naturally occurring Transcription Factor IIIA molecule, Taxonomic identifier 9606 [NCBI] (TFIIIA9606) found at http://www.uniprot.org/uniprot/Q92664. The TFIIIA TI9606 protein is 365 amino acids in length.

The human TFIIIA (TI 9606) polypeptide is 365 amino acids in length. There are nine zinc fingers in the structure moving from the 5' (NH2) to 3' (COOH) end of the molecule designated as zinc finger 1, zinc finger 2, zinc finger 3, zinc finger 4, zinc finger 5, zinc finger 6, zinc finger 7, zinc finger 8, and zinc finger 9. There is a nucleus location sequence (NLS) near the terminal portion of the molecule at the 3' end. To create a modified TFIIIA polypeptide to seek out the poly uracil tail of a negative-sense viral genome the native human TFIIIA amino acid sequence would be recoded as follows:

The following table summarizes the changes to the TFIIIA polypeptide amino acid sequencing:

ZINC FINGER	Original Amino Acid Sequence	Modified Amino Acid Sequence
1	SANYSKAWKLDA	SSSKSKSKKSKK
2	GKAFIRDYHLSR	KKSKKSSKSSSK
3	DQKFNTKSNLKK	KSKKKSKSSSKK
4	KKTFKKHQQLKI	KKSKKKSKSSKK
5	GKHFASPSKLKR	KKSKKSSSKSKK
6	SFVAKTWTELLK	SSSKKSSKSSKK
7	RKTFKRKDYLKQ	ATTFTATDYLTQ
8	PREGCGRTYTTVFNLQS	PAAGCGATYTTVFALQA
9	GKTFAMKQSLTR	GTTFAMTQALTA

Table 4

Modifying the zinc fingers of TFIIIA to combat COVID-19.

Zinc finger 1 is considered to include amino acids 40 to 64. Within zinc finger 1, the amino acids 48 to 59 'SANYSKAWKLDA' are changed to the amino acid sequence 'SSSKSKSKKSKK'.

Zinc finger 2 is considered to include amino acids 70 to 94. Within zinc finger 2, amino acids 78 to 89 'GKAFIRDYHLSR' are changed to the amino acid sequence 'KKSKKSSKSSSK'.

Zinc finer 3 is considered to include amino acids 100 to 125. Within zinc finger 3, amino acids 108 to 119 'DQKFNTKSNLKK' are changed to the amino acid sequence 'KSKKKSKSSSKK'.

Zinc finger 4 is considered to include amino acids 132 to 154. Within zinc finger 4, amino acids 140 to 151 'KKTFKKHQQLKI' are changed to the amino acid sequence 'KKSKKKSKSSKK'.

Zinc finger 5 is considered to include amino acids 162 to 186. Within zinc finger 5, amino acids 170 to 181 'GKHFASPSKLKR' are changed to the amino acid sequence 'KKSKKSSSKSKK'.

Zinc finger 6 is considered to include amino acids 189 to 213.
Zinc finger 6, amino acids 196 to 207 'SFVAKTWTELLK' are changed to the amino acid sequence 'SSSKKSSKSSKK'.

Zinc finger 7 is considered to include amino acids 217 to 239.
Within zinc finger 7, amino acids 223 TO 234 'RKTFKRKDYLKQ' are changed to the amino acid sequence 'ATTFTATDYLTQ'.

Zinc finger 8 is considered to include amino acids 246 to 271.
Within zinc finger 8, amino acids 249 to 265 'PREGCGRTYTTVFNLQS' are changed to the amino acid sequence 'PAAGCGATYTTVFALQA'.

Zinc finger 9 is considered to include the amino acids 277 to 301.
Within zinc finger 9, amino acids 285 TO 296 'GKTFAMKQSLTR' are changed to the amino acid sequence 'GTTFAMTQALTA'.

The cell restricts flow of molecules which enter into the nucleus from the cytoplasm. In the cycle of protein production, messenger RNAs are generated in the nucleus as a result of transcription complexes decoding the DNA. The mRNAs travel from the nucleus to the cytoplasm, where the mRNAs are translated by ribosomes and polypeptides are created. A portion of the polypeptides generated in the translation process are required to enter the nucleus to perform duties required by cell metabolism and to satisfy the structural requirements of the cell's nuclear architecture. Polypeptides destined to enter the nucleus are labeled with a particular sequence of amino acids termed the nuclear location sequence (NLS). The gateways through the nuclear membrane separating the cytoplasm from the inner chamber of the nucleus recognize the NLS coded into the structure of the polypeptide and grant access to polypeptides which possess the proper NLS.

The amino acid sequence 'PDKKKMKLK' present in the 3' tail of the native TFIIIA polypeptide (TI9606) from amino acid 303 to 311 acts as the nuclear location sequence, giving the molecule access to the translocate from the cell's cytoplasm to the nucleus of the cell.[18] It is desirable to maintain the modified TFIIIA in the cytoplasm and prevent the polypeptide from entering into the nucleus. In order to trap the modified TFIIIA polypeptide in the cytoplasm of a cell to optimize the molecule's effectiveness, the lysine amino acids of the native NSL are changed to threonine. The modified TFIIIA polypeptide is to possess the modified amino acid sequence of amino acids 303 to 311 as described as 'PDTTTMTLT'.

The modified form of the TFIIIA molecule is as follows with the original amino acid sequence comprising the molecule modified as mentioned above and the new amino acid sequences appearing in their defined position and underlined for clarity.

```
1         10         20         30         40         50         60
 MDPPAVVAES VSSLTIADAF IAAGESSAPT PPRPALPRRF ICSFPDCSSS KSKSKKSKKH
         70         80         90        100        110        120
 LCKHTGERPF VCDYEGCKKS KKSSKSSSKH ILTHTGEKPF VCAANGCKSK KKSKSSSKKH
        130        140        150        160        170        180
 FERKHENQQK QYICSFEDCK KSKKKSKSSK KHQCQHTNEP LFKCTQEGCK KSKKSSSKSK
        190        200        210        220        230        240
 KHAKAHEGYV CQKGCSSSKK SSKSSKKHVR ETHKEEILCE VCATTFTATD YLTQHMKTHA
        250        260        270        280        290        300
 PERDVCRCPA AGCGATYTTV FALQAHILSF HEESRPFVCE HAGCGTTFAM TQALTAHAVV
        310        320        330        340        350        360
 HDPDTTTMTL TVKKSREKRS LASHLSGYIP PKRKQGQGLS LCQNGESPNC VEDKMLSTVA
 365
VLTLG
```

Coronavirus replicates its RNA genome in the cytoplasm of the host cell and passes a copy of the genetic code onto the next generation of virus virions. Once constructed with a copy of the viral code, the coronavirus virion exits the host cell and travels to other potential host cells to repeat the replication process. The TFIIIA polypeptide reconstructed in the above manner will transform this modified TFIIIA polypeptide into a medically therapeutic agent that will seek out and bind to the poly uracil tail of the negative-sense coronavirus genome or other similar negative-sense RNA viral genome. Once the modified TFIIIA polypeptide has attached itself to the poly uracil tail of the negative-sense coronavirus genome or other similar negative-sense RNA viral genome, the presence of the modified TFIIIA polypeptide attached to the viral genome will interfere with the replication process meant to copy the virus's genome.

If the viral genome is prevented from being replicated by the physical attachment of TFIIIA to the virus's genome, there will be no copies of the viral genome to pass on to the next generation and the infectious nature of the virus is neutralized. The impotent viral genome will be broken down and destroyed cellular enzymes.

Targeting the unique poly uracil tail of the negative-sense coronavirus genome with a modified TFIIIA polypeptide as described should not affect other native mRNAs, nor the translation of native mRNAs.

It can be assumed that there may be variation in the arrangement of the amino acid construct used in the zinc fingers to facilitate the lysine (K) amino acids to bind to the uracil tail. Various configurations of the zinc fingers, as dictated by variance in the amino acid construct of the zinc fingers, may induce more optimal binding to the negative-sense coronavirus genome or on the other hand, create less binding with other nontarget molecules in the cell's cytoplasm. The modified TFIIIA polypeptide as presented is likely not the only possible therapeutic amino acid sequence.

Likely other specific segments of viral RNA, in addition to the poly uracil tail, can be determined to be unique target sequences, which modified TNFIIIA polypeptides can be constructed to seek out and bind to in order to neutralize coronavirus or other RNA viruses.

Translation of a messenger RNA (mRNA) generates a polypeptide molecule. To create the said modified TFIIIA polypeptide to neutralize COVID19, a mRNA needs to be designed. In order to design a proper mRNA, the nucleotide sequence of the original native human mRNA, which is responsible for the native TFIIIA polypeptide, needs to be recoded in order that when the modified mRNA is translated the said modified TFIIIA polypeptide described herein will be generated.

Would like to celebrate and honor the hard work and dedication of the many researchers whose efforts made accessing this information on the NCBI website possible, so that the study and understanding of human genetics could advance toward a cure for a variety of challenging diseases.

The original nucleotide coding for the mRNA of the native TFIIIA polypeptide is as follows:

Taken from the NCBI website:

```
COMMENT  REFSEQ INFORMATION: The reference sequence is identical
                             to CM000675.2.
    On Feb 3, 2014 this sequence version replaced NC _000013.10.
    Assembly Name: GRCh38.p13 Primary Assembly
    The DNA sequence is composed of genomic sequence, primarily
    finished clones that were sequenced as part of the Human
    Genome Project. PCR products and WGS shotgun sequence have
    been added where necessary to fill gaps or correct errors.
    All such additions are manually curated by GRC staff. For more
    information see: https://genomereference.org.

    ##Genome-Annotation-Data-START##
    Annotation Provider          :: NCBI
    Annotation Status            :: Updated annotation
    Annotation Name              :: Homo sapiens Updated Annotation
                                    Release 109.20200228
    Annotation Version           :: 109.20200228
    Annotation Pipeline          :: NCBI eukaryotic genome
                                    annotation pipeline
    Annotation Software Version :: 8.3
    Annotation Method            :: Best-placed RefSeq; propagated
                                    RefSeq model
    Features Annotated           :: Gene; mRNA; CDS; ncRNA
    ##Genome-Annotation-Data-END##


FEATURES     Location/Qualifiers
   source      1..11205
             /organism="Homo sapiens"
             /mol _type="genomic DNA"
             /db _xref="taxon:9606"
             /chromosome="13"
   gene        1..11205
             /gene="GTF3A"
             /gene _synonym="AP2; TFIIIA"
             /note="general transcription factor IIIA; Derived by
             automated computational analysis using gene prediction
             method: BestRefSeq."
             /db _xref="GeneID:2971"
             /db _xref="HGNC:HGNC:4662"
             /db _xref="MIM:600860"

   mRNA        join(1..320,2474..2574,5252..5348,5915..6003,8113..8186,
             9521..9601,10187..10416,10515..10574,10815..11205)
             /gene="GTF3A"
             /gene _synonym="AP2; TFIIIA"
             /product="general transcription factor IIIA"
             /note="Derived by automated computational analysis using
             gene prediction method: BestRefSeq."
             /transcript _id="NM _002097.3"
             /db _xref="GeneID:2971"
             /db _xref="HGNC:HGNC:4662"
             /db _xref="MIM:600860"

   CDS         join(120..320,2474..2574,5252..5348,5915..6003,8113..8186,
             9521..9601,10187..10416,10515..10574,10815..10979)
             /gene="GTF3A"
             /gene _synonym="AP2; TFIIIA"
             /note="non-AUG (CUG) translation initiation codon; Derived
```

by automated computational analysis using gene prediction method: BestRefSeq."
/codon _start=1
/product="transcription factor IIIA"
/protein _id="NP _002088.2"
/db _xref="CCDS:CCDS45019.1"
/db _xref="GeneID:2971"
/db _xref="HGNC:HGNC:4662"
/db _xref="MIM:600860"
/translation="MDPPAVVAESVSSLTIADAFIAAGESSAPTPPRPALPRRFICSF
PDCSANYSKAWKLDAHLCKHTGERPFVCDYEGCGKAFIRDYHLSRHILTHTGEKPFVC
AANGCDQKFNTKSNLKKHFERKHENQQKQYICSFEDCKKTFKKHQQLKIHQCQHTNEP
LFKCTQEGCGKHFASPSKLKRHAKAHEGYVCQKGCSFVAKTWTELLKHVRETHKEEIL
CEVCRKTFKRKDYLKQHMKTHAPERDVCRCPREGCGRTYTTVFNLQSHILSFHEESRP
FVCEHAGCGKTFAMKQSLTRHAVVHDPDKKKMKLKVKKSREKRSLASHLSGYIPPKRK
QGQGLSLCQNGESPNCVEDKMLSTVAVLTLG"

join
1..320
2474..2574
5252..5348
5915..6003
8113..8186
9521..9601
10187..10416
10515..10574
10815..11205

Note: letters which are struck through are not included in the mRNA coding.

ORIGIN
1..320

1 aagtgtgccg gcgtcgcgcg aaggttcagc agggagccgt gggccgggcg cgccggttcc
61 cggcacgtgt ctcggcacgt ggcagcgcgc ctggccctgg gcttggaggc gccggcgccc
121 tggatccgcc ggccgtggtc gccgagtcgg tgtcgtcctt gaccatcgcc gacgcgttca
181 ttgcagccgg cgagagctca gctccgaccc cgccgcgccc cgcgcttccc aggaggttca
241 tctgctcctt ccctgactgc agcgccaatt acagcaaagc ctggaagctt gacgcgcacc
301 tgtgcaagca cacgggggag

2474..2574

2461 ~~tttttcctgc tag~~agaccat ttgtttgtga ctatgaaggg tgtggcaagg ccttcatcag
2521 ggactaccat ctgagccgcc acattctgac tcacacagga gaaaagccgt ttgt~~gtaagt~~

5252..5348

5221 ~~ttaatatttt ggtttatata acttcttaca~~ gttgtgcagc caatggctgt gatcaaaaat
5281 tcaacacaaa atcaaacttg aagaaacatt ttgaacgcaa acatgaaaat caacaaaaac
5341 aatatata~~gt aagtatgatt ttatatgctt aaattttttg agtattttta cacttactgc~~

5915..6003

5881 ~~tccataagac taacgagcct ttacaattta acag~~tgcagt tttgaagact gtaagaagac
5941 ctttaagaaa catcagcagc tgaaaatcca tcagtgccag cataccaatg aacctctatt
6001 caa~~gtaggta cttcatgtgg ctgaaaatgc ctggattcta ggtgtgaata agattggaaa~~

8113..8186

8101 ~~ttgccaatgc ag~~gtgtaccc aggaaggatg tgggaaacac tttgcatcac ccagcaagct
8161 gaaacgacat gccaaggccc acgagg~~tgt gtacggatag cctgggtgtg ctccgagggg~~

9521..9601

9481 ~~tgagtattca tgacagacaa tgcaccaatt tttttaatag~~ gctatgtatg tcaaaaagga
9541 tgttcctttg tggcaaaaac atggacggaa cttctgaaac atgtgagaga aacccataaa
9601 g~~gtaaggcag gcatgaatgg caggcatggt gtaaatgttt gtccccacag aactgattta~~

10187..10416

10141 ~~gtaatatctg gggaaatttg tgaaatttgt ctgtctgtcc caccag~~agga aatactatgt
10201 gaagtatgcc ggaaaacatt taaacgcaaa gattacctta agcaacacat gaaaactcat
10261 gccccagaaa gggatgtatg tcgctgtcca agagaaggct gtggaagaac ctatacaact
10321 gtgtttaatc tccaaagcca tatcctctcc ttccatgagg aaagccgccc ttttgtgtgt
10381 gaacatgctg gctgtggcaa aacatttgca atgaaa~~gtaa gcactcaccc tcatactcat~~

10515..10574

10501 ~~ctcttttcatt gtag~~caaagt ctcactaggc atgctgttgt acatgatcct gacaagaaga
10561 aaatgaagct caaa~~gtaagt tgaaactact taggcaagct tagttttcaa gtggaaattg~~

10815..11205

10801 ~~ccttattccc aaag~~gtcaaa aaatctcgtg aaaaacggag tttggcctct catctcagtg
10861 gatatatccc tcccaaaagg aaacaagggc aaggcttatc tttgtgtcaa aacggagagt
10921 cacccaactg tgtggaagac aagatgctct cgacagttgc agtacttacc cttggctaag
10981 aactgcactg ctttgtttaa aggactgcag accaaggagc gagctttctc tcagagcatg
11041 cttttcttta ttaaaattac tgatgcagaa catttgattc cttatcattt ccatggtctt
11101 tgttcaaagt gtctctttcc tgggtctctt gagtttcttt atatgccttc tcctcatttt
11161 tgctgaaagc acgaagaaca cacattaaag cttttcctcc ttgaa
//

June 16, 2020 version of TFIIIA and mRNA is presented in Appendix IV.

To accomplish the task of generating a modified TFIIIA polypeptide which will seek out and bind to a coronavirus negative-sense uracil tail, a modified mRNA is constructed. Likely how an amino acid is oriented to the polypeptide is crucial for the stereochemistry of the molecule, which translates into the functionality of the molecule. Codon codes are three letters. The first two letters likely dictate the identity of the amino acid. The third letter of the codon code is likely the 360-degree orientation of the 'R' chain of the amino acid, with four different orientations about an axis possible including, 0 degrees, 90 degrees, 180 degrees and 270 degrees. Additional study will be necessary to properly spatially orient amino acids to amino acid sequences. The coding used in the table below is an attempt to preserve the orientation of the amino acids to coincide replaced amino acid with the orientation of the original amino acid. Note this is a mRNA, but t's are used to represent the uracil (u) nucleotides.

Amino Acid	Segment	ZF/N	Orig AA	DNA code	Δ	Insert AA	DNA code	Change to Zinc Fingers of the native mRNA coding
48	261-263	1/1	S	agc	=	S	agc	No change in S
49	264-266	1/2	A	gcc	>>	S	tcc	S spacer; orient 'c'
50	267-269	1/3	N	aat	>>	S	tct	S spacer; orient 't'
51	270-272	1/4	Y	tac	>>	K	aag	K binder #1; orient 'g'
52	273-275	1/5	S	agc	=	S	agc	No change in S
53	276-278	1/6	K	aaa	=	K	aaa	K binder #2; no change
54	279-281	1/7	A	gcc	>>	S	tcc	S spacer; orient 'c'
55	282-284	1/8	W	tgg	>>	K	aag	K binder #3; orient 'g'
56	285-287	1/9	K	aag	=	K	aag	K binder #4; orient 'g'
57	288-290	1/10	L	ctt	>>	S	tct	S spacer; orient 't'
58	291-293	1/11	D	gac	>>	K	aag	K binder #5; orient 'g'
59	294-296	1/12	A	gcg	>>	K	aag	K binder #6; orient 'g'
78	2504-2506	2/1	G	ggc	>>	K	aag	K binder #7; orient 'g'
79	2507-2509	2/2	K	aag	=	K	aag	K binder #8; no change
80	2510-2512	2/3	A	gcc	>>	S	tcc	S spacer; orient 'c'
81	2513-2515	2/4	F	ttc	>>	K	aag	K binder #9; orient 'g'
82	2516-2518	2/5	I	atc	>>	K	aag	K binder #10; orient 'g'
83	2519-2521	2/6	R	agg	>>	S	tcg	S spacer; orient 'g'
84	2522-2524	2/7	D	gac	>>	S	tcc	S spacer; orient 'c'
85	2525-2527	2/8	Y	tac	>>	K	aag	K binder #11; orient 'g'
86	2528-2530	2/9	H	cat	>>	S	tct	S spacer; orient 't'
87	2531-2533	2/10	L	ctg	>>	S	tcg	S spacer; orient 'g'
88	2534-2536	2/11	S	agc	=	S	agc	No change in S
89	2537-2539	2/12	R	cgc	>>	K	aag	K binder #12; orient 'g'
108	5271-5273	3/1	D	gat	>>	K	aaa	K binder #13
109	5274-5276	3/2	Q	caa	>>	S	tca	S spacer; orient 'a'
110	5277-5279	3/3	K	aaa	=	K	aaa	K binder #14; no change
111	5280-5282	3/4	F	ttc	>>	K	aag	K binder #15; orient 'g'
112	5283-5285	3/5	N	aac	>>	K	aag	K binder #16; orient 'g'
113	5286-5288	3/6	T	aca	>>	S	tca	S spacer; orient 'a'
114	5289-5291	3/7	K	aaa	=	K	aaa	K binder #17; no change
115	5292-5294	3/8	S	tca	=	S	tca	No change in S
116	5295-5297	3/9	N	aac	>>	S	tcc	S spacer; orient 'c'
117	5298-5300	3/10	L	ttg	>>	S	tcg	S spacer; orient 'g'
118	5301-5303	3/11	K	aag	=	K	aag	K binder #18; no change

Amino Acid	Segment	ZF/N	Orig AA	DNA code	Δ	Insert AA	DNA code	Change to Zinc Fingers of the native mRNA coding
119	5304-5306	3/12	K	aaa	=	K	aaa	K binder #19; no change
140	5933-5935	4/1	K	aag	=	K	aag	K binder #20; no change
141	5936-5938	4/2	K	aag	=	K	aag	K binder #21; no change
142	5939-5941	4/3	T	acc	>>	S	tcc	S spacer; orient 'c'
143	5942-5944	4/4	F	ttt	>>	K	aaa	K binder #22; orient 'a'
144	5945-5947	4/5	K	aag	=	K	aag	K binder #23; no change
145	5948-5950	4/6	K	aaa	=	K	aaa	K binder #24; no change
146	5951-5953	4/7	H	cat	>>	S	tct	S spacer; orient 't'
147	5954-5956	4/8	Q	cag	>>	K	aag	K binder #25; orient 'g'
148	5957-5959	4/9	Q	cag	>>	S	tcg	S spacer; orient 'g'
149	5960-5962	4/10	L	ctg	>>	S	tcg	S spacer; orient 'g'
150	5963-5965	4/11	K	aaa	=	K	aaa	K binder #26; no change
151	5966-5968	4/12	I	atc	>>	K	aag	K binder #27; orient 'g'
170	8132-8134	5/1	G	ggg	>>	K	aag	K binder #28; orient 'g'
171	8135-8137	5/2	K	aaa	=	K	aaa	K binder #29; no change
172	8138-8140	5/3	H	cac	>>	S	tcc	S spacer; orient 'g'
173	8141-8143	5/4	F	ttt	>>	K	aaa	K binder #30; orient 'a'
174	8144-8146	5/5	A	gca	>>	K	aaa	K binder #31; orient 'a'
175	8147-8149	5/6	S	tca	=	S	tca	S spacer; orient 'a'
176	8150-8152	5/7	P	ccc	>>	S	tcc	S spacer; orient 'c'
177	8153-8155	5/8	S	agc	=	S	agc	No change in S
178	8156-8158	5/9	K	aag	=	K	aag	K binder #32; no change
179	8159-8161	5/10	L	ctg	>>	S	tcg	S spacer; orient 'g'
180	8162-8164	5/11	K	aaa	=	K	aaa	K binder #33; no change
181	8165-8167	5/12	R	cga	>>	K	aag	K binder #34; orient 'g'
196	9544-9546	6/1	S	tcc	=	S	tcc	No change in S
197	9547-9549	6/2	F	ttt	>>	S	tct	S spacer; orient 't'
198	9550-9552	6/3	V	gtg	>>	S	tcg	S spacer; orient 'g'
199	9553-9555	6/4	A	gca	>>	K	aaa	K binder #35; orient 'a'
200	9556-9558	6/5	K	aaa	=	K	aaa	K binder #36; orient 'a'
201	9559-9561	6/6	T	aca	>>	S	tca	S spacer; orient 'a'
202	9562-9564	6/7	W	tgg	>>	S	tcg	S spacer; orient 'g'
203	9565-9567	6/8	T	acg	>>	K	aag	K binder #37; orient 'g'
204	9568-9570	6/9	E	gaa	>>	S	tca	S spacer; orient 'a'
205	9571-9573	6/10	L	ctt	>>	S	tct	S spacer; orient 't'
206	9574-9576	6/11	L	ctg	>>	K	aag	K binder #38; orient 'g'
207	9577-9579	6/12	K	aaa	=	K	aaa	K binder #39; no change
223	10210-10212	7/1	R	cgg	>>	A	gcg	'A' substitute for 'R' orient 'g'
224	10213-10215	7/2	K	aaa	>>	T	aca	'T' substitute for 'K' orient 'a'
225	10216-10218	7/3	T	aca	>>	T	aca	Original coding
226	10219-10221	7/4	F	ttt	=	F	ttt	Original coding
227	10222-10224	7/5	K	aaa	>>	T	aca	'T' substitute for 'K' orient 'a'
228	10225-10227	7/6	R	cgc	>>	A	gcc	'A' substitute for 'R' orient 'c'
229	10228-10230	7/7	K	aaa	>>	T	aca	'T' substitute for 'K' orient 'a'
230	10231-10233	7/8	D	gat	=	D	gat	Original coding
231	10234-10236	7/9	Y	tac	=	Y	tac	Original coding
232	10237-10239	7/10	L	ctt	=	L	ctt	Original coding
233	10240-10242	7/11	K	aag	>>	T	acg	'T' substitute for 'K' orient 'g'
234	10243-10245	7/12	Q	caa	=	Q	caa	Original coding
249	10288-10290	8/1	P	cca	=	P	cca	Original coding
250	10291-10293	8/2	R	aga	>>	A	gca	'A' substitute for 'R' orient 'a'
251	10294-10296	8/3	E	gaa	>>	A	gca	'A' substitute for 'E' orient 'a'
252	10297-10299	8/4	G	ggc	=	G	ggc	Original coding
253	10300-10302	8/5	C	tgt	=	C	tgt	Original coding

Amino Acid	Segment	ZF/N	Orig AA	DNA code	Δ	Insert AA	DNA code	Change to Zinc Fingers of the native mRNA coding
254	10303-10305	8/6	G	gga	=	G	gga	Original coding
255	10306-10308	8/7	R	aga	>>	A	gca	'A' substitute for 'R' using 'a'
256	10309-10311	8/8	T	acc	=	T	acc	Original coding
257	10312-10314	8/9	Y	tat	=	Y	tat	Original coding
258	10315-10317	8/10	T	aca	=	T	aca	Original coding
259	10318-10320	8/11	T	act	=	T	act	Original coding
260	10321-10323	8/12	V	gtg	=	V	gtg	Original coding
261	10324-10326	8/13	F	ttt	=	F	ttt	Original coding
262	10327-10329	8/14	N	aat	>>	A	gct	'A' substitute for 'N' orient 't'
263	10330-10332	8/15	L	ctc	=	L	ctc	Original coding
364	10334-10336	8/16	Q	caa	=	Q	caa	Original coding
265	10337-10339	8/17	S	agc	>>	A	gcc	'A' substitute for 'S' orient 'c'
285	10396-10398	9/1	G	ggc	=	G	ggc	Original coding
286	10399-10401	9/2	K	aaa	>>	T	aca	'T' substitute for 'K' orient 'a'
287	10402-10404	9/3	T	aca	=	T	aca	Original coding
288	10405-10407	9/4	F	ttt	=	F	ttt	Original coding
289	10408-10410	9/5	A	gca	=	A	gca	Original coding
290	10411-10413	9/6	M	atg	=	M	atg	Original coding
291	10414-10416	9/7	K	aaa	>>	T	aca	'T' substitute for 'K' orient 'a'
292	10515-10517	9/8	Q	caa	=	Q	caa	Original coding
293	10518-10520	9/9	S	agt	>>	A	gct	'A' substitute for 'S' orient 't'
294	10521-10523	9/10	L	ctc	=	L	ctc	Original coding
295	10524-10526	9/11	T	act	=	T	act	Original coding
296	10527-10529	9/12	R	agg	>>	A	gcg	'A' substitute for 'R' orient 'g'
303	10548-10550	10/1	P	cct	=	P	cct	Original coding
304	10551-10553	10/2	D	gac	=	D	gac	Original coding
305	10554-10556	10/3	K	aag	>>	T	acg	'T' substitute for 'K' orient 'g'
306	10557-10559	10/4	K	aag	>>	T	acg	'T' substitute for 'K' orient 'g'
307	10561-10563	10/5	K	aaa	>>	T	aca	'T' substitute for 'K' orient 'a'
308	10564-10566	10/6	M	atg	=	M	atg	Original coding
309	10567-10569	10/7	K	aag	>>	T	acg	'T' substitute for 'K' orient 'g'
310	10570-10572	10/8	L	ctc	=	L	ctc	Original coding
311	10573-10575	10/9	K	aaa	>>	T	aca	'T' substitute for 'K' orient 'a'

Table 5

Detailed changes to the amino acids to properly construct the mRNA to combat COVID-19.

Sequence for the modified mRNA to generate the said modified TFIIIA protein is as follows. The amino acids which have been changed are underlined for clarity. Note this is a mRNA, but t's are used to represent the uracil (u) nucleotides.

5' end

1 aagtgtgccg gcgtcgcgcg aaggttcagc agggagccgt gggccgggcg cgccggttcc 60
61 cggcacgtgt ctcggcacgt ggcagcgcgc ctggccctgg gcttggaggc gccggcgcc 119

(*Note the first amino acid is coded as an L (ctg) rather than the expected M (atg).)

120/1 (nucleotide # / amino acid #) 179/20

L D P P A V V A E S V S S L T I A D A F

ctg gat ccg ccg gcc gtg gtc gcc gag tcg gtg tcg tcc ttg acc atc gcc gac gcg ttc

180/21 239/40

I A A G E S S A P T P P R P A L P R R F

att gca gcc ggc gag agc tca gct ccg acc ccg ccg cgc ccc gcg ctt ccc agg agg ttc

240/41 299/60

I C S F P D C S S S K S K S K K S K K H

atc tgc tcc ttc cct gac tgc agc tcc tct aag agc aaa tcc aag aag tct aag aag cac

300/61 359/80

L C K H T G E R P F V C D Y E G C K K S

ctg tgc aag cac acg ggg gag aga cca ttt gtt tgt gac tat gaa ggg tgt aag aag tcc

360/81 419/100

K K S S K S S S K H I L T H T G E K P F

aag aag tcg tcc aag tct tcg acg aag cac att ctg act cac aca gga gaa aag ccg ttt

420/101 479/120

V C A A N G C K S K K K S K S S S K K H

gtt tgt gca gcc aat ggc tgt aaa tca aaa aag aag tca aaa tca tcc tcg aag aaa cat

480/121 539/140

F E R K H E N Q Q K Q Y I C S F E D C K

ttt gaa cgc aaa cat gaa aat caa caa aaa caa tat ata tgc agt ttt gaa gac tgt aag

540/141 599/160

K S K K K S K S S K K H Q C Q H T N E P

aag tcc aaa aag aaa tct aag tcg tcg aaa aag cat cag tgc cag cat acc aat gaa cct

600/161 659/180

L F K C T Q E G C K K S K K S S S K S K

cta ttc aag tgt acc cag gaa gga tgt aag aaa tcc aaa aaa tca tcc agc aag tcg aaa

660/181 719/200

K H A K A H E G Y V C Q K G C S S S K K

aag cat gcc aag gcc cac gag ggc tat gta tgt caa aaa gga tgt tcc tct tcg aaa aaa

720/201 779/220

S S K S S K K H V R E T H K E E I L C E

tca tcg aag tca tct aag aaa cat gtg aga gaa acc cat aaa gag gaa ata cta tgt gaa

780/221 839/240
Y C A T T F T A T D Y L T Q H M K T H A
gta tgc gcg aca aca ttt aca gcc aca gat tac ctt acg caa cac atg aaa act cat gcc

840/241 899/260
P E R D V C R C P A A G C G A T Y T T V
cca gaa agg gat gta tgt cgc tgt cca gca gca ggc tgt gga gca acc tat aca act gtg

900/261 959/280
F A L Q A H I L S F H E E S R P F V C E
ttt gct ctc caa gcc cat atc ctc tcc ttc cat gag gaa agc cgc cct ttt gtg tgt gaa

960/281 1019/300
H A G C G T T F A M T Q A L T A H A V V
cat gct ggc tgt ggc aca aca ttt gca atg aca caa gct ctc act gcg cat gct gtt gta

1020/301 1079/320
H D P D T T T M T L T V K K S R E K R S
cat gat cct gac acg acg aca atg acg ctc aca gtc aaa aaa tct cgt gaa aaa cgg agt

1080/321 1139/340
L A S H L S G Y I P P K R K Q G Q G L S
ttg gcc tct cat ctc agt gga tat atc cct ccc aaa agg aaa caa ggg caa ggc tta tct

1140/341 1199/360
L C Q N G E S P N C V E D K M L S T V A
ttg tgt caa aac gga gag tca ccc aac tgt gtg gaa gac aag atg ctc tcg aca gtt gca

1214/365 STOP
V L T L G ◎
gta ctt acc ctt ggc taa

3' end

1218 gaactgcact gctttgttta aaggactgca gaccaaggag cgagctttct ctcagagcat 1277
1278 gcttttcttt attaaaatta ctgatgcaga acatttgatt ccttatcatt tccatggtct 1337
1338 ttgttcaaag tgtctctttc ctgggtctct tgagtttctt tatatgcctt ctcctcattt 1397
1398 ttgctgaaag cacgaagaac acacattaaa gcttttcctc cttgaa 1443

The modified mRNA is 1443 nucleotides long, though the final length depends upon the number of adenosine nucleotides comprising the 3' tail of the mRNA.

CONCLUSION

The human race cannot allow a misguided scrap of malignant bio-programming code to ravage the world's population without being heatedly contested by our best efforts at innovation and invention. We must capitalize on the advancements in the knowledge of how the DNA is decoded, the construct of transcription factors and how mRNAs are translated. A modified mRNA could generate, through the process of cellular translation, a modified TFIIIA polypeptide designed to seek out the poly uracil tail of a negative-sense version of the coronavirus offers a practical virus-specific means to neutralize the current coronavirus global pandemic threat.

CHAPTER TWELVE

USING CD8A CELL SURFACE RECEPTOR mRNA TO CONSTRUCT A VACCINE TO PREVENT CORONAVIRUS INFECTION

ABSTRACT

A modified version of the human CD8A cell surface glycoprotein messenger ribonucleic acid molecule is designed so that, when translated, will produce a 'S' (spike) protein (probe) to be mounted on the surface of the human cell which translates the messenger ribonucleic acid. The 'S' probe architecture is highly conserved, thus a desirable target for the human immune system to recognize and react to in order to prevent or manage a coronavirus infection. An artificial CD8A cell surface glycoprotein mRNA vaccine carrying the nucleotide instructions to enact a cell to construct a coronavirus 'S' probe and mount the 'S' probe on the surface of the said cell, in order to alert the human immune system to generate immunity against coronavirus, offers a practical virus-specific means to neutralize the current coronavirus global pandemic threat.

BACKGROUND OF THE INVENTION

FIELD OF THE INVENTION

This invention relates to any medical device intended to generate a polypeptide using a messenger ribonucleic acid as the template for construction, that will act as a cell surface receptor or a cell surface probe or a cell surface glycoprotein on a eukaryote cell.

SUMMARY DESCRIPTION

The coronavirus places a 'S' probe or sometimes referred to as a 'spike' protein on the surface of the virion.[19,20] The 'S' probe can be utilized by the human immune system to uniquely identify the coronavirus. In order to artificially alert the human immune system to be aware of the coronavirus, the CD8A mRNA is used to carry the coronavirus 'S' probe. Normally, the native human CD8A mRNA would be translated by intracellular ribosomes and produce a CD8A glycoprotein on the surface of a human cell. In this case, the nucleotide sequencing coding for the native human CD8A has been modified. The nucleotide sequencing coding for the native human CD8A glycoprotein cell surface receptor has been replaced by the nucleotide coding sequence of the coronavirus 'S' probe.

The construct of this mRNA coronavirus vaccine is comprised of: 5' leader nucleotide sequence of a native human mRNA for CD8A glycoprotein cell surface receptor, attached to the nucleotide coding sequence for coronavirus 'S' probe, attached to the 'taa' STOP code codon, attached to the 3' terminal end nucleotide sequence of a native human mRNA coding for CD8A glycoprotein cell surface receptor, attached to a sequence of adenine nucleotides comprising the tail of the molecule.

Native Human CD8A CSR 5' Leader End Region:

```
  1 cucuguaaaa uaaaugcgcu gggccggauc uuuucugagu ucucuucucc ccuacgaauu
 61 cuagaucccu ccucuguccu cccugcgcca gggaccuucg ggcgacccuu cccuguaccc
121 ccaccccacc cucucuggac cccguuucug ccucaguacg gcgcgcugag cucugccccc
181 ugcccaggcc cugaccccu caggagccgc gguuuccugg gguaacagug ggaaacgugu
241 cggccgucuc cgcucaggcg cuugcugugu acagaaag
279 gcugau ucaggcacac cggcucucgu cgccuuggug gcccucccca
325 gcccuccucc gcgccugcuc cggguggcgc uccgcugggc uccucgugcg ccuguccgcg
385 accgcaccca ccucauccug gcaccccau cguggcauca cguguucccu caucuguccu
445 cauggcuggc gugccccucu gcggugagac cugcagaaca ggaauuggug ccgggucagc
505 agccggcgau gaagccggac gaagccugca aaccccaccc auacgccagc uucacauagc
565 uccuauccau ugcacagcag cguggggaag caccguucuc uacccuccaa
615 a caaaagcaug aaccaggugc aguggcucac gucuguaauc
```

```
656 ccagcauuuu ggaggccaag guggauggau ggauuccuug aguccaggag uucaagacca
716 gccugggcaa cauggugaac ccccaucucu acaaaaauuu agccag
```

CORONAVIRUS Wuhan-Hu-1 'S' Protein Probe nucleic acid coding:

```
 762 auguuugu uuuucuuguu uuauugccac uagucucuag
 800 ucaguguguu aaucuuacaa ccagaacuca auuacccccu gcauacacua auucuuucac
 860 acgugguguu uauuacccug acaaaguuuu cagauccuca guuuuacauu caacucagga
 920 cuuguucuua ccuuucuuuu ccaauguuac uugguuccau gcuauacaug ucucugggac
 980 caaugguacu aagagguuug auaacccugu ccuaccauuu aaugauggug uuuauuuugc
1040 uuccacugag aagucuaaca uaauaagagg cuggauuuuu gguacuacuu uagauucgaa
1100 gacccagucc cuacuuauug uuaauaacgc uacuaauguu guuauuaaag ucugugaauu
1160 ucaauuuugu aaugauccau uuuugggugu uuauuaccac aaaaacaaca aaaguuggau
1220 ggaaagugag uucagaguuu auucuagugc gaauaauugc acuuuugaau augucucuca
1280 gccuuuucuu auggaccuug aaggaaaaca ggguaauuuc aaaaaucuua gggaauuugu
1340 guuuaagaau auugaugguu auuuuaaaau auauucuaag cacacgccua uuaauuuagu
1400 gcgugaucuc ccucaggguu uuucggcuuu agaaccauug guagauuugc caauagguau
1460 uaacaucacu agguuucaaa cuuuacuugc uuuacauaga aguuauuuga cuccugguga
1520 uucuucuuca gguuggacag cuggugcugc agcuuauuau gugguuauc uucaaccuag
1580 gacuuuucua uuaaaauaua augaaaaugg aaccauuaca gaugcuguag acugugcacu
1640 ugacccucuc ucagaaacaa aguguacguu gaaauccuuc acuguagaaa aaggaaucua
1700 ucaaacuucu aacuuuagag uccaaccaac agaaucuauu guuagauuuc cuaauauuac
1760 aaacuugugc ccuuuuggug aaguuuuuaa cgccaccaga uuugcaucug uuuaugcuug
1820 gaacaggaag agaaucagca acuguguugc ugauuauucu guccuauaua auuccgcauc
1880 auuuuccacu uuuaaguguu auggaguguc uccuacuaaa uuaaaugauc ucugcuuuac
1940 uaaugucuau gcagauucau uuguaauuag aggugaugaa gucagacaaa ucgcuccagg
2000 gcaaacugga aagauugcug auuauaauua uaaauuacca gaugauuuua caggcugcgu
2060 uauagcuugg aauucuaaca aucuugauuc uaagguuggu gguaauuaua auuaccugua
2120 uagauuguuu aggaagucua aucucaaacc uuuugagaga gauauuucaa cugaaaucua
2180 ucaggccggu agcacaccuu guaauggugu ugaagguuuu aauuguuacu uuccuuuaca
2240 aucauauggu uuccaaccca cuaauggugu ugguuaccaa ccauacagag uaguaguacu
2300 uucuuuugaa cuucuacaug caccagcaac uguuugugga ccuaaaaagu cuacuaauuu
2360 gguuaaaaac aaauguguca auuucaacuu caaugguuua acaggcacag guguucuuac
2420 ugagucuaac aaaaaguuuc ugccuuucca acaauuuggc agagacauug cugacacuac
2480 ugaugcuguc cgugauccac agacacuuga gauucuugac auuacaccau guucuuuugg
2540 uggugucagu guuauaacac caggaacaaa uacuucuaac cagguugcug uucuuuauca
2600 ggauguuaac ugcacagaag ucccuguugc uauucaugca gaucaacuua cuccuacuug
2660 gcguguuuau ucuacagguu cuaauguuuu ucaaacacgu gcaggcuguu uaauaggggc
2720 ugaacauguc aacaacucau augagugugа cauacccauu ggugcaggua uaugcgcuag
2780 uuaucagacu cagacuaauu cuccucggcg ggcacguagu guagcuaguc aauccaucau
2840 ugccuacacu augucacuug gugcagaaaa uucaguugcu uacucuaaua acucuauugc
2900 cauacccaca aauuuuacua uuaguguuac cacagaaauu cuaccagugu cuaugaccaa
2960 gacaucagua gauuguacaa uguacauuug uggugauuca acugaaugca gcaaucuuuu
3020 guugcaauau ggcaguuuuu guacacaauu aaaccgugcu uuaacuggaa uagcuguuga
3080 acaagacaaa aacacccaag aaguuuuugc acaagucaaa caaauuuaca aaacaccacc
3140 aauuaaagau uuugguggu uuaauuuuuc acaaauauua ccagauccau caaaaccaag
3200 caagagguca uuuauugaag aucuacuuuu caacaaagug acacuugcag augcuggcuu
3260 caucaaacaa uaugguggauu gccuuggugа uauugcugcu agagaccuca uuugugcaca
3320 aaaguuuaac ggccuuacug uuuugccacc uuugcucaca gaugaaauga uugcucaaua
3380 cacuucugca cuguuagcgg guacaaucac uucugguugg accuuuggug caggugcugc
3440 auuacaaaua ccauuugcua ugcaaauggc uuauagguuu aaugguauug gaguuacaca
3500 gaauguucuc uaugagaacc aaaaauugau ugccaaccaa uuuaauagug cuauuggcaa
3560 aauucaagac ucacuuucuu ccacagcaag ugcacuugga aaacuucaag augugguсaa
3620 ccaaaaugca caagcuuuaa acacgcuugu uaaacaacuu agcuccaauu uuggugcaau
3680 uucaaguguu uuaaaugaua uccuuucacg ucuugacaaa guugaggcug aagugcaaau
3740 ugauagguug aucacaggca gacuucaaag uuugcagaca uaugugacuc aacaauuaau
3800 uagagcugca gaaaucagag cuucugcuaa ucuugcugcu acuaaaaugu cagagugugu
3860 acuuggacaa ucaaaaagag uugauuuuug uggaaagggc uaucaucuua uguccuuccc
```

```
3920 ucagucagca ccucauggug uagucuucuu gcaugugacu uauguccug cacaagaaaa
3980 gaacuucaca acugcuccug ccauuuguca ugauggaaaa gcacacuuuc cucgugaagg
4040 ugucuuuguu ucaaauggca cacacugguu uguaacacaa aggaauuuuu augaaccaca
4100 aaucauuacu acagacaaca cauuugugug ugguaacugu gauguuguaa uaggaauugu
4160 caacaacaca guuuaugauc cuuugcaacc ugaauuagac ucauucaagg aggaguuaga
4220 uaaauauuuu aagaaucaua caucaccaga uguugauuua ggugacaucu cuggcauuaa
4280 ugcuucaguu guaaacauuc aaaaagaaau ugaccgccuc aaugagguug ccaagaauuu
4340 aaaugaaucu cucaucgauc uccaagaacu uggaaaguau gagcaguaua uaaaauggcc
4400 augguacauu uggcuagguu uuauagcugg cuugauugcc auaguaaugg ugacaauuau
4460 gcuuugcugu augaccaguu gcuguaguug ucucaagggc uguuguucuu guggauccug
4520 cugcaaauuu gaugaagacg acucugagcc agugcucaaa ggagucaaau uacauuacac
4580 a

4581 uaa
```

Note: nucleotides 4581-4583 is 'uaa' which is a STOP codon.[14,15]

Native Human CD8A CSR 3' Terminal End Region:

```
4584 ccc ugugcaacag ccacuacauu
4607 acuucaaacu gagauccuuc cuuuugaggg agcaaguccu ucccuuucau uuuuuccagu
4667 cuuccucccu guguauucau ucucaugauu auuauuuuag uggggggcggg gugggaaaga
4727 uuacuuuuuc uuuauguguu ugacgggaaa caaaacuagg uaaaaucuac aguacaccac
4787 aagggucaca auacuguugu gcgcacaucg cgguagggcg uggaaagggg caggccagag
4847 cuacccgcag aguucucaga aucaugcuga gagagcugga ggcacccaug ccaucucaac
4907 cucuuccccg cccguuuuac aaagggggag gcuaaagccc agagacagcu ugaucaaagg
4967 cacacagcaa gucaggguug gagcaguagc uggagggacc uugucuccca gcucagggcu
5027 cuuuccucca caccauucag gucuuucuuu ccgaggcccc ugucucaggg ugaggugcuu
5087 gagucuccaa cggcaaggga acaaguacuu cuugauaccu gggauacugu gcccagagcc
5147 ucgaggaggu aaugaauuaa agaagagaac ugccuuuggc agaguucuau aauguaaaca
5207 auaucagacu uuuuuuuuuu auaaucaagc cuaaaauugu auagaccuaa aauaaaauga
5267 aguggugagc uuaacccugg aaaaugaauc ccucuaucuc uaaagaaaau cucugugaaa
5327 ccccuaugug gaggcggaau ugcucuccca gcccuugcau ugcagagggg cccaugaaag
5387 aggacaggcu accccuuuac aaauagaauu ugagcaucag ugagguuaaa cuaaggcccu
5447 cuugaaucuc ugaauuugag auacaaacau guuccuggga ucacugauga cuuuuuauac
5507 uuuguaaaga caauuguugg agagccccuc acacagcccu ggccucugcu caacuagcag
5567 auacagggau gaggcagacc ugacucucuu aaggaggcug agagcccaaa cugcuguccc
5627 aaacaugcac uuccuugcuu aagguauggu acaagcaaug ccugcccauu ggagagaaaa
5687 aacuuaagua gauaaggaaa uaagaaccac ucauaauucu ucaccuuagg aauaaucucc
5747 uguuaauaug guguacauuc uuccugauua uuucuacac auacauguaa aauaugucuu
5807 ucuuuuuuaa auaggguugu acuaugcugu uaugaguggc uuuaaugaau aaacauuugu
5867 agcauccucu uuaaugggua aacagcaucc g
```

Poly adenine nucleotide tail

5898 a**aaaaaaaaa aaaaaaaaa aaaaaaaaa aaa** //

DETAILED DESCRIPTION

The gene for the CD8 refers to 'Cluster of Differentiation' 8 gene. The CD8 gene produces a messenger ribonucleic acid (mRNA) which codes for the CD8 cell surface glycoprotein, which may also be referred to as an antigen. The CD8 antigen can be comprised of two differing chains, one alpha chain and one beta chain, or the CD8 antigen can be comprised of two like chains, two alpha chains. CD8 antigen acts as a coreceptor. The CD8 antigen can be found on most cytotoxic T lymphocytes. The CD8 coreceptor functions to interact with the T-cell receptor on a T-lymphocyte to recognize antigens displayed by an antigen presenting cell.[21,22]

For clarity, in the context of this text, in reference to the CD8A, the terms 'cell surface receptor' and 'coreceptor' and 'antigen' and 'cell surface glycoprotein' all mean the same concept.

The CD8A cell surface receptor gene discussed in this application is identified at the National Center for Biotechnology Information (NCBI), NC_000002, 23792 bp, DNA linear CON 02-MAR-2020.[23,24]

The CD8A cell surface receptor gene description can be used to locate the CD8A mRNA description, which codes for the CD8A cell surface glycoprotein. The 5' leader nucleotide sequence of the CD8A cell surface receptor (CSR) mRNA can be taken from the CD8A cell surface receptor gene. The 5' leader nucleotide sequence of the native human CD8A mRNA can be attached to a nucleotide sequence coding for a desired polypeptide, which can be then be attached to the 3' nucleotide terminal end sequence of the native human CD8A mRNA. See Figure 25.

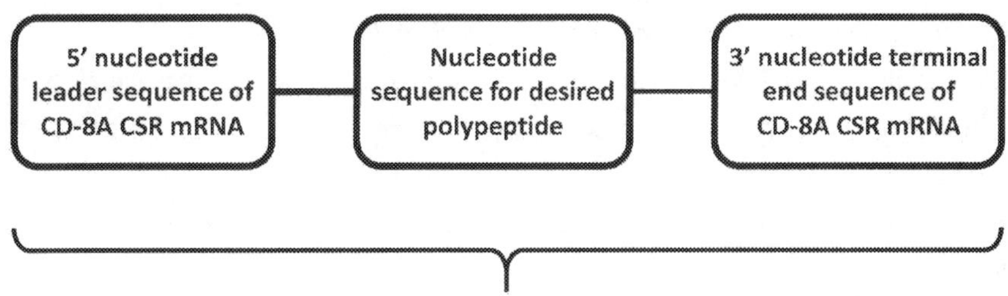

Figure 25

Construct of mRNA to prevent and manage COVID-19.

The CD8A cell surface receptor gene description can be used to locate the CD8A mRNA description, which codes for the CD8A cell surface glycoprotein. The 5' leader nucleotide sequence of the CD8A cell surface receptor (CSR) mRNA can be taken from the CD8A cell surface receptor gene. The 5' leader nucleotide sequence of the native human CD8A mRNA can be attached to a nucleotide sequence coding for a desired polypeptide, which can be then be attached to the 3' nucleotide terminal end sequence of the native human CD8A mRNA. See Figure 26.

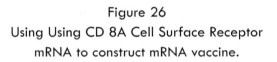

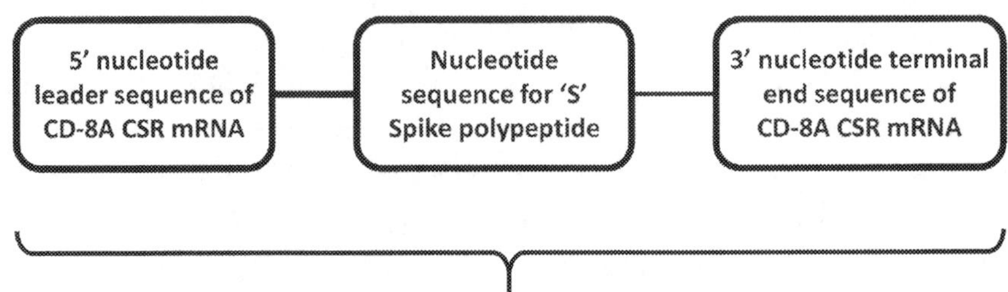

Figure 26
Using Using CD 8A Cell Surface Receptor mRNA to construct mRNA vaccine.

'S' protein probe or 'Spike' protein nucleotide code associated with the Wuhan-Hu -1 version of the coronavirus MN908947.[10]

Would like to celebrate and honor the hard work and dedication of the many researchers whose efforts made accessing this information on the NCBI website possible, so that the study and understanding of human genetics could advance toward a cure for a variety of challenging diseases.

NCBI Website: https://www.ncbi.nlm.nih.gov/nuccore/MN908947

```
LOCUS          MN908947    29903 bp ss-RNA    linear  VRL 11-FEB-2020
DEFINITION     Severe acute respiratory syndrome coronavirus 2
               isolate Wuhan-Hu-1, complete genome.
ACCESSION      MN908947
VERSION        MN908947.3
KEYWORDS       .
SOURCE         Severe acute respiratory syndrome coronavirus 2
               (SARS-CoV-
  ORGANISM     Severe acute respiratory syndrome coronavirus 2
```

```
            Viruses; Riboviria; Nidovirales; Cornidovirineae;
            Coronaviridae;
            Orthocoronavirinae; Betacoronavirus; Sarbecovirus.
REFERENCE   1  (bases 1 to 29903)
AUTHORS     Wu, F., Zhao, S., Yu, B., Chen, Y.M., Wang, W., Song,
            Z.G., Hu, Y., Tao, Z.W., Tian, J.H., Pei, Y.Y., Yuan,
            M.L., Zhang, Y.L., Dai, F.H., Liu, Y., Wang, Q.M.,
            Zheng, J.J., Xu, L., Holmes, E.C. and Zhang, Y.Z.
TITLE       A new coronavirus associated with human respiratory
            disease in China
JOURNAL     Nature (2020) In press
PUBMED      32015508
REMARK      Publication Status: Available-Online prior to print
REFERENCE   2  (bases 1 to 29903)
AUTHORS     Wu, F., Zhao, S., Yu, B., Chen, Y.-M., Wang, W., Hu,
            Y., Song, Z.-G., Tao, Z.-W., Tian, J.-H., Pei, Y.-Y.,
            Yuan, M.L., Zhang, Y.-L., Dai, F.-H., Liu, Y., Wang,
            Q.-M., Zheng, J.-J., Xu, L., Holmes, E.C. and Zhang,
            Y.-Z.
TITLE       Direct Submission
JOURNAL     Submitted (05-JAN-2020) Shanghai Public Health
            Clinical Center & School of Public Health, Fudan
            University, Shanghai, China
COMMENT     On Jan 17, 2020 this sequence version replaced
            MN908947.2.

            ##Assembly-Data-START##
            Assembly Method       :: Megahit v. V1.1.3
            Sequencing Technology :: Illumina
            ##Assembly-Data-END##
FEATURES    Location/Qualifiers
     source 1..29903
            /organism="Severe acute respiratory syndrome
            coronavirus 2"
            /mol _type="genomic RNA"
            /isolate="Wuhan-Hu-1"
            /host="Homo sapiens"
            /db _xref="taxon:2697049"
            /country="China"
            /collection _date="Dec-2019"


     gene   21563..25384
            /gene="S"
     CDS    21563..25384
            /gene="S"
            /note="structural protein"
            /codon _start=1
            /product="surface glycoprotein"
            /protein _id="QHD43416.1"
```

```
/translation="MFVFLVLLPLVSSQCVNLTTRTQLPPAYTNSFTRGVYYPDKVFR
SSVLHSTQDLFLPFFSNVTWFHAIHVSGTNGTKRFDNPVLPFNDGVYFASTEKSNIIR
GWIFGTTLDSKTQSLLIVNNATNVVIKVCEFQFCNDPFLGVYYHKNNKSWMESEFRVY
SSANNCTFEYVSQPFLMDLEGKQGNFKNLREFVFKNIDGYFKIYSKHTPINLVRDLPQ
GFSALEPLVDLPIGINITRFQTLLALHRSYLTPGDSSSGWTAGAAAYYVGYLQPRTFL
LKYNENGTITDAVDCALDPLSETKCTLKSFTVEKGIYQTSNFRVQPTESIVRFPNITN
LCPFGEVFNATRFASVYAWNRKRISNCVADYSVLYNSASFSTFKCYGVSPTKLNDLCF
TNVYADSFVIRGDEVRQIAPGQTGKIADYNYKLPDDFTGCVIAWNSNNLDSKVGGNYN
YLYRLFRKSNLKPFERDISTEIYQAGSTPCNGVEGFNCYFPLQSYGFQPTNGVGYQPY
RVVVLSFELLHAPATVCGPKKSTNLVKNKCVNFNFNGLTGTGVLTESNKKFLPFQQFG
RDIADTTDAVRDPQTLEILDITPCSFGGVSVITPGTNTSNQVAVLYQDVNCTEVPVAI
HADQLTPTWRVYSTGSNVFQTRAGCLIGAEHVNNSYECDIPIGAGICASYQTQTNSPR
RARSVASQSIIAYTMSLGAENSVAYSNNSIAIPTNFTISVTTEILPVSMTKTSVDCTM
YICGDSTECSNLLLQYGSFCTQLNRALTGIAVEQDKNTQEVFAQVKQIYKTPPIKDFG
GFNFSQILPDPSKPSKRSFIEDLLFNKVTLADAGFIKQYGDCLGDIAARDLICAQKFN
GLTVLPPLLTDEMIAQYTSALLAGTITSGWTFGAGAALQIPFAMQMAYRFNGIGVTQN
VLYENQKLIANQFNSAIGKIQDSLSSTASALGKLQDVVNQNAQALNTLVKQLSSNFGA
ISSVLNDILSRLDKVEAEVQIDRLITGRLQSLQTYVTQQLIRAAEIRASANLAATKMS
ECVLGQSKRVDFCGKGYHLMSFPQSAPHGVVFLHVTYVPAQEKNFTTAPAICHDGKAH
FPREGVFVSNGTHWFVTQRNFYEPQIITTDNTFVSGNCDVVIGIVNNTVYDPLQPELD
SFKEELDKYFKNHTSPDVDLGDISGINASVVNIQKEIDRLNEVAKNLNESLIDLQELG
KYEQYIKWPWYIWLGFIAGLIAIVMVTIMLCCMTSCCSCLKGCCSCGSCCKFDEDDSE
PVLKGVKLHYT"
```

21541 ~~cttgttaaca actaaacgaa ca~~atgtttgt ttttcttgtt ttattgccac tagtctctag
21601 tcagtgtgtt aatcttacaa ccagaactca attaccccct gcatacacta attctttcac
21661 acgtggtgtt tattaccctg acaaagtttt cagatcctca gttttacatt caactcagga
21721 cttgttctta cctttctttt ccaatgttac ttggttccat gctatacatg tctctgggac
21781 caatggtact aagaggtttg ataaccctgt cctaccattt aatgatggtg tttattttgc
21841 ttccactgag aagtctaaca taataagagg ctggattttt ggtactactt tagattcgaa
21901 gacccagtcc ctacttattg ttaataacgc tactaatgtt gttattaaag tctgtgaatt
21961 tcaattttgt aatgatccat ttttgggtgt ttattaccac aaaaacaaca aaagttggat
22021 ggaaagtgag ttcagagttt attctagtgc gaataattgc acttttgaat atgtctctca
22081 gccttttctt atggaccttg aaggaaaaca gggtaatttc aaaaatctta gggaatttgt
22141 gtttaagaat attgatggtt attttaaaat atattctaag cacacgccta ttaatttagt
22201 gcgtgatctc cctcagggtt tttcggcttt agaaccattg gtagatttgc caataggtat
22261 taacatcact aggtttcaaa ctttacttgc tttacataga agttatttga ctcctggtga
22321 ttcttcttca ggttggacag ctggtgctgc agcttattat gtgggttatc ttcaacctag
22381 gacttttcta ttaaaatata atgaaaatgg aaccattaca gatgctgtag actgtgcact
22441 tgaccctctc tcagaaacaa agtgtacgtt gaaatccttc actgtagaaa aaggaatcta
22501 tcaaacttct aactttagag tccaaccaac agaatctatt gttagatttc ctaatattac
22561 aaacttgtgc ccttttggtg aagtttttaa cgccaccaga tttgcatctg tttatgcttg
22621 gaacaggaag agaatcagca actgtgttgc tgattattct gtcctatata attccgcatc
22681 attttccact tttaagtgtt atggagtgtc tcctactaaa ttaaatgatc tctgctttac
22741 taatgtctat gcagattcat ttgtaattag aggtgatgaa gtcagacaaa tcgctccagg
22801 gcaaactgga aagattgctg attataatta taaattacca gatgatttta caggctgcgt
22861 tatagcttgg aattctaaca atcttgattc taaggttggt ggtaattata attacctgta
22921 tagattgttt aggaagtcta atctcaaacc ttttgagaga gatatttcaa ctgaaatcta
22981 tcaggccggt agcacacctt gtaatggtgt tgaaggtttt aattgttact ttcctttaca
23041 atcatatggt ttccaaccca ctaatggtgt tggttaccaa ccatacagag tagtagtact
23101 ttcttttgaa cttctacatg caccagcaac tgtttgtgga cctaaaaagt ctactaattt
23161 ggttaaaaac aaatgtgtca atttcaactt caatggttta acaggcacag gtgttcttac
23221 tgagtctaac aaaaagtttc tgcctttcca acaatttggc agagacattg ctgacactac
23281 tgatgctgtc cgtgatccac agacacttga gattcttgac attacaccat gttcttttgg
23341 tggtgtcagt gttataacac caggaacaaa tacttctaac caggttgctg ttctttatca
23401 ggatgttaac tgcacagaag tccctgttgc tattcatgca gatcaactta ctcctacttg

```
23461 gcgtgtttat tctacaggtt ctaatgtttt tcaaacacgt gcaggctgtt taatagggc
23521 tgaacatgtc aacaactcat atgagtgtga catacccatt ggtgcaggta tatgcgctag
23581 ttatcagact cagactaatt ctcctcggcg ggcacgtagt gtagctagtc aatccatcat
23641 tgcctacact atgtcacttg gtgcagaaaa ttcagttgct tactctaata actctattgc
23701 catacccaca aattttacta ttagtgttac cacagaaatt ctaccagtgt ctatgaccaa
23761 gacatcagta gattgtacaa tgtacatttg tggtgattca actgaatgca gcaatctttt
23821 gttgcaatat ggcagttttt gtacacaatt aaaccgtgct ttaactggaa tagctgttga
23881 acaagacaaa aacacccaag aagtttttgc acaagtcaaa caaatttaca aaacaccacc
23941 aattaaagat tttggtggtt ttaatttttc acaaatatta ccagatccat caaaaccaag
24001 caagaggtca tttattgaag atctactttt caacaaagtg acacttgcag atgctggctt
24061 catcaaacaa tatggtgatt gccttggtga tattgctgct agagacctca tttgtgcaca
24121 aaagtttaac ggccttactg ttttgccacc tttgctcaca gatgaaatga ttgctcaata
24181 cacttctgca ctgttagcgg gtacaatcac ttctggttgg acctttggtg caggtgctgc
24241 attacaaata ccatttgcta tgcaaatggc ttataggttt aatggtattg gagttacaca
24301 gaatgttctc tatgagaacc aaaaattgat tgccaaccaa tttaatagtg ctattggcaa
24361 aattcaagac tcactttctt ccacagcaag tgcacttgga aaacttcaag atgtggtcaa
24421 ccaaaatgca caagctttaa acacgcttgt taaacaactt agctccaatt ttggtgcaat
24481 ttcaagtgtt ttaaatgata tcctttcacg tcttgacaaa gttgaggctg aagtgcaaat
24541 tgataggttg atcacaggca gacttcaaag tttgcagaca tatgtgactc aacaattaat
24601 tagagctgca gaaatcagag cttctgctaa tcttgctgct actaaaatgt cagagtgtgt
24661 acttggacaa tcaaaaagag ttgatttttg tggaaagggc tatcatctta tgtccttccc
24721 tcagtcagca cctcatggtg tagtcttctt gcatgtgact tatgtccctg cacaagaaaa
24781 gaacttcaca actgctcctg ccatttgtca tgatggaaaa gcacactttc ctcgtgaagg
24841 tgtctttgtt tcaaatggca cacactggtt tgtaacacaa aggaattttt atgaaccaca
24901 aatcattact acagacaaca catttgtgtc tggtaactgt gatgttgtaa taggaattgt
24961 caacaacaca gtttatgatc ctttgcaacc tgaattagac tcattcaagg aggagttaga
25021 taaatatttt aagaatcata catcaccaga tgttgattta ggtgacatct ctggcattaa
25081 tgcttcagtt gtaaacattc aaaaagaaat tgaccgcctc aatgaggttg ccaagaattt
25141 aaatgaatct ctcatcgatc tccaagaact tggaaagtat gagcagtata taaaatggcc
25201 atggtacatt tggctaggtt ttatagctgg cttgattgcc atagtaatgg tgacaattat
25261 gctttgctgt atgaccagtt gctgtagttg tctcaagggc tgttgttctt gtggatcctg
25321 ctgcaaattt gatgaagacg actctgagcc agtgctcaaa ggagtcaaat tacattacac
25381 ataaacgaac ttatggattt gtttatgaga atcttcacaa ttggaactgt aactttgaag
```

Nucleotide code for the CD8A cell surface glycoprotein.[23]

NCBI Website: https://www.ncbi.nlm.nih.gov/nuccore/NC_000002.12?report=genbank&from=86784605&to=86808396&strand=true

In this text, the terms cell surface receptor (CSR) and cell surface glycoprotein have the same meaning.

Would like to celebrate and honor the hard work and dedication of the many researchers whose efforts made accessing this information on the NCBI website possible, so that the study and understanding of human genetics could advance toward a cure for a variety of challenging diseases.

CD8A Cell Surface Receptor Genome

```
LOCUS          NC _000002 23792 bp DNA linear CON 02-MAR-2020
```

```
DEFINITION    Homo sapiens chromosome 2, GRCh38.p13 Primary Assembly.
ACCESSION     NC_000002 REGION: complement(86784605..86808396)
VERSION       NC_000002.12
DBLINK        BioProject: PRJNA168
              Assembly: GCF_000001405.39
KEYWORDS      RefSeq.
SOURCE        Homo sapiens (human)
  ORGANISM    Homo sapiens
              Eukaryota; Metazoa; Chordata; Craniata; Vertebrata;
              Euteleostomi; Mammalia; Eutheria; Euarchontoglires;
              Primates; Haplorrhini; Catarrhini; Hominidae; Homo.
REFERENCE     1 (bases 1 to 23792)
AUTHORS       Hillier, L.W., Graves, T.A., Fulton, R.S., Fulton, L.A.,
              Pepin, K.H., Minx, P., Wagner-McPherson, C., Layman,
              D., Wylie, K., Sekhon, M., Becker, M.C., Fewell, G.A.,
              Delehaunty, K.D., Miner, T.L., Nash, W.E., Kremitzki,
              C., Oddy, L., Du, H., Sun, H., Bradshaw-Cordum, H., Ali,
              J., Carter, J., Cordes, M., Harris, A., Isak, A., van
              Brunt, A., Nguyen, C., Du, F., Courtney, L., Kalicki,
              J., Ozersky, P., Abbott, S., Armstrong, J., Belter,
              E.A., Caruso, L., Cedroni, M., Cotton, M., Davidson,
              T., Desai, A., Elliott, G., Erb, T., Fronick, C., Gaige,
              T., Haakenson, W., Haglund, K., Holmes, A., Harkins,
              R., Kim, K., Kruchowski, S.S., Strong, C.M., Grewal, N.,
              Goyea, E., Hou, S., Levy, A., Martinka, S., Mead, K.,
              McLellan, M.D., Meyer, R., Randall-Maher, J., Tomlinson,
              C., Dauphin-Kohlberg, S., Kozlowicz-Reilly, A., Shah,
              N., Swearengen-Shahid, S., Snider, J., Strong, J.T.,
              Thompson, J., Yoakum, M., Leonard, S., Pearman, C.,
              Trani, L., Radionenko, M., Waligorski, J.E., Wang, C.,
              Rock, S.M., Tin-Wollam, A.M., Maupin, R., Latreille, P.,
              Wendl, M.C., Yang, S.P., Pohl, C., Wallis, J.W., Spieth,
              J., Bieri, T.A., Berkowicz, N., Nelson, J.O., Osborne,
              J., Ding, L., Meyer, R., Sabo, A., Shotland, Y.,
              Sinha, P., Wohldmann, P.E., Cook, L.L., Hickenbotham,
              M.T., Eldred, J., Williams, D., Jones, T.A., She, X.,
              Ciccarelli, F.D., Izaurralde, E., Taylor, J., Schmutz,
              J., Myers, R.M., Cox, D.R., Huang, X., McPherson, J.D.,
              Mardis, E.R., Clifton, S.W., Warren, W.C., Chinwalla,
              A.T., Eddy, S.R., Marra, M.A., Ovcharenko, I., Furey,
              T.S., Miller, W., Eichler, E.E., Bork, P., Suyama, M.,
              Torrents, D., Waterston, R.H. and Wilson, R.K.
TITLE         Generation and annotation of the DNA sequences of
              human chromosomes 2 and 4
JOURNAL       Nature 434 (7034), 724-731 (2005)
PUBMED        15815621
REFERENCE     2 (bases 1 to 23792)
CONSRTM       International Human Genome Sequencing Consortium
TITLE         Finishing the euchromatic sequence of the human genome
JOURNAL       Nature 431 (7011), 931-945 (2004)
PUBMED        15496913
REFERENCE     3 (bases 1 to 23792)
```

AUTHORS Lander, E.S., Linton, L.M., Birren, B., Nusbaum, C., Zody, M.C., Baldwin, J., Devon, K., Dewar, K., Doyle, M., FitzHugh, W., Funke, R., Gage, D., Harris, K., Heaford, A., Howland, J., Kann, L., Lehoczky, J., LeVine, R., McEwan, P., McKernan, K., Meldrim, J., Mesirov, J.P., Miranda, C., Morris, W., Naylor, J., Raymond, C., Rosetti, M., Santos, R., Sheridan, A., Sougnez, C., Stange-Thomann, N., Stojanovic, N., Subramanian, A., Wyman, D., Rogers, J., Sulston, J., Ainscough, R., Beck, S., Bentley, D., Burton, J., Clee, C., Carter, N., Coulson, A., Deadman, R., Deloukas, P., Dunham, A., Dunham, I., Durbin, R., French, L., Grafham, D., Gregory, S., Hubbard, T., Humphray, S., Hunt, A., Jones, M., Lloyd, C., McMurray, A., Matthews, L., Mercer, S., Milne, S., Mullikin, J.C., Mungall, A., Plumb, R., Ross, M., Shownkeen, R., Sims, S., Waterston, R.H., Wilson, R.K., Hillier, L.W., McPherson, J.D., Marra, M.A., Mardis, E.R., Fulton, L.A., Chinwalla, A.T., Pepin, K.H., Gish, W.R., Chissoe, S.L., Wendl, M.C., Delehaunty, K.D., Miner, T.L., Delehaunty, A., Kramer, J.B., Cook, L.L., Fulton, R.S., Johnson, D.L., Minx, P.J., Clifton, S.W., Hawkins, T., Branscomb, E., Predki, P., Richardson, P., Wenning, S., Slezak, T., Doggett, N., Cheng, J.F., Olsen, A., Lucas, S., Elkin, C., Uberbacher, E., Frazier, M., Gibbs, R.A., Muzny, D.M., Scherer, S.E., Bouck, J.B., Sodergren, E.J., Worley, K.C., Rives, C.M., Gorrell, J.H., Metzker, M.L., Naylor, S.L., Kucherlapati, R.S., Nelson, D.L., Weinstock, G.M., Sakaki, Y., Fujiyama, A., Hattori, M., Yada, T., Toyoda, A., Itoh, T., Kawagoe, C., Watanabe, H., Totoki, Y., Taylor, T., Weissenbach, J., Heilig, R., Saurin, W., Artiguenave, F., Brottier, P., Bruls, T., Pelletier, E., Robert, C., Wincker, P., Smith, D.R., Doucette-Stamm, L., Rubenfield, M., Weinstock, K., Lee, H.M., Dubois, J., Rosenthal, A., Platzer, M., Nyakatura, G., Taudien, S., Rump, A., Yang, H., Yu, J., Wang, J., Huang, G., Gu, J., Hood, L., Rowen, L., Madan, A., Qin, S., Davis, R.W., Federspiel, N.A., Abola, A.P., Proctor, M.J., Myers, R.M., Schmutz, J., Dickson, M., Grimwood, J., Cox, D.R., Olson, M.V., Kaul, R., Raymond, C., Shimizu, N., Kawasaki, K., Minoshima, S., Evans, G.A., Athanasiou, M., Schultz, R., Roe, B.A., Chen, F., Pan, H., Ramser, J., Lehrach, H., Reinhardt, R., McCombie, W.R., de la Bastide, M., Dedhia, N., Blocker, H., Hornischer, K., Nordsiek, G., Agarwala, R., Aravind, L., Bailey, J.A., Bateman, A., Batzoglou, S., Birney, E., Bork, P., Brown, D.G., Burge, C.B., Cerutti, L., Chen, H.C., Church, D., Clamp, M., Copley, R.R., Doerks, T., Eddy, S.R., Eichler, E.E., Furey, T.S., Galagan, J., Gilbert, J.G., Harmon, C., Hayashizaki, Y.,Haussler, D., Hermjakob, H., Hokamp, K., Jang, W., Johnson, L.S., Jones, T.A., Kasif, S., Kaspryzk, A.,Kennedy, S.,

```
            Kent, W.J., Kitts, P., Koonin, E.V., Korf, I., Kulp,
            D., Lancet, D., Lowe, T.M., McLysaght, A., Mikkelsen,
            T.,Moran, J.V., Mulder, N., Pollara, V.J., Ponting, C.P.,
            Schuler, G., Schultz, J., Slater, G., Smit, A.F., Stupka,
            E., Szustakowski, J., Thierry-Mieg, D., Thierry-Mieg,
            J., Wagner, L., Wallis, J., Wheeler, R., Williams,
            A., Wolf, Y.I., Wolfe, K.H., Yang, S.P., Yeh, R.F.,
            Collins, F., Guyer, M.S., Peterson, J., Felsenfeld, A.,
            Wetterstrand, K.A., Patrinos, A., Morgan, M.J., de Jong,
            P., Catanese, J.J., Osoegawa, K., Shizuya, H., Choi, S.
            and Chen, Y.J.
CONSRTM     International Human Genome Sequencing Consortium
TITLE       Initial sequencing and analysis of the human genome
JOURNAL     Nature 409 (6822), 860-921 (2001)
PUBMED      11237011
REMARK      Erratum:[Nature 2001 Aug 2;412(6846):565]
COMMENT     REFSEQ INFORMATION: The reference sequence is
            identical to CM000664.2.
            On Feb 3, 2014 this sequence version replaced NC_
            000002.11.
            Assembly Name: GRCh38.p13 Primary Assembly
            The DNA sequence is composed of genomic sequence,
            primarily finished clones that were sequenced as part
            of the Human Genome Project. PCR products and WGS
            shotgun sequence have been added where necessary to
            fill gaps or correct errors. All such additions are
            manually curated by GRC staff. For more information
            see: https://genomereference.org.

            ##Genome-Annotation-Data-START##
            Annotation Provider          :: NCBI
            Annotation Status            :: Updated annotation
            Annotation Name              :: Homo sapiens Updated
                                            Annotation Release
                                            109.20200228
            Annotation Version           :: 109.20200228
            Annotation Pipeline          :: NCBI eukaryotic genome
                                            annotation pipeline
            Annotation Software Version  :: 8.3
            Annotation Method            :: Best-placed RefSeq;
                                            propagated RefSeq model
            Features Annotated           :: Gene; mRNA; CDS; ncRNA
            ##Genome-Annotation-Data-END##
FEATURES             Location/Qualifiers
     source          1..23792
                     /organism="Homo sapiens"
                     /mol _type="genomic DNA"
                     /db _xref="taxon:9606"
                     /chromosome="2"
     gene            1..23792
                     /gene="CD8A"
                     /gene _synonym="CD8; Leu2; p32"
                     /note="CD8a molecule; Derived by automated
                     computational
                     analysis using gene prediction method:
                     BestRefSeq."
```

/db _xref="GeneID:925"
/db _xref="HGNC:HGNC:1706"
/db _xref="MIM:186910"

mRNA

join(1..278,615..950,6740..6886,17302..17620,17716.
.18069, 18647..18757,18964..19074,19837..19867,2242
6..23792)
/gene="CD8A"
/gene _synonym="CD8; Leu2; p32"
/product="CD8a molecule, transcript variant 3"
/note="Derived by automated computational
analysis using
gene prediction method: BestRefSeq."
/transcript _id="NM_001145873.1"
/db _xref="GeneID:925"
/db _xref="HGNC:HGNC:1706"
/db _xref="MIM:186910"

CD8A CSR 5' Region:

Section 1: 1..278,

Section 2: 615..950,

Section 3: 6740..6886

Note: letters which are struck through are not included in the mRNA coding.

Section 1:
1..278

ORIGIN

1 ctctgtaaaa taaatgcgct gggccggatc ttttctgagt tctcttctcc cctacgaatt
61 ctagatccct cctctgtcct ccctgcgcca gggaccttcg ggcgaccctt ccctgtaccc
121 ccaccccacc ctctctggac cccgtttctg cctcagtacg gcgcgctgag ctctgccccc
181 tgcccaggcc ctgacccccct caggagccgc ggtttcctgg ggtaacagtg ggaaacgtgt
241 cggccgtctc cgctcaggcg cttgctgtgt acagaaag~~gt~~ ~~gaattcatgg~~ ~~gaaaggtggc~~

Section 2:
615..950

601 ~~tccgtctcct~~ ~~ttag~~gctgat tcaggcacac cggctctcgt cgccttggtg gccctcccca
661 gccctcctcc gcgcctgctc cgggtggcgc tccgctgggc tcctcgtgcg cctgtccgcg
721 accgcaccca cctcatcctg gcacccccat cgtggcatca cgtgttccct catctgtcct
781 catggctggc gtgcccctct gcggtgagac ctgcagaaca ggaattggtg ccgggtcagc
841 agccggcgat gaagccggac gaagcctgca aaccccaccc atacgccagc ttcacatagc
901 tcctatccat tgcacagcag cgtggggaag caccgttctc taccctccaa ~~gtaagaagct~~

Section 3:
6740..6886

6721 ~~tccttttttt ttcaaaaag~~a caaaagcatg aaccaggtgc agtggctcac gtctgtaatc
6781 ccagcatttt ggaggccaag gtggatggat ggattccttg agtccaggag ttcaagacca
6841 gcctgggcaa catggtgaac cccatctct acaaaaattt agccag~~gtat gatggtgtgc~~

CD8A CSR 3' Region:

22478-23792

22441 ~~gggagacaag cccagccttt cggcgagata cgtctaa~~ccc tgtgcaacag ccactacatt
22501 acttcaaact gagatccttc cttttgaggg agcaagtcct tccctttcat tttttccagt
22561 cttcctccct gtgtattcat tctcatgatt attattttag tgggggcggg gtgggaaaga
22621 ttactttttc tttatgtgtt tgacgggaaa caaaactagg taaaatctac agtacaccac
22681 aagggtcaca atactgttgt gcgcacatcg cggtagggcg tggaaagggg caggccagag
22741 ctacccgcag agttctcaga atcatgctga gagagctgga ggcacccatg ccatctcaac
22801 ctcttccccg cccgttttac aaagggggag gctaaagccc agagacagct tgatcaaagg
22861 cacacagcaa gtcagggttg gagcagtagc tggagggacc ttgtctccca gctcagggct
22921 ctttcctcca caccattcag gtctttcttt ccgaggcccc tgtctcaggg tgaggtgctt
22981 gagtctccaa cggcaaggga acaagtactt cttgatacct gggatactgt gcccagagcc
23041 tcgaggaggt aatgaattaa agaagagaac tgcctttggc agagttctat aatgtaaaca
23101 atatcagact tttttttttt ataatcaagc ctaaaattgt atagacctaa aataaaatga
23161 agtggtgagc ttaaccctgg aaaatgaatc cctctatctc taaagaaaat ctctgtgaaa
23221 cccctatgtg gaggcggaat tgctctccca gcccttgcat tgcagagggg cccatgaaag
23281 aggacaggct accccctttac aaatagaatt tgagcatcag tgaggttaaa ctaaggccct
23341 cttgaatctc tgaatttgag atacaaacat gttcctggga tcactgatga ctttttatac
23401 tttgtaaaga caattgttgg agagcccctc acacagccct ggcctctgct caactagcag
23461 atacagggat gaggcagacc tgactctctt aaggaggctg agagcccaaa ctgctgtccc
23521 aaacatgcac ttccttgctt aaggtatggt acaagcaatg cctgcccatt ggagagaaaa
23581 aacttaagta gataaggaaa taagaaccac tcataattct tcaccttagg aataatctcc
23641 tgttaatatg gtgtacattc ttcctgatta ttttctacac atacatgtaa aatatgtctt
23701 tcttttttaa atagggttgt actatgctgt tatgagtggc tttaatgaat aaacatttgt
23761 agcatcctct ttaatgggta aacagcatcc g

Poly adenine nucleotide tail

a **aaaaaaaaaaaaaa**
//

Consolidating the CD8A cell surface glycoprotein mRNA nucleotide code for the 5' region and 3' region:

Native Human CD8A CSR 5' Leader End Region:

1 ctctgtaaaa taaatgcgct gggccggatc ttttctgagt tctcttctcc cctacgaatt
61 ctagatccct cctctgtcct ccctgcgcca gggaccttcg ggcgaccctt ccctgtaccc
121 ccaccccacc ctctctggac cccgtttctg cctcagtacg gcgcgctgag ctctgccccc
181 tgcccaggcc ctgacccccct caggagccgc ggtttcctgg ggtaacagtg ggaaacgtgt
241 cggccgtctc cgctcaggcg cttgctgtgt acagaaag
615 gctgat tcaggcacac cggctctcgt cgccttggtg gccctcccca

```
 661 gccctcctcc gcgcctgctc cgggtggcgc tccgctgggc tcctcgtgcg cctgtccgcg
 721 accgcaccca cctcatcctg gcacccccat cgtggcatca cgtgttccct catctgtcct
 781 catggctggc gtgcccctct gcggtgagac ctgcagaaca ggaattggtg ccgggtcagc
 841 agccggcgat gaagccggac gaagcctgca aaccccaccc atacgccagc ttcacatagc
 901 tcctatccat tgcacagcag cgtggggaag caccgttctc taccctccaa
6740 a caaaagcatg aaccaggtgc agtggctcac gtctgtaatc
6781 ccagcatttt ggaggccaag gtggatggat ggattccttg agtccaggag ttcaagacca
6841 gcctgggcaa catggtgaac ccccatctct acaaaaattt agccag
```

Note: INSERT BETWEEN CD8A CSR 5' leader end region and CD8A terminal 3' terminal end region DESIRED POLYPEPTIDE NUCLEOTIDE CODING SEQUENCE

```
taa
```

Note 'taa' is a STOP codon.[14,15]

Native Human CD8A CSR 3' Terminal End Region:

```
22478 ccc tgtgcaacag ccactacatt
22501 acttcaaact gagatccttc cttttgaggg agcaagtcct tccctttcat tttttccagt
22561 cttcctccct gtgtattcat tctcatgatt attattttag tgggggcggg gtgggaaaga
22621 ttactttttc tttatgtgtt tgacgggaaa caaaactagg taaaatctac agtacaccac
22681 aagggtcaca atactgttgt gcgcacatcg cggtagggcg tggaaagggg caggccagag
22741 ctacccgcag agttctcaga atcatgctga gagagctgga ggcacccatg ccatctcaac
22801 ctcttccccg cccgttttac aaagggggag gctaaagccc agagacagct tgatcaaagg
22861 cacacagcaa gtcagggttg gagcagtagc tggagggacc ttgtctccca gctcagggct
22921 ctttcctcca caccattcag gtctttcttt ccgaggcccc tgtctcaggg tgaggtgctt
22981 gagtctccaa cggcaaggga acaagtactt cttgatacct gggatactgt gcccagagcc
23041 tcgaggaggt aatgaattaa agaagagaac tgcctttggc agagttctat aatgtaaaca
23101 atatcagact tttttttttt ataatcaagc ctaaaattgt atagacctaa aataaaatga
23161 agtggtgagc ttaaccctgg aaaatgaatc cctctatctc taaagaaaat ctctgtgaaa
23221 cccctatgtg gaggcggaat tgctctccca gcccttgcat tgcagagggg cccatgaaag
23281 aggacaggct acccctttac aaatagaatt tgagcatcag tgaggttaaa ctaaggccct
23341 cttgaatctc tgaatttgag atacaaacat gttcctggga tcactgatga ctttttatac
23401 tttgtaaaga caattgttgg agagcccctc acacagccct ggcctctgct caactagcag
23461 atacagggat gaggcagacc tgactctctt aaggaggctg agagcccaaa ctgctgtccc
23521 aaacatgcac ttccttgctt aaggtatggt acaagcaatg cctgcccatt ggagagaaaa
23581 aacttaagta gataaggaaa taagaaccac tcataattct tcaccttagg aataatctcc
23641 tgttaatatg gtgtacattc ttcctgatta ttttctacac atacatgtaa aatatgtctt
23701 tctttttttaa atagggttgt actatgctgt tatgagtggc tttaatgaat aaacatttgt
23761 agcatcctct ttaatgggta aacagcatcc g
```

Poly adenine nucleotide tail

a **aaaaaaaaaaaaaa**
//

CONSTRUCTING mRNA CD8A VACCINE to place COVID-19 virion surface probe on cell surface of human cell:

Consolidating CD8A CSR 5' region and 3' region and adding the Coronavirus 'S' protein nucleic acid coding:

Native Human CD8A CSR 5' Leader End Region:

```
  1 ctctgtaaaa taaatgcgct gggccggatc ttttctgagt tctcttctcc cctacgaatt
 61 ctagatccct cctctgtcct ccctgcgcca gggaccttcg ggcgaccctt ccctgtaccc
121 ccaccccacc ctctctggac cccgtttctg cctcagtacg gcgcgctgag ctctgccccc
181 tgcccaggcc ctgacccccct caggagccgc ggtttcctgg ggtaacagtg ggaaacgtgt
241 cggccgtctc cgctcaggcg cttgctgtgt acagaaag
279 gctgat tcaggcacac cggctctcgt cgccttggtg gccctcccca
325 gccctcctcc gcgcctgctc cgggtggcgc tccgctgggc tcctcgtgcg cctgtccgcg
385 accgcaccca cctcatcctg gcacccccat cgtggcatca cgtgttccct catctgtcct
445 catggctggc gtgcccctct gcggtgagac ctgcagaaca ggaattggtg ccgggtcagc
505 agccggcgat gaagccggac gaagcctgca aaccccaccc atacgccagc ttcacatagc
565 tcctatccat tgcacagcag cgtggggaag caccgttctc taccctccaa
615 a caaaagcatg aaccaggtgc agtggctcac gtctgtaatc
656 ccagcatttt ggaggccaag gtggatggat ggattccttg agtccaggag ttcaagacca
716 gcctgggcaa catggtgaac cccatctct acaaaaattt agccag
```

CORONAVIRUS Wuhan-Hu-1 'S' Protein Probe nucleic acid coding:

```
 762 atgtttgt ttttcttgtt ttattgccac tagtctctag
 800 tcagtgtgtt aatcttacaa ccagaactca attaccccct gcatacacta attctttcac
 860 acgtggtgtt tattaccctg acaaagtttt cagatcctca gttttacatt caactcagga
 920 cttgttctta cctttctttt ccaatgttac ttggttccat gctatacatg tctctgggac
 980 caatggtact aagaggtttg ataaccctgt cctaccattt aatgatggtg tttattttgc
1040 ttccactgag aagtctaaca taataagagg ctggattttt ggtactactt tagattcgaa
1100 gacccagtcc ctacttattg ttaataacgc tactaatgtt gttattaaag tctgtgaatt
1160 tcaattttgt aatgatccat ttttgggtgt ttattaccac aaaaacaaca aaagttggat
1220 ggaaagtgag ttcagagttt attctagtgc gaataattgc acttttgaat atgtctctca
1280 gccttttctt atggaccttg aaggaaaaca gggtaatttc aaaaatctta gggaatttgt
1340 gtttaagaat attgatggtt attttaaaat atattctaag cacacgccta ttaatttagt
1400 gcgtgatctc cctcagggtt tttcggcttt agaaccattg gtagatttgc caataggtat
1460 taacatcact aggtttcaaa ctttacttgc tttacataga agttatttga ctcctggtga
1520 ttcttcttca ggttggacag ctggtgctgc agcttattat gtgggttatc ttcaacctag
1580 gacttttcta ttaaaatata atgaaaatgg aaccattaca gatgctgtag actgtgcact
1640 tgaccctctc tcagaaacaa agtgtacgtt gaaatccttc actgtagaaa aaggaatcta
1700 tcaaacttct aactttagag tccaaccaac agaatctatt gttagatttc ctaatattac
1760 aaacttgtgc ccttttggtg aagtttttaa cgccaccaga tttgcatctg tttatgcttg
1820 gaacaggaag agaatcagca actgtgttgc tgattattct gtcctatata attccgcatc
1880 attttccact tttaagtgtt atggagtgtc tcctactaaa ttaaatgatc tctgctttac
1940 taatgtctat gcagattcat ttgtaattag aggtgatgaa gtcagacaaa tcgctccagg
2000 gcaaactgga aagattgctg attataatta taaattacca gatgatttta caggctgcgt
2060 tatagcttgg aattctaaca atcttgattc taaggttggt ggtaattata attacctgta
2120 tagattgttt aggaagtcta atctcaaacc ttttgagaga gatatttcaa ctgaaatcta
2180 tcaggccggt agcacacctt gtaatggtgt tgaaggtttt aattgttact ttcctttaca
2240 atcatatggt ttccaaccca ctaatggtgt tggttaccaa ccatacagag tagtagtact
2300 ttcttttgaa cttctacatg caccagcaac tgtttgtgga cctaaaaagt ctactaattt
2360 ggttaaaaac aaatgtgtca atttcaactt caatggttta acaggcacag gtgttcttac
2420 tgagtctaac aaaaagtttc tgcctttcca acaatttggc agagacattg ctgacactac
```

```
2480 tgatgctgtc cgtgatccac agacacttga gattcttgac attacaccat gttcttttgg
2540 tggtgtcagt gttataacac caggaacaaa tacttctaac caggttgctg ttctttatca
2600 ggatgttaac tgcacagaag tccctgttgc tattcatgca gatcaactta ctcctacttg
2660 gcgtgtttat tctacaggtt ctaatgtttt tcaaacacgt gcaggctgtt taataggggc
2720 tgaacatgtc aacaactcat atgagtgtga catacccatt ggtgcaggta tatgcgctag
2780 ttatcagact cagactaatt ctcctcggcg ggcacgtagt gtagctagtc aatccatcat
2840 tgcctacact atgtcacttg gtgcagaaaa ttcagttgct tactctaata actctattgc
2900 catacccaca aattttacta ttagtgttac cacagaaatt ctaccagtgt ctatgaccaa
2960 gacatcagta gattgtacaa tgtacatttg tggtgattca actgaatgca gcaatctttt
3020 gttgcaatat ggcagttttt gtacacaatt aaaccgtgct ttaactggaa tagctgttga
3080 acaagacaaa aacacccaag aagtttttgc acaagtcaaa caaatttaca aaacaccacc
3140 aattaaagat tttggtggtt ttaatttttc acaaatatta ccagatccat caaaaccaag
3200 caagaggtca tttattgaag atctactttt caacaaagtg acacttgcag atgctggctt
3260 catcaaacaa tatggtgatt gccttggtga tattgctgct agagacctca tttgtgcaca
3320 aaagtttaac ggccttactg ttttgccacc tttgctcaca gatgaaatga ttgctcaata
3380 cacttctgca ctgttagcgg gtacaatcac ttctggttgg acctttggtg caggtgctgc
3440 attacaaata ccatttgcta tgcaaatggc ttataggttt aatggtattg gagttacaca
3500 gaatgttctc tatgagaacc aaaaattgat tgccaaccaa tttaatagtg ctattggcaa
3560 aattcaagac tcactttctt ccacagcaag tgcacttgga aaacttcaag atgtggtcaa
3620 ccaaaatgca caagctttaa acacgcttgt taaacaactt agctccaatt ttggtgcaat
3680 ttcaagtgtt ttaaatgata tcctttcacg tcttgacaaa gttgaggctg aagtgcaaat
3740 tgataggttg atcacaggca gacttcaaag tttgcagaca tatgtgactc aacaattaat
3800 tagagctgca gaaatcagag cttctgctaa tcttgctgct actaaaatgt cagagtgtgt
3860 acttggacaa tcaaaaagag ttgatttttg tggaaagggc tatcatctta tgtccttccc
3920 tcagtcagca cctcatggtg tagtcttctt gcatgtgact tatgtccctg cacaagaaaa
3980 gaacttcaca actgctcctg ccatttgtca tgatggaaaa gcacactttc ctcgtgaagg
4040 tgtctttgtt tcaaatggca cacactggtt tgtaacacaa aggaattttt atgaaccaca
4100 aatcattact acagacaaca catttgtgtc tggtaactgt gatgttgtaa taggaattgt
4160 caacaacaca gtttatgatc ctttgcaacc tgaattagac tcattcaagg aggagttaga
4220 taaatatttt aagaatcata catcaccaga tgttgattta ggtgacatct ctggcattaa
4280 tgcttcagtt gtaaacattc aaaaagaaat tgaccgcctc aatgaggttg ccaagaattt
4340 aaatgaatct ctcatcgatc tccaagaact tggaaagtat gagcagtata taaaatggcc
4400 atggtacatt tggctaggtt ttatagctgg cttgattgcc atagtaatgg tgacaattat
4460 gctttgctgt atgaccagtt gctgtagttg tctcaagggc tgttgttctt gtggatcctg
4520 ctgcaaattt gatgaagacg actctgagcc agtgctcaaa ggagtcaaat tacattacac
4580 a
4581 taa
```

Note: nucleotides 4581-4583 is 'taa', which is a STOP codon. [14,15]

Native Human CD8A 3' Terminal End Region:

```
4584 ccc tgtgcaacag ccactacatt
4607 acttcaaact gagatccttc cttttgaggg agcaagtcct tccctttcat tttttccagt
4667 cttcctccct gtgtattcat tctcatgatt attattttag tgggggcggg gtgggaaaga
4727 ttactttttc tttatgtgtt tgacgggaaa caaaactagg taaaatctac agtacaccac
4787 aagggtcaca atactgttgt gcgcacatcg cggtagggcg tggaaagggg caggccagag
4847 ctacccgcag agttctcaga atcatgctga gagagctgga ggcacccatg ccatctcaac
4907 ctcttccccg cccgttttac aaagggggag gctaaagccc agagacagct tgatcaaagg
4967 cacacagcaa gtcagggttg gagcagtagc tggagggacc ttgtctccca gctcagggct
5027 ctttcctcca caccattcag gtctttcttt ccgaggcccc tgtctcaggg tgaggtgctt
5087 gagtctccaa cggcaaggga acaagtactt cttgatacct gggatactgt gcccagagcc
5147 tcgaggaggt aatgaattaa agaagagaac tgcctttggc agagttctat aatgtaaaca
5207 atatcagact tttttttttt ataatcaagc ctaaaattgt atagacctaa aataaaatga
5267 agtggtgagc ttaaccctgg aaaatgaatc cctctatctc taaagaaaat ctctgtgaaa
5327 cccctatgtg gaggcggaat tgctctccca gcccttgcat tgcagagggg cccatgaaag
5387 aggacaggct acccctttac aaatagaatt tgagcatcag tgaggttaaa ctaaggccct
```

```
5447 cttgaatctc tgaatttgag atacaaacat gttcctggga tcactgatga ctttttatac
5507 tttgtaaaga caattgttgg agagcccctc acacagccct ggcctctgct caactagcag
5567 atacagggat gaggcagacc tgactctctt aaggaggctg agagcccaaa ctgctgtccc
5627 aaacatgcac ttccttgctt aaggtatggt acaagcaatg cctgcccatt ggagagaaaa
5687 aacttaagta gataaggaaa taagaaccac tcataattct tcaccttagg aataatctcc
5747 tgttaatatg gtgtacattc ttcctgatta ttttctacac atacatgtaa aatatgtctt
5807 tctttttaa atagggttgt actatgctgt tatgagtggc tttaatgaat aaacatttgt
5867 agcatcctct ttaatgggta aacagcatcc g
```

Poly adenine nucleotide tail

```
5898 aaaaaaaaaa aaaaaaaaaa aaaaaaaaaa aaa     //
```

The modified mRNA to function as a COVID-19 RNA vaccine is 5888 nucleotides long, though the final length depends upon the number of adenine nucleotides comprising the 3' tail of the mRNA. Above mRNA is shown with 33 adenine nucleotides comprising the tail, similar to the positive-sense coronavirus mRNA. Number of adenine nucleotides in the 3' tail is a function of the optimal performance of the mRNA inside a target cell.

To summarize, the construct of this mRNA coronavirus vaccine is comprised of: 5' leader nucleotide sequence of a native human mRNA for CD8A glycoprotein cell surface receptor, attached to the nucleotide coding sequence for coronavirus 'S' probe, attached to the 'taa' STOP code codon, attached to the 3' terminal end nucleotide sequence of a native human mRNA coding for CD8A glycoprotein cell surface receptor, attached to a sequence of adenine nucleotides comprising the tail of the molecule.

To code like a mRNA, the COVID-19 mRNA vaccine nucleotide coding with t's replaced by u's as by convention the construct of a messenger ribonucleic acid.

Native Human CD8A CSR 5' Leader End Region:

```
  1 cucuguaaaa uaaaugcgcu gggccggauc uuuucugagu ucucuucucc ccuacgaauu
 61 cuagaucccu ccucuguccu cccugcgcca gggaccuucg ggcgacccuu cccuguaccc
121 ccaccccacc cucucuggac cccguuucug ccucaguacg gcgcgcugag cucugccccc
181 ugcccaggcc cugacccccu caggagccgc gguuuccugg gguaacagug ggaaacgugu
241 cggccgucuc cgcucaggcg cuugcugugu acagaaag
279 gcugau ucaggcacac cggcucucgu cgccuuggug gcccucccca
325 gcccuccucc gcgccugcuc cgggcggcgc uccgcugggc uccucgugcg ccuguccgcg
385 accgcaccca ccucauccug gcacccccau cguggcauca cguguucccu caucuguccu
445 cauggcuggc gugccccucu gcggugagac cugcagaaca ggaauuggug ccgggucagc
505 agccggcgau gaagccggac gaagccugca aaccccaccc auacgccagc uucacauagc
```

```
565 uccuauccau ugcacagcag cguggggaag caccguucuc uacccuccaa
615 a caaaagcaug aaccaggugc aguggcucac gucuguaauc
656 ccagcauuuu ggaggccaag guggauggau ggauuccuug aguccaggag uucaagacca
716 gccugggcaa cauggugaac ccccaucucu acaaaaauuu agccag
```

CORONAVIRUS Wuhan-Hu-1 'S' Protein Probe nucleic acid coding:

```
 762 auguuugu uuuucuuguu uuauugccac uagucucuag
 800 ucaguguguu aaucuuacaa ccagaacuca auuacccccu gcauacacua auucuuucac
 860 acgugguguu uauuacccug acaaaguuuu cagauccuca guuuuacauu caacucagga
 920 cuuguucuua ccuuucuuuu ccaauguuac uugguuccau gcuauacaug ucucugggac
 980 caaugguacu aagagguuug auaacccugu ccuaccauuu aaugauggug uuuauuuugc
1040 uuccacugag aagucuaaca uaauaagagg cuggauuuuu gguacuacuu uagauucgaa
1100 gacccagucc cuacuuauug uuaauaacgc uacuaauguu guuauuaaag ucugugaauu
1160 ucaauuuugu aaugauccau uuuugggugu uuauuaccac aaaaacaaca aaaguuggau
1220 ggaaagugag uucagaguuu auucuagugc gaauaauugc acuuuugaau augucucuca
1280 gccuuuucuu auggaccuug aaggaaaaca ggguaauuuc aaaaaucuua gggaauuugu
1340 guuuaagaau auugaugguu auuuuaaaau auauucuaag cacacgccua uuaauuuagu
1400 gcgugaucuc ccucaggguu uuucggcuuu agaaccauug guagauuugc caauagguau
1460 uaacaucacu agguuucaaa cuuuacuugc uuuacauaga aguuauuuga cuccugguga
1520 uucuucuuca gguuggacag cuggugcugc agcuuauuau gugguuauc uucaaccuag
1580 gacuuuucua uuaaaauaua augaaaaugg aaccauuaca gaugcuguag acugugcacu
1640 ugacccucuc ucagaaacaa aguguacguu gaaauccuuc acuguagaaa aaggaaucua
1700 ucaaacuucu aacuuuagag uccaaccaac agaaucuauu guuagauuuc cuaauauuac
1760 aaacuugugc ccuuuuggug aaguuuuuaa cgccaccaga uuugcaucug uuuaugcuug
1820 gaacaggaag agaaucagca acuguguugc ugauuauucu guccuauaua auuccgcauc
1880 auuuuccacu uuuaaguguu auggaguguc uccuacuaaa uuaaaugauc ucugcuuuac
1940 uaaugucuau gcagauucau uuguaauuag aggugaugaa gucagacaaa ucgcuccagg
2000 gcaaacugga aagauugcug auuauaauua uaaauuacca gaugauuuua caggcugcgu
2060 uauagcuugg aauucuaaca aucuugauuc uaagguuggu gguaauuaua auuaccugua
2120 uagauuguuu aggaagucua aucucaaacc uuuugagaga gauauuucaa cugaaaucua
2180 ucaggccggu agcacaccuu guaauggugu ugaagguuuu aauuguuacu uuccuuuaca
2240 aucauauggu uuccaaccca cuaauggugu ugguuaccaa ccauacagag uaguaguacu
2300 uucuuuugaa cuucuacaug caccagcaac uguuugugga ccuaaaaagu cuacuaauuu
2360 gguuaaaaac aaauguguca auuucaacuu caaugguuua acaggcacag guguucuuac
2420 ugagucuaac aaaaaguuuc ugccuuucca acaauuuggc agagacauug cugacacuac
2480 ugaugcuguc cgugauccac agacacuuga gauucuugac auuacaccau guucuuuugg
2540 uggugucagu guuauaacac caggaacaaa uacuucuaac cagguugcug uucuuuauca
2600 ggauguuaac ugcacagaag ucccuguugc uauucaugca gaucaacuua cuccuacuug
2660 gcguguuuau ucuacagguu cuaauguuuu ucaaacacgu gcaggcuguu uaauaggggc
2720 ugaacauguc aacaacucau augaguguga cauacccauu ggugcaggua uaugcgcuag
2780 uuaucagacu cagacuaauu cuccucggcg ggcacguagu guagcuaguc aauccaucau
2840 ugccuacacu augucacuug gugcagaaaa uucaguugcu uacucuaaua acucuauugc
2900 cauacccaca aauuuuacua uuaguguuac cacagaaauu cuaccagugu cuaugaccaa
2960 gacaucagua gauuguacaa uguacauuug uggugauuca acugaaugca gcaaucuuuu
3020 guugcaauau ggcaguuuuu guacacaauu aaaccgugcu uuaacuggaa uagcuguuga
3080 acaagacaaa aacacccaag aaguuuuugc acaagucaaa caaauuuaca aaacaccacc
3140 aauuaaagau uuuggugguu uuaauuuuuc acaaauauua ccagauccau caaaaccaag
3200 caagagguca uuuauugaag aucuacuuuu caacaaagug acacuugcag augcuggcuu
3260 caucaaacaa uauggugauu gccuugguga uauugcugcu agagaccuca uuugugcaca
3320 aaaguuuaac ggccuuacug uuuugccacc uuugcucaca gaugaaauga uugcucaaua
3380 cacuucugca cuguuagcgg guacaaucac uucugguugg accuuuggug caggugcugc
3440 auuacaaaua ccauuugcua ugcaaauggc uuauagguuu aaugguauug gaguuacaca
3500 gaauguucuc uaugagaacc aaaaauugau ugccaaccaa uuuaauagug cuauuggcaa
3560 aauucaagac ucacuuucuu ccacagcaag ugcacuugga aaacuucaag auguggucaa
3620 ccaaaaugca caagcuuuaa acacgcuugu uaaacaacuu agcuccaauu uuggugcaau
3680 uucaaguguu uuaaaugaua uccuuucacg ucuugacaaa guugaggcug aagugcaaau
3740 ugauagguug aucacaggca gacuucaaag uuugcagaca uaugugacuc aacaauuaau
```

```
3800 uagagcugca gaaaucagag cuucugcuaa ucuugcugcu acuaaaaugu cagagugugu
3860 acuuggacaa ucaaaaagag uugauuuuug uggaaagggc uaucaucuua uguccuuccc
3920 ucagucagca ccucauggug uagucuucuu gcaugugacu uauguccug cacaagaaaa
3980 gaacuucaca acugcuccug ccauuuguca ugauggaaaa gcacacuuuc cucgugaagg
4040 ugucuuuguu ucaaauggca cacacugguu uguaacacaa aggaauuuuu augaaccaca
4100 aaucauuacu acagacaaca cauuuguguc ugguaacugu gauguuguaa uaggaauugu
4160 caacaacaca guuuaugauc cuuugcaacc ugaauuagac ucauucaagg aggaguuaga
4220 uaaauauuuu aagaaucaua caucaccaga uguugauuua ggugacaucu cuggcauuaa
4280 ugcuucaguu guaaacauuc aaaaagaaau ugaccgccuc aaugagguug ccaagaauuu
4340 aaaugaaucu cucaucgauc uccaagaacu uggaaaguau gagcaguaua uaaaauggcc
4400 augguacauu uggcuagguu uuauagcugg cuugauugcc auaguaaugg ugacaauuau
4460 gcuuugcugu augaccaguu gcuguaguug ucucaagggc uguuguucuu guggauccug
4520 cugcaaauuu gaugaagacg acucugagcc agugcucaaa ggagucaaau uacauuacac
4580 a

4581 uaa
```

Note: nucleotides 4581-4583 is ‘uaa’, which is a STOP codon.[14,15]

Native Human CD8A CSR 3’ Terminal End Region:

```
4584 ccc ugugcaacag ccacuacauu
4607 acuucaaacu gagauccuuc cuuuugaggg agcaaguccu ucccuuucau uuuuuccagu
4667 cuuccucccu guguauucau ucucaugauu auuauuuuag ugggggcggg gugggaaaga
4727 uuacuuuuuc uuuauguguu ugacgggaaa caaaacuagg uaaaaucuac aguacaccac
4787 aagggucaca auacuguugu gcgcacaucg cgguagggcg uggaaagggg caggccagag
4847 cuacccgcag aguucucaga aucaugcuga gagagcugga ggcacccaug ccaucucaac
4907 cucuuccccg cccguuuuac aaagggggag gcuaaagccc agagacagcu ugaucaaagg
4967 cacacagcaa gucaggguug gagcaguagc uggagggacc uugucuccca gcucagggcu
5027 cuuuccucca caccauucag gucuuucuuu ccgaggcccc ugucucaggg ugaggugcuu
5087 gagucuccaa cggcaaggga acaaguacuu cuugauaccu gggauacugu gcccagagcc
5147 ucgaggaggu aaugaauuaa agaagagaac ugccuuuggc agaguucuau aauguaaaca
5207 auaucagacu uuuuuuuuuu auaaucaagc cuaaaauugu auagaccuaa aauaaaauga
5267 aguggugagc uuaacccugg aaaaugaauc ccucuaucuc uaaagaaaau cucugugaaa
5327 ccccuaugug gaggcggaau ugcucuccca gcccuugcau ugcagagggg cccaugaaag
5387 aggacaggcu accccuuuac aaauagaauu ugagcaucag ugagguuaaa cuaaggcccu
5447 cuugaaucuc ugaauuugag auacaaacau guuccuggga ucacugauga cuuuuuauac
5507 uuuguaaaga caauuguugg agagccccuc acacagcccu ggccucugcu caacuagcag
5567 auacagggau gaggcagacc ugacucucuu aaggaggcug agagcccaaa cugcuguccc
5627 aaacaugcac uuccuugcuu aagguauggu acaagcaaug ccugcccauu ggagagaaaa
5687 aacuuaagua gauaaggaaa uaagaaccac ucauaauucu ucaccuuagg aauaaucucc
5747 uguuaauaug guguacauuc uuccugauua uuuucuacac auacauguaa aauaugucuu
5807 ucuuuuuuaa auaggguugu acuaugcugu uaugaguggc uuuaaugaau aaacauuugu
5867 agcauccucu uuaaugggua aacagcaucc g
```

Poly adenine nucleotide tail

```
5898 aaaaaaaaaa aaaaaaaaaa aaaaaaaaaa aaa      //
```

SUMMARY

The human race cannot allow a misguided scrap of malignant bio-programming code to ravage the world's population without being heatedly contested by our best efforts at innovation and invention. We must capitalize on the advancements in the knowledge of how mRNAs are constructed and coded. A modified mRNA could generate, through the process of cellular translation, a vaccine against coronavirus by place an 'S' probe on the surface of the cell to act as a means to alert the immune system of the construct of a unique feature of the construct of the coronavirus virion. The 'S' probe architecture is highly conserved, so thus a desirable target. An effective mRNA vaccine offering immunity against coronavirus offers a practical virus-specific means to neutralize the current coronavirus global pandemic threat.

CHAPTER THIRTEEN

USING -UAA- AS A JOINER TO BUILD A DUAL VACCINE AGAINST BOTH THE WUHAN AND MOSCOW VERSIONS OF THE COVID-19 'S' PROTEIN

ABSTRACT

The functional aspect of the concept described in this text is the use of one artificial messenger RNA to produce two cell surface receptors consisting of the 'S' (spike) protein (probe) for the Wuhan-Hu-1 coronavirus and the 'S' (spike) protein (probe) for the Moscow coronavirus. Given there are three different stop codons to choose from, in the case of an artificial messenger ribonucleic acid constructed to generate multiple polypeptides in a single reading of the messenger ribonucleic acid, the UAA stop code is chosen to facilitate the task. The use of the nucleotide codon UAA as an AND function to act as a joiner between two polypeptide nucleotide sequences in an artificial messenger ribonucleic acid molecule such that the first nucleotide sequence is translated to create a polypeptide and because of the presence of the UAA codon between the two nucleotide sequences, subsequently the second nucleotide sequence is translated by the ribosome reading complex to generate another polypeptide during a single translation event cycle of the artificial messenger ribonucleic acid.

FIELD OF THE INVENTION

This invention relates to any medical device intended to generate a polypeptide in a eukaryote cell using a messenger ribonucleic acid as the template for construction.

THE ROLE OF THE THREE STOP CODE CODONS

As written for RNA, the START codon 'AUG' signals initiation of the translation process. Written for RNA the three STOP codes are codons 'UGA', 'UAA' and 'UAG' or 'uga', 'uaa' and 'uag'; written for DNA the same three STOP codes are codons 'TGA', 'TAA' and 'TAG' or 'tga', 'taa' and 'tag'. The three STOP codons 'UGA', 'UAA' and 'UAG' signal termination of the translation process, but in addition to terminating the translation process, each STOP codon exhibits other unique behaviors as described below.[14,15]

As written for RNA, the 'UGA' represents the three nucleotide codon uracil-guanine-adenine or represented as the three nucleotide codon code uracil-guanine-adenine or 'uga' when referring to the construct of a ribonucleic acid (RNA). At times in the science literature when 'thymine' or 't' is used in place of 'uracil' or otherwise 'u', then 'UGA' may be represented as 'TGA' or 'tga'. In the context of deoxynucleic acid (DNA) the four nucleotides used in the construct of the DNA include the nucleotides adenine (a), cytosine (c), guanine (g) and thymine (t). In the context and construction of DNA, the 'UGA' stop code codon is represented as 'TGA' representing the nucleotides 'thymine-guanine-adenine'. DNA is the template origin that native RNAs are generated from during the process of transcription.

The 'UGA' STOP codon present in a mature mRNA molecule is found in prokaryote mRNAs and viral mRNAs. The UGA STOP codon signals that once the ribosome translating the mRNA reaches this point in mRNA's codon sequence, the ribosome is to stop linking amino acids to the protein molecule, the ribosome is to disassemble, and the protein generated by the translation process is to be released. The UGA STOP codon does not alter the 3' end of the mRNA molecule. [14,15]

As written for RNA, the 'UAA' represents the three nucleotide codon uracil-adenine-adenine or represented as the three nucleotide codon code uracil-adenine-adenine or 'uaa' when referring to the construct of a ribonucleic acid (RNA). At times in the science literature when 'thymine' or 't' is used in place of 'uracil' or 'u', then 'UAA' may be represented as 'TAA' or 'taa'. In the context of deoxynucleic acid (DNA) the four nucleotides used in the construct of the DNA include the nucleotides adenine (a), cytosine (c), guanine (g) and thymine (t). In the context and construction of DNA, the 'UAA' stop code codon is represented as 'TAA' representing the nucleotides 'thymine-adenine-adenine'. DNA is the template origin that native RNAs are generated from during the process of transcription.

The 'UAA' STOP codon is present in prokaryote mRNAs, eukaryote mRNAs and viral mRNAs. The UAA STOP codon specifies to the ribosome reading the mRNA that it is to stop translating the mRNA at that point, release the protein that has been generated, remain assembled, and continue reading the mRNA's code and seek out another START codon to restart the translation process on the same mRNA molecule. Though 'UAA' is considered a STOP code codon, this codon actually acts like an AND function, directing the cell's nucleotide decoding machinery to complete one function and then seek out another subsequent function. An mRNA may contain multiple translatable segments and when translated, may produce more than one differing protein per mRNA molecule. The UAA STOP codon is utilized to specify the end of each protein's code, except for the last protein produced by transcribing a mRNA, which requires a 'UGA' STOP codon or a UAG STOP codon. [14,15]

As written for RNA, the 'UAG' represents the three nucleotide codon uracil-adenine-guanine or represented as the three nucleotide codon code uracil-adenine-guanine or 'uag' when referring to the construct of a ribonucleic acid (RNA). At times in the science literature when 'thymine' or 't' is used in place of 'uracil' or 'u' then 'UAG' may be represented as 'TAG' or 'tag'. In the context of deoxynucleic acid (DNA) the four nucleotides used in the construct of the DNA include the nucleotides adenine (a), cytosine (c), guanine (g) and thymine (t). In the context and construction of DNA, the 'UAG' stop code codon is represented as 'TAG' representing the nucleotides 'thymine-adenine-guanine'. DNA is the template origin that native RNAs are generated from during the process of transcription.

The UAG STOP codon is present in the human mRNAs, other eukaryote mRNAs and viral mRNAs. The UAG STOP codon specifies to the ribosome reading the mRNA to terminate the translation process, disassemble and creates a signal to remove one or more adenine monophosphate molecules from the multiple adenine tail, often referred to as the Poly (A) tail, attached to the mRNA 3' terminal end of the molecule being translated. Once enough adenine monophosphate molecules have been removed from the mRNA's Poly (A) tail, the mRNA molecule is enzymatically terminated. [14,15]

The 'UAA' STOP codon is unique in that it is recognized in the science literature as a STOP codon, but in fact, functionally the UAA codon exhibits an 'AND' function. Of the three recognized STOP codons, UGA, UAA and UAG, the codon UAA directs the ribosome reader of the mRNA to stop adding amino acids on to the polypeptide being generated, but to continue downstream toward the 3' end of the mRNA in search of other segments nucleotide sequencing to decode. Thus, if an artificial mRNA is constructed for the purposes of a medical treatment, and one or more polypeptides are intended to be the product of the translation of the said artificial mRNA, then the use of a specific 'UAA' STOP codon, rather than one of the other two STOP codons, is deliberate and a necessary part of the construction of the said mRNA in order to generate two or more separate polypeptides during a single translation event cycle of the said artificial mRNA. The 'UAA' STOP codon would be required to be present between two segments of nucleotide sequencing, each coding for the same polypeptide or a different polypeptide. The 'UAA' STOP codon would be required to be present between the nucleotide sequencing coding for one or more polypeptides and the 3' terminal end of the mRNA.

Coronavirus is also referred to as COVID-19 and also referred to as Severe Acute Respiratory Syndrome (SARS) coronavirus with COVID-19 being the version of the virus which mutated and first infected humans in 2019. Coronavirus infection often results in a lung infection, though the virus can be found present in other parts of the body. Coronavirus utilizes the 'S' probe, mounted on the exterior of the virion which carries virus's genetic information, to seek out and engage human cells, which it targets for the purpose of infection and replication. The 'S' protein probe appears to be highly conserved, with little variation in the amino acid structure of the protein probe.[19,20,24,25]

There are two different versions of the coronavirus 'S' spike protein known to date related to the COVID-19 form of coronavirus. Examples of the two known variations can be found as the 'S' protein probe from the Wuhan-Hu-1 (MN908947) strain of the virus and the 'S' protein probe from the Moscow (MT510643.1) strain of the virus. The Wuhan-Hu-1 version coronavirus 'S' (spike) protein (probe) has an aspartic acid 'D' at amino acid position 614, where the 'S' (spike) protein (probe) for the Moscow coronavirus version has a glycine 'G' at amino acid position 614.

SUMMARY DESCRIPTION

When artificial mRNAs are constructed for the purposes of a medical treatment, and one or more polypeptides are intended to be the product of the translation of the said artificial mRNA, then the use of a 'UAA' STOP codon is deliberate and a necessary part of the construction of the said mRNA. The 'UAA' STOP codon would be required to be present between two segments of nucleotide sequencing, each coding for the same polypeptide or a different polypeptide. The 'UAA' STOP codon would be required to be present between the nucleotide sequencing coding for one or more polypeptides and the 3' terminal end of the mRNA.

The coronavirus places a 'S' probe or sometimes referred to as a 'spike' protein on the surface of the virion. The 'S' probe can be utilized by the human immune system to uniquely identify the coronavirus. In order to artificially alert the human immune system to be aware of the coronavirus, the CD8A mRNA is used to carry the coronavirus 'S' probe. Normally, the native human CD8A mRNA would be translated by intracellular ribosomes and produce a CD8A glycoprotein on the surface of a human cell. In this case, the nucleotide sequencing coding for the native human CD8A has been modified. The nucleotide sequencing coding for the native human CD8A glycoprotein cell surface receptor has been replaced by the nucleotide coding sequence of the coronavirus 'S' probe.

Using -UAA- as a Joiner to Build a Dual Vaccine Against Both the Wuhan and Moscow Versions of the COVID-19 'S' Protein

The coronavirus's 'S' protein is highly conserved. The Wuhan-Hu-1 coronavirus 'S' (spike) protein (probe) and the 'S' (spike) protein (probe) for the Moscow coronavirus vary in one amino acid.[10,25] The Wuhan-Hu-1 version coronavirus 'S' (spike) protein (probe) has a aspartic acid 'D' at amino acid position 614, where the 'S' (spike) protein (probe) for the Moscow coronavirus version has a glycine 'G' at amino acid position 614. This variation could be enough to make ineffective a vaccine designed against the Wuhan-Hu-1 coronavirus 'S' probe. Though, as an example of how important one nucleotide can be, sickle cell anemia is the result of one nucleotide mutation, with glutamic acid being substituted by valine due to the GAG codon being changed to GTG in the beta-globulin gene at position 6; the mutation described as E6V. In order to account for the variation between the Wuhan-Hu-1 coronavirus 'S' probe and the Moscow version of the coronavirus 'S' probe, a mRNA is constructed which would carry the nucleotide coding sequences to mount copies of both 'S' probes on the surface of the human cell which has translated the mRNA. The two nucleotide coding sequences the Wuhan-Hu-1 version coronavirus 'S' (spike) protein and the Moscow coronavirus version would be separated by a UAA codon code. The second nucleotide coding sequence, the Moscow coronavirus version would also be separated from the 3' terminal end of the mRNA by a UAA codon code.

The construct of this polyvalent mRNA coronavirus vaccine is comprised of: 5' leader nucleotide sequence of a native human mRNA for CD8A glycoprotein cell surface receptor, attached to the nucleotide coding sequence for coronavirus Wuhan-Hu-1 coronavirus 'S' (spike) protein (probe), attached to the 'taa' STOP code codon, Moscow coronavirus 'S' (spike) protein (probe), attached to the 'taa' STOP code codon, attached to the 3' terminal end nucleotide sequence of a native human mRNA coding for CD8A glycoprotein cell surface receptor, attached to a sequence of adenine nucleotides comprising the tail of the molecule. The nucleotide coding of the mRNA is in the four RNA nucleotides adenine, cytosine, guanine and uracil.

Native Human CD8A CSR 5' Leader End Region:

```
 1 cucuguaaaa uaaaugcgcu gggccggauc uuuucugagu ucucuucucc ccuacgaauu
61 cuagaucccu ccucuguccu cccugcgcca gggaccuucg ggcgacccuu cccuguaccc
```

121 ccaccccacc cucucuggac cccguuucug ccucaguacg gcgcgcugag cucugccccc
181 ugcccaggcc cugacccccu caggagccgc gguuuccugg gguaacagug ggaaacgugu
241 cggccgucuc cgcucaggcg cuugcugugu acagaaag
279 gcugau ucaggcacac cggcucucgu cgccuuggug gcccuccccca
325 gcccuccucc gcgccugcuc cggguggcgc uccgcugggc uccucgugcg ccuguccgcg
385 accgcaccca ccucauccug gcacccccau cguggcauca cguguucccu caucuguccu
445 cauggcuggc gugccccucu gcggugagac cugcagaaca ggaauuggug ccgggucagc
505 agccggcgau gaagccggac gaagccugca aaccccaccc auacgccagc uucacauagc
565 uccuauccau ugcacagcag cguggggaag caccguucuc uacccuccaa
615 a caaaagcaug aaccaggugc aguggcucac gucuguaauc
656 ccagcauuuu ggaggccaag guggauggau ggauuccuug aguccaggag uucaagacca
716 gccugggcaa cauggugaac ccccaucucu acaaaaauuu agccag

CORONAVIRUS Wuhan-Hu-1 'S' Protein Probe nucleic acid coding:

762 auguuugu uuuucuuguu uuauugccac uagucucuag
800 ucaguguguu aaucuuacaa ccagaacuca auuacccccu gcauacacua auucuuucac
860 acgugguguu uauuacccug acaaaguuuu cagauccuca guuuuacauu caacucagga
920 cuuguucuua ccuuucuuuu ccaauguuac uugguuccau gcuauacaug ucucugggac
980 caaugguacu aagagguuug auaacccugu ccuaccauuu aaugauggug uuuauuuugc
1040 uuccacugag aagucuaaca uaauaagagg cuggauuuuu gguacuacuu uagauucgaa
1100 gacccagucc cuacuuauug uuaauaacgc uacuaauguu guuauuaaag ucugugaauu
1160 ucaauuuugu aaugauccau uuuugggugu uuauuaccac aaaaacaaca aaaguuggau
1220 ggaaagugag uucagaguuu auucuagugc gaauaauugc acuuugaau augucucuca
1280 gccuuuucuu auggaccuug aaggaaaaca ggguaauuuc aaaaaucuua gggaauuugu
1340 guuuaagaau auugaugguu auuuuaaaau auauucuaag cacacgccua uuaauuuagu
1400 gcgugaucuc ccucaggguu uuucggcuuu agaaccauug guagauuugc caauagguau
1460 uaacaucacu agguuucaaa cuuuacuugc uuuacauaga aguuauuuga cuccugguga
1520 uucuucuuca gguuggacag cuggugcugc agcuuauuau gugguuauc uucaaccuag
1580 gacuuuucua uuaaaauaua augaaaaugg aaccauuaca gaugcuguag acugugcacu
1640 ugacccucuc ucagaaacaa aguguacguu gaaauccuuc acuguagaaa aaggaaucua
1700 ucaaacuucu aacuuuagag uccaaccaac agaaucuauu guuagauuuc cuaauauuac
1760 aaacuugugc ccuuuuggug aaguuuuuaa cgccaccaga uuugcaucug uuuaugcuug
1820 gaacaggaag agaaucagca acuguguugc ugauuauucu guccuauaua auuccgcauc
1880 auuuuccacu uuuaaguguu auggaguguc uccuacuaaa uuaaaugauc ucugcuuuac
1940 uaaugucuau gcagauucau uuguaauuag aggugaugaa gucagacaaa ucgcuccagg
2000 gcaaacugga aagauugcug auuauaauua uaaauuacca gaugauuuua caggcugcgu
2060 uauagcuugg aauucuaaca aucuugauuc uaagguuggu gguaauuaua auuaccugua
2120 uagauuguuu aggaagucua aucucaaacc uuuugagaga gauauuucaa cugaaaucua
2180 ucaggccggu agcacaccuu guaauggugu ugaagguuuu aauuguuacu uuccuuuaca
2240 aucauauggu uuccaaccca cuaauggugu ugguuaccaa ccauacagag uaguaguacu
2300 uucuuuugaa cuucuacaug caccagcaac uguuugugga ccuaaaaagu cuacuaauuu
2360 gguuaaaaac aaauguguca auuucaacuu caaugguuua acaggcacag guguucuuac
2420 ugagucuaac aaaaaguuuc ugccuuucca acaauuuggc agagacauug cugacacuac
2480 ugaugcuguc cgugauccac agacacuuga gauucuugac auuacaccau guucuuuugg
2540 uggugucagu guuauaacac caggaacaaa uacuucuaac cagguugcug uucuuuauca
2600 ggauguuaac ugcacagaag ucccuguugc uauucaugca gaucaacuua cuccuacuug
2660 gcguguuuau ucuacagguu cuaauguuuu ucaaacacgu gcaggcuguu uaauaggggc
2720 ugaacauguc aacaacucau augaguguga cauacccauu ggugcaggua uaugcgcuag
2780 uuaucagacu cagacuaauu cuccucggcg ggcacguagu guagcuaguc aauccaucau
2840 ugccuacacu augucacuug gugcagaaaa uucaguugcu uacucuaaua acucuauugc
2900 cauacccaca aauuuuacua uuaguguuac cacagaaauu cuaccagugu cuaugaccaa
2960 gacaucagua gauuguacaa uguacauuug uggugauuca acugaaugca gcaaucuuuu
3020 guugcaauau ggcaguuuuu guacacaauu aaaccgugcu uuaacuggaa uagcuguuga
3080 acaagacaaa aacacccaag aaguuuuugc acaagucaaa caaauuuaca aaacaccacc
3140 aauuaaagau uuuggugguu uuaauuuuuc acaaauauua ccagauccau caaaaccaag
3200 caagagguca uuuauugaag aucuacuuuu caacaaagug acacuugcag augcuggcuu
3260 caucaaacaa uauggugauu gccuugguga uauugcugcu agagaccuca uuugugcaca

```
3320 aaaguuuaac ggccuuacug uuuugccacc uuugcucaca gaugaaauga uugcucaaua
3380 cacuucugca cuguuagcgg guacaaucac uucugguugg accuuuggug caggugcugc
3440 auuacaaaua ccauuugcua ugcaaauggc uuauagguuu aaugguauug gaguuacaca
3500 gaauguucuc uaugagaacc aaaaauugau ugccaaccaa uuuaauagug cuauuggcaa
3560 aauucaagac ucacuuucuu ccacagcaag ugcacuugga aaacuucaag auguggucaa
3620 ccaaaaugca caagcuuuaa acacgcuugu uaaacaacuu agcuccaauu uuggugcaau
3680 uucaaguguu uuaaaugaua uccuuucacg ucuugacaaa guugaggcug aagugcaaau
3740 ugauagguug aucacaggca gacuucaaag uuugcagaca uaugugacuc aacaauuaau
3800 uagagcugca gaaaucagag cuucugcuaa ucuugcugcu acuaaaaugu cagagugugu
3860 acuuggacaa ucaaaaagag uugauuuuug uggaaagggc uaucaucuua uguccuuccc
3920 ucagucagca ccucauggug uagucuucuu gcaugugacu uaugucccug cacaagaaaa
3980 gaacuucaca acugcuccug ccauuuguca ugauggaaaa gcacacuuuc cucgugaagg
4040 ugucuuuguu ucaaauggca cacacugguu uguaacacaa aggaauuuuu augaaccaca
4100 aaucauuacu acagacaaca cauuuguguc ugguaacugu gauguuguaa uaggaauugu
4160 caacaacaca guuuaugauc cuuugcaacc ugaauuagac ucauucaagg aggaguuaga
4220 uaaauauuuu aagaaucaua caucaccaga uguugauuua ggugacaucu cuggcauuaa
4280 ugcuucaguu guaaacauuc aaaaagaaau ugaccgccuc aaugagguug ccaagaauuu
4340 aaaugaaucu cucaucgauc uccaagaacu uggaaaguau gagcaguaua uaaaauggcc
4400 augguacauu uggcuagguu uuauagcugg cuugauugcc auaguaaugg ugacaauuau
4460 gcuuugcugu augaccaguu gcuguaguug ucucaagggc uguuguucuu guggauccug
4520 cugcaaauuu gaugaagacg acucugagcc agugcucaaa ggagucaaau uacauuacac
4580 a

4581 uaa
```

Note: nucleotides 4581-4583 is 'uaa', which is functioning as a STOP/ AND codon.[14,15]

CORONAVIRUS Moscow 'S' Protein Probe nucleic acid coding:

```
4584 augu uuguuuuucu uguuuuauug ccacuagucu cuagucagug
4628 uguuaaucuu acaaccagaa cucaauuacc cccugcauac acuaauucuu ucacacgugg
4688 uguuuauuac ccugacaaag uuuucagauc cucaguuuua cauucaacuc aggacuuguu
4748 cuuaccuuuc uuuuccaaug uuacuugguu ccaugcuaua caugucucug ggaccaaugg
4808 uacuaagagg uuugauaacc cuguccuacc auuuaaugau gguguuuauu uugcuuccac
4868 ugagaagucu aacauaauaa gaggcuggau uuuugguacu acuuuagauu cgaagaccca
4928 gucccuacuu auuguuaaua acgcuacuaa uguuguuauu aaagucugug aauuucaauu
4988 uuguaaugau ccauuuuugg guguuuauua ccacaaaaac aacaaaaguu ggauggaaag
5048 ugaguucaga guuuauucua gugcgaauaa uugcacuuuu gaauaugucu cucagccuuu
5108 ucuuauggac cuugaaggaa aacaggguaa uuucaaaaau cuuagggaau uuguguuuaa
5168 gaauauugau gguuauuuua aaauauauuc uaagcacacg ccuauuaauu uagugcguga
5228 ucucccucag gguuuuucgg cuuuagaacc auugguagau uugccaauag guauuaacau
5288 cacuagguuu caaacuuuac uugcuuuaca uagaaguuau uugacuccug gugauucuuc
5348 uucagguugg acagcuggug cugcagcuua uuaugugggu uaucuucaac cuaggacuuu
5408 ucuauuaaaa uauaaugaaa auggaaccau uacagaugcu guagacugug cacuugaccc
5468 ucucucagaa acaaagugua cguugaaauc cuucacugua gaaaaaggaa ucuaucaaac
5528 uucuaacuuu agaguccaac caacagaauc uauuguuaga uuuccuaaua uuacaaacuu
5588 gugcccuuuu ggugaaguuu uuaacgccac cagauuugca ucuguuuaug cuuggaacag
5648 gaagagaauc agcaacugug uugcugauua uucuguccua uauaauuccg caucauuuuc
5708 cacuuuuaag uguuauggag ugucuccuac uaaauuaaau gaucucugcu uuacuaaugu
5768 cuaugcagau ucauuuguaa uuagaggugа ugaagucaga caaaucgcuc cagggcaaac
5828 uggaaagauu gcugauuaua auuauaaauu accagaugau uuuacaggcu gcguuauagc
5888 uuggaauucu aacaaucuug auucuaaggu ugguggua au uauaauuacc uguauagauu
5948 guuuaggaag ucuaaucuca aaccuuuuga gagagauauu ucaacugaaa ucuaucaggc
6008 cgguagcaca ccuuguaaug guguugaagg uuuuaauugu uacuuuccuu uacaaucaua
6068 ugguuuccaa cccacuaaug guguugguua ccaaccauac agaguaguag uacuuucuuu
6128 ugaacuucua caugcaccag caacuguuug uggaccuaaa aagucuacua auuugguuaa
```

```
6188 aaacaaaugu gucaauuuca acuucaaugg uuuaacaggc acagguguuc uuacugaguc
6248 uaacaaaaag uuucugccuu uccaacaauu uggcagagac auugcugaca cuacugaugc
6308 uguccgugau ccacagacac uugagauucu ugacauuaca ccauguucuu uuggugugu
6368 caguguuaua acaccaggaa caaauacuuc uaaccagguu gcuguucuuu aucagggugu
6428 uaacugcaca gaaguccug uugcuauuca ugcagaucaa cuuacuccua cuuggcgugu
6488 uuauucuaca gguucuaaug uuuuucaaac acgugcaggc uguuuaauag ggcugaaca
6548 ugucaacaac ucauaugagu gugacauacc cauuggugca gguauaugcg cuaguuauca
6608 gacucagacu aauucuccuc ggcgggcacg uaguguagcu agucaaucca ucauugccua
6668 cacuauguca cuuggugcag aaaauucagu ugcuuacucu aauaacucua uugccauacc
6728 cacaaauuuu acuauuagug uuaccacaga aauucuacca gugucuauga ccaagacauc
6788 aguagauugu acaauguaca uuuguggguga uucaacugaa ugcagcaauc uuuuguugca
6848 auauggcagu uuuuguacac aauuaaaccg ugcuuuaacu ggaauagcug uugaacaaga
6908 caaaaacacc caagaaguuu uugcacaagu caaacaaauu uacaaaacac caccaauuaa
6968 agauuuuggu gguuuuaauu uuucacaaau auuaccagau ccaucaaaac caagcaagag
7028 gucauuuauu gaagaucuac uuuucaacaa agugacacuu gcagaugcug gcuucaucaa
7088 acaauauggu gauugccuug gugauauugc ugcuagagac cucauuugug cacaaaaguu
7148 uaacggccuu acuguuuugc caccuuugcu cacagaugaa augauugcuc aauacacuuc
7208 ugcacuguua gcggguacaa ucacuucugg uuggaccuuu ggugcaggug cugcauuaca
7268 aauaccauuu gcuaugcaaa uggcuuauag guuuaauggu auuggaguua cacagaaugu
7328 ucucuaugag aaccaaaaau ugauugccaa ccaauuuaau agugcuauug gcaaaauuca
7388 agacucacuu ucuuccacag caagugcacu uggaaaacuu caagaugugg ucaaccaaaa
7448 ugcacaagcu uuaaacacgc uuguuaaaca acuuagcucc aauuuuggug caauuucaag
7508 uguuuuaaau gauauccuuu cacgucuuga caaaguugag gcugaagugc aaauugauag
7568 guugaucaca ggcagacuuc aaaguuugca gacauaugug acucaacaau uaauuagagc
7628 ugcagaaauc agagcuucug cuaaucuugc ugcuacuaaa augucagagu guguacuugg
7688 acaaucaaaa agaguugauu uuuguggaaa gggcuaucau cuuauguccu ucccucaguc
7748 agcaccucau gguguagucu ucuugcaugu gacuuauguc ccugcacaag aaaagaacuu
7808 cacaacugcu ccugccauuu gucaugaugg aaaagcacac uuuccucgug aaggugucuu
7868 uguuucaaau ggcacacacu gguuuguaac acaaaggaau uuuuaugaac cacaaaucau
7928 uacuacagac aacacauuug ugucugguaa cugugauguu guaauaggaa uugucaacaa
7988 cacaguuuau gauccuuugc aaccugaauu agacucauuc aaggaggagu uagauaaaua
8048 uuuuaagaau cauacaucac cagauguuga uuuaggugac aucucuggca uuaaugcuuc
8108 aguuguaaac auucaaaaag aaauugaccg ccucaaugag guugccaaga auuuaaauga
8168 aucucucauc gaucuccaag aacuuggaaa guaugagcag uauauaaaau ggccauggua
8228 cauuuggcua gguuuuauag cuggcuugau ugccauagua auggugacaa uuaugcuuug
8288 cuguaugacc aguugcugua guugucucaa gggcuguugu ucuuguggau ccugcugcaa
8348 auuugaugaa gacgacucug agccagugcu caaaggaguc aaauuacauu acaca

8403 uaa
```

Note nucleotides 8403-8405 is 'uaa', which is a STOP codon.[14,15]

Native Human CD8A CSR 3' Terminal End Region:

```
8406 ccc ugugcaacag ccacuacauu
8429 acuucaaacu gagauccuuc cuuuugaggg agcaaguccu ucccuuucau uuuuuccagu
8489 cuuccucccu guguauucau ucucaugauu auuauuuuag ugggggcggg gugggaaaga
8549 uuacuuuuuc uuuauguguu ugacgggaaa caaaacuagg uaaaaucuac aguacaccac
8609 aagggucaca auacuguugu gcgcacaucg cgguagggcg uggaaagggg caggccagag
8669 cuacccgcag aguucucaga aucaugcuga gagagcugga ggcacccaug ccaucucaac
8729 cucuuccccg cccguuuuac aaagggggag gcuaaagccc agagacagcu ugaucaaagg
8789 cacacagcaa gucaggguug gagcaguagc uggagggacc uugucuccca gcucagggcu
8849 cuuuccucca caccauucag gucuuucuuu ccgaggcccc ugucucaggg ugaggugcuu
8909 gagucuccaa cggcaaggga acaaguacuu cuugauaccu gggauacugu gcccagagcc
8969 ucgaggaggu aaugaauuaa agaagagaac ugccuuuggc agaguucuau aauguaaaca
9029 auaucagacu uuuuuuuuuu auaaucaagc cuaaaauugu auagaccuaa aauaaaauga
9089 aguggugagc uuaacccugg aaaaugaauc ccucuaucuc uaaagaaaau cucugugaaa
```

```
9149 ccccuaugug gaggcggaau ugcucuccca gcccuugcau ugcagagggg cccaugaaag
9209 aggacaggcu accccuuuac aaauagaauu ugagcaucag ugagguuaaa cuaaggcccu
9269 cuugaaucuc ugaauuugag auacaaacau guuccuggga ucacugauga cuuuuuauac
9329 uuuguaaaga caauuguugg agagccccuc acacagcccu ggccucugcu caacuagcag
9389 auacagggau gaggcagacc ugacucucuu aaggaggcug agagcccaaa cugcuguccc
9449 aaacaugcac uuccuugcuu aagguauggu acaagcaaug ccugcccauu ggagagaaaa
9509 aacuuaagua gauaaggaaa uaagaaccac ucauaauucu ucaccuuagg aauaaucucc
9569 uguuaauaug guguacauuc uuccugauua uuuucuacac auacauguaa aauaugucuu
9629 ucuuuuuuaa auagguugu acuaugcugu uaugaguggc uuuaaugaau aaacauuugu
9689 agcauccucu uuaaugggua aacagcaucc g
9720 aaaaaaaaaa aaaaaaaaaa aaaaaaaaaa aaaa     //
```

DETAILED DESCRIPTION

In the event an artificial mRNA is constructed for the purposes of a medical treatment, and one or more polypeptides are intended to be the product of the translation of the said artificial mRNA, then the use of a 'UAA' STOP codon is deliberate and a necessary part of the construction of the said mRNA. The 'UAA' STOP codon would be required to be present between two segments of nucleotide sequencing, each coding for the same polypeptide or a different polypeptide. See Figure 27.

Demonstrates use of the nucleotide codon 'uaa' as a joiner between two nucleotide sequences coded to produce polypeptides in a manmade messenger ribonucleic acid

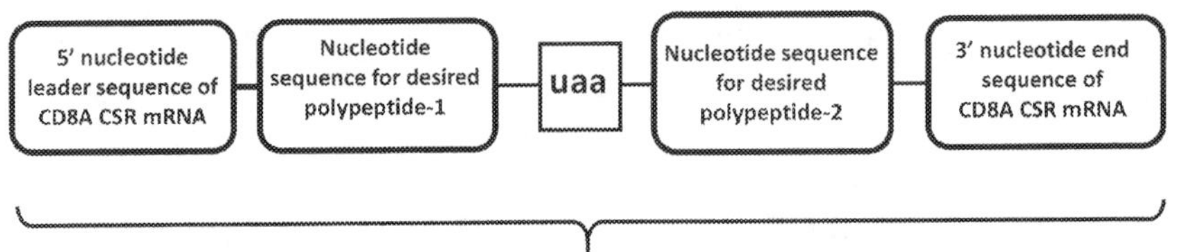

Artificial messenger ribonucleic acid coded for two polypeptide products using 'uaa' to join polypeptide-1 and polypeptide-2 nucleotide sequences

Figure 27
Construct of mRNA to code for two different polypeptides.

In the event an artificial mRNA is constructed for the purposes of a medical treatment, and one or more polypeptides are intended to be the product of the translation of the said artificial mRNA, then the use of a 'UAA' STOP codon is deliberate and a necessary part of the construction of the said mRNA. The 'UAA' STOP codon would be required to be present between two segments of nucleotide sequencing, each coding for the same polypeptide or a different polypeptide. The 'UAA' STOP codon would be required to be present between the nucleotide sequencing coding for one or more polypeptides and the 3' terminal end of the mRNA.

The coronavirus's 'S' protein is highly conserved. The Wuhan-Hu-1 coronavirus 'S' (spike) protein (probe) and the 'S' (spike) protein (probe) for the Moscow coronavirus vary in one amino acid. The Wuhan-Hu-1 version coronavirus 'S' (spike) protein (probe) has an aspartic acid 'D' at amino acid position 614, where the 'S' (spike) protein (probe) for the Moscow coronavirus version has a glycine 'G' at amino acid position 614. This variation could be enough to make ineffective a vaccine designed against the Wuhan-Hu-1 coronavirus 'S' probe. In order to account for the variation between the Wuhan-Hu-1 coronavirus 'S' probe and the Moscow version of the coronavirus 'S' probe, an mRNA is constructed which would mount copies of both 'S' probes on the surface of the human cell which has translated the mRNA.

As an example, an RNA vaccine intended to protect a patient from coronavirus by generating through translation of the mRNA, the 'S' protein probe from the Wuhan-Hu-1 (MN908947) strain of the virus and the 'S' protein probe from the Moscow (MT510643.1) strain of the virus would appear as the illustration in Figure 28.[10,25] The 'uaa' codon would be position between the nucleotide sequence for the Wuhan-Hu-1 'S' polypeptide and the Moscow 'S' polypeptide. The 'uaa' codon would also be positioned between the Moscow version of the 'S' polypeptide nucleotide coding sequence and the 3' terminal end of the mRNA.

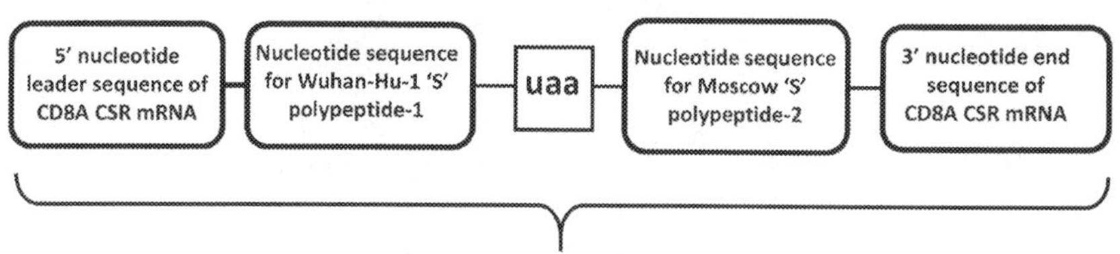

Figure 28
Illustration of a mRNA to code for both the Wuhan-1 and Moscow 'S' proteins.

The 'S' structural protein information taken from the gene for the Wuhan-Hu-1 (MN908947) coronavirus as described on the NCBI website.

Would like to celebrate and honor the hard work and dedication of the many researchers whose efforts made accessing this information on the NCBI website possible, so that the study and understanding of human genetics could advance toward a cure for a variety of challenging diseases.

NCBI Website: https://www.ncbi.nlm.nih.gov/nuccore/MN908947

```
LOCUS           MN908947 29903 bp ss-RNA linear VRL 11-FEB-2020
DEFINITION      Severe acute respiratory syndrome coronavirus 2 isolate
                Wuhan-Hu-1, complete genome.
ACCESSION       MN908947
VERSION         MN908947.3
KEYWORDS        .
SOURCE          Severe acute respiratory syndrome coronavirus 2
                (SARS-CoV-2)
ORGANISM        Severe acute respiratory syndrome coronavirus 2
                Viruses; Riboviria; Nidovirales; Cornidovirineae;
                Coronaviridae; Orthocoronavirinae; Betacoronavirus;
                Sarbecovirus.
REFERENCE       1 (bases 1 to 29903)
AUTHORS         Wu, F., Zhao, S., Yu, B., Chen, Y.M., Wang, W., Song,
                Z.G., Hu, Y., Tao, Z.W., Tian, J.H., Pei, Y.Y., Yuan,
                M.L., Zhang, Y.L., Dai, F.H., Liu, Y., Wang, Q.M., Zheng,
                J.J., Xu, L., Holmes, E.C. and Zhang, Y.Z.
TITLE           A new coronavirus associated with human respiratory
                disease in China
JOURNAL         Nature (2020) In press
PUBMED          32015508
REMARK          Publication Status: Available-Online prior to print
REFERENCE       2 (bases 1 to 29903)
AUTHORS         Wu, F., Zhao, S., Yu, B., Chen, Y.-M., Wang, W., Hu, Y.,
                Song, Z.-G., Tao, Z.-W., Tian, J.-H., Pei, Y.-Y., Yuan,
                M.L., Zhang, Y.-L., Dai, F.-H., Liu, Y., Wang, Q.-M.,
                Zheng, J.-J., Xu, L., Holmes, E.C. and Zhang, Y.-Z.
TITLE           Direct Submission
JOURNAL         Submitted (05-JAN-2020) Shanghai Public Health Clinical
                Center & School of Public Health, Fudan University,
                Shanghai, China
COMMENT         On Jan 17, 2020 this sequence version replaced MN908947.2.

                ##Assembly-Data-START##
                Assembly Method       :: Megahit v. V1.1.3
                Sequencing Technology :: Illumina
                ##Assembly-Data-END##


FEATURES                 Location/Qualifiers
     source              1..29903
                         /organism="Severe acute respiratory syndrome
                         coronavirus 2"
```

```
                    /mol _type="genomic RNA"
                    /isolate="Wuhan-Hu-1"
                    /host="Homo sapiens"
                    /db _xref="taxon:2697049"
                    /country="China"
                    /collection _date="Dec-2019"

     gene           21563..25384
                    /gene="S"
     CDS            21563..25384
                    /gene="S"
                    /note="structural protein"
                    /codon _start=1
                    /product="surface glycoprotein"
                    /protein _id="QHD43416.1"
/translation="MFVFLVLLPLVSSQCVNLTTRTQLPPAYTNSFTRGVYYPDKVFR
SSVLHSTQDLFLPFFSNVTWFHAIHVSGTNGTKRFDNPVLPFNDGVYFASTEKSNIIR
GWIFGTTLDSKTQSLLIVNNATNVVIKVCEFQFCNDPFLGVYYHKNNKSWMESEFRVY
SSANNCTFEYVSQPFLMDLEGKQGNFKNLREFVFKNIDGYFKIYSKHTPINLVRDLPQ
GFSALEPLVDLPIGINITRFQTLLALHRSYLTPGDSSSGWTAGAAAYYVGYLQPRTFL
LKYNENGTITDAVDCALDPLSETKCTLKSFTVEKGIYQTSNFRVQPTESIVRFPNITN
LCPFGEVFNATRFASVYAWNRKRISNCVADYSVLYNSASFSTFKCYGVSPTKLNDLCF
TNVYADSFVIRGDEVRQIAPGQTGKIADYNYKLPDDFTGCVIAWNSNNLDSKVGGNYN
YLYRLFRKSNLKPFERDISTEIYQAGSTPCNGVEGFNCYFPLQSYGFQPTNGVGYQPY
RVVVLSFELLHAPATVCGPKKSTNLVKNKCVNFNFNGLTGTGVLTESNKKFLPFQQFG
RDIADTTDAVRDPQTLEILDITPCSFGGVSVITPGTNTSNQVAVLYQDVNCTEVPVAI
HADQLTPTWRVYSTGSNVFQTRAGCLIGAEHVNNSYECDIPIGAGICASYQTQTNSPR
RARSVASQSIIAYTMSLGAENSVAYSNNSIAIPTNFTISVTTEILPVSMTKTSVDCTM
YICGDSTECSNLLLQYGSFCTQLNRALTGIAVEQDKNTQEVFAQVKQIYKTPPIKDFG
GFNFSQILPDPSKPSKRSFIEDLLFNKVTLADAGFIKQYGDCLGDIAARDLICAQKFN
GLTVLPPLLTDEMIAQYTSALLAGTITSGWTFGAGAALQIPFAMQMAYRFNGIGVTQN
VLYENQKLIANQFNSAIGKIQDSLSSTASALGKLQDVVNQNAQALNTLVKQLSSNFGA
ISSVLNDILSRLDKVEAEVQIDRLITGRLQSLQTYVTQQLIRAAEIRASANLAATKMS
ECVLGQSKRVDFCGKGYHLMSFPQSAPHGVVFLHVTYVPAQEKNFTTAPAICHDGKAH
FPREGVFVSNGTHWFVTQRNFYEPQIITTDNTFVSGNCDVVIGIVNNTVYDPLQPELD
SFKEELDKYFKNHTSPDVDLGDISGINASVVNIQKEIDRLNEVAKNLNESLIDLQELG
KYEQYIKWPWYIWLGFIAGLIAIVMVTIMLCCMTSCCSCLKGCCSCGSCCKFDEDDSE
PVLKGVKLHYT"
```

Note: The letters which are shown to be struck through are not included in the final mRNA product.

21541 ~~cttgttaaca actaaacgaa ca~~atgtttgt ttttcttgtt ttattgccac tagtctctag
21601 tcagtgtgtt aatcttacaa ccagaactca attacccct gcatacacta attctttcac
21661 acgtggtgtt tattaccctg acaaagtttt cagatcctca gttttacatt caactcagga
21721 cttgttctta cctttctttt ccaatgttac ttggttccat gctatacatg tctctgggac
21781 caatggtact aagaggtttg ataaccctgt cctaccattt aatgatggtg tttattttgc
21841 ttccactgag aagtctaaca taataagagg ctggattttt ggtactactt tagattcgaa
21901 gacccagtcc ctacttattg ttaataacgc tactaatgtt gttattaaag tctgtgaatt
21961 tcaattttgt aatgatccat ttttgggtgt ttattaccac aaaaacaaca aaagttggat
22021 ggaaagtgag ttcagagttt attctagtgc gaataattgc acttttgaat atgtctctca
22081 gcctttcctt atggaccttg aaggaaaaca gggtaatttc aaaaatctta gggaatttgt
22141 gtttaagaat attgatggtt attttaaaat atattctaag cacacgccta ttaatttagt
22201 gcgtgatctc cctcagggtt tttcggcttt agaaccattg gtagatttgc caataggtat
22261 taacatcact aggtttcaaa ctttacttgc tttacataga agttatttga ctcctggtga

22321 ttcttcttca ggttggacag ctggtgctgc agcttattat gtgggttatc ttcaacctag
22381 gacttttcta ttaaaatata atgaaaatgg aaccattaca gatgctgtag actgtgcact
22441 tgaccctctc tcagaaacaa agtgtacgtt gaaatccttc actgtagaaa aaggaatcta
22501 tcaaacttct aactttagag tccaaccaac agaatctatt gttagatttc ctaatattac
22561 aaacttgtgc ccttttggtg aagtttttaa cgccaccaga tttgcatctg tttatgcttg
22621 gaacaggaag agaatcagca actgtgttgc tgattattct gtcctatata attccgcatc
22681 attttccact tttaagtgtt atggagtgtc tcctactaaa ttaaatgatc tctgctttac
22741 taatgtctat gcagattcat ttgtaattag aggtgatgaa gtcagacaaa tcgctccagg
22801 gcaaactgga aagattgctg attataatta taaattacca gatgatttta caggctgcgt
22861 tatagcttgg aattctaaca atcttgattc taaggttggt ggtaattata attacctgta
22921 tagattgttt aggaagtcta atctcaaacc ttttgagaga gatatttcaa ctgaaatcta
22981 tcaggccggt agcacacctt gtaatggtgt tgaaggtttt aattgttact ttcctttaca
23041 atcatatggt ttccaaccca ctaatggtgt tggttaccaa ccatacagag tagtagtact
23101 ttcttttgaa cttctacatg caccagcaac tgtttgtgga cctaaaaagt ctactaattt
23161 ggttaaaaac aaatgtgtca atttcaactt caatggttta acaggcacag gtgttcttac
23221 tgagtctaac aaaaagtttc tgcctttcca acaatttggc agagacattg ctgacactac
23281 tgatgctgtc cgtgatccac agacacttga gattcttgac attacaccat gttcttttgg
23341 tggtgtcagt gttataacac caggaacaaa tacttctaac caggttgctg ttctttatca
23401 ggatgttaac tgcacagaag tccctgttgc tattcatgca gatcaactta ctcctacttg
23461 gcgtgtttat tctacaggtt ctaatgtttt tcaaacacgt gcaggctgtt taataggggc
23521 tgaacatgtc aacaactcat atgagtgtga catacccatt ggtgcaggta tatgcgctag
23581 ttatcagact cagactaatt ctcctcggcg ggcacgtagt gtagctagtc aatccatcat
23641 tgcctacact atgtcacttg gtgcagaaaa ttcagttgct tactctaata actctattgc
23701 catacccaca aattttacta ttagtgttac cacagaaatt ctaccagtgt ctatgaccaa
23761 gacatcagta gattgtacaa tgtacatttg tggtgattca actgaatgca gcaatctttt
23821 gttgcaatat ggcagttttt gtacacaatt aaaccgtgct ttaactggaa tagctgttga
23881 acaagacaaa aacacccaag aagtttttgc acaagtcaaa caaatttaca aaacaccacc
23941 aattaaagat tttggtggtt ttaatttttc acaaatatta ccagatccat caaaaccaag
24001 caagaggtca tttattgaag atctactttt caacaaagtg acacttgcag atgctggctt
24061 catcaaacaa tatggtgatt gccttggtga tattgctgct agagacctca tttgtgcaca
24121 aaagtttaac ggccttactg ttttgccacc tttgctcaca gatgaaatga ttgctcaata
24181 cacttctgca ctgttagcgg gtacaatcac ttctggttgg acctttggtg caggtgctgc
24241 attacaaata ccatttgcta tgcaaatggc ttataggttt aatggtattg gagttacaca
24301 gaatgttctc tatgagaacc aaaaattgat tgccaaccaa tttaatagtg ctattggcaa
24361 aattcaagac tcactttctt ccacagcaag tgcacttgga aaacttcaag atgtggtcaa
24421 ccaaaatgca caagctttaa acacgcttgt taaacaactt agctccaatt ttggtgcaat
24481 ttcaagtgtt ttaaatgata tcctttcacg tcttgacaaa gttgaggctg aagtgcaaat
24541 tgataggttg atcacaggca gacttcaaag tttgcagaca tatgtgactc aacaattaat
24601 tagagctgca gaaatcagag cttctgctaa tcttgctgct actaaaatgt cagagtgtgt
24661 acttggacaa tcaaaaagag ttgattttg tggaaagggc tatcatctta tgtccttccc
24721 tcagtcagca cctcatggtg tagtcttctt gcatgtgact tatgtccctg cacaagaaaa
24781 gaacttcaca actgctcctg ccatttgtca tgatggaaaa gcacactttc ctcgtgaagg
24841 tgtctttgtt tcaaatggca cacactggtt tgtaacacaa aggaattttt atgaaccaca
24901 aatcattact acagacaaca catttgtgtc tggtaactgt gatgttgtaa taggaattgt
24961 caacaacaca gtttatgatc ctttgcaacc tgaattagac tcattcaagg aggagttaga
25021 taaatatttt aagaatcata catcaccaga tgttgattta ggtgacatct ctggcattaa
25081 tgcttcagtt gtaaacattc aaaaagaaat tgaccgcctc aatgaggttg ccaagaattt
25141 aaatgaatct ctcatcgatc tccaagaact tggaaagtat gagcagtata taaaatggcc
25201 atggtacatt tggctaggtt ttatagctgg cttgattgcc atagtaatgg tgacaattat
25261 gctttgctgt atgaccagtt gctgtagttg tctcaagggc tgttgttctt gtggatcctg
25321 ctgcaaattt gatgaagacg actctgagcc agtgctcaaa ggagtcaaat tacattacac
25381 ataa~~acgaac ttatggattt gtttatgaga atcttcacaa ttggaactgt aactttgaag~~

The 'S' structural protein information taken from the gene for the Moscow (MT510643.1) coronavirus as described on the NCBI website.

NCBI Website: https://www.ncbi.nlm.nih.gov/nuccore/MT510643.1.

Severe acute respiratory syndrome coronavirus 2 isolate SARS-CoV-2/human/RUS/SCPM-O-cDNA-01/2020 ORF1ab polyprotein (ORF1ab), ORF1a polyprotein (ORF1ab), surface glycoprotein (S), ORF3a protein (ORF3a), envelope protein (E), membrane glycoprotein (M), ORF6 pro...

GenBank: MT510643.1
FASTA Graphics

Go to:

```
LOCUS           MT510643 29544 bp RNA linear VRL 26-MAY-2020
DEFINITION      Severe acute respiratory syndrome coronavirus 2
                isolate SARS-CoV-2/human/RUS/SCPM-O-cDNA-01/2020
                ORF1ab polyprotein (ORF1ab), ORF1a polyprotein
                (ORF1ab), surface glycoprotein (S), ORF3a
                protein (ORF3a), envelope protein (E), membrane
                glycoprotein (M), ORF6 protein (ORF6), ORF7a protein
                (ORF7a), ORF7b (ORF7b), ORF8 protein (ORF8), and
                nucleocapsid phosphoprotein (N) genes, complete
                cds; and ORF10 protein (ORF10) gene, partial cds.
ACCESSION       MT510643
VERSION         MT510643.1
DBLINK          BioSample: SAMN15009583
KEYWORDS        .
SOURCE          Severe acute respiratory syndrome coronavirus 2
                (SARS-CoV-2)
  ORGANISM      Severe acute respiratory syndrome coronavirus 2
                Viruses; Riboviria; Orthornavirae; Pisuviricota;
                Pisoniviricetes; Nidovirales; Cornidovirineae;
                Coronaviridae; Orthocoronavirinae; Betacoronavirus;
                Sarbecovirus.

REFERENCE       1 (bases 1 to 29544)
AUTHORS         Dyatlov, I., Shemyakin, I., Khramov, M., Bogun, A.,
                Kislichkina, A., Frolov, V., Shishkina, L., Sizova, A.,
                Chekan, L., Blagodatskikh, S., Podkopaev, Y., Kosilova,
                I., Koroleva-Ushakova, A., Tyurin, E., Galkina,
                E., Slukina, N., Shaikhutdinova, R., Kalmantayev,
                T., Kalmantayeva, O., Fursova, N., Silkina, M.,
                Gorbatov, A., Titareva, G., Firstova, V., Makarova,
                M., Gapelchenkova, T., Solovieva, A., Slukin, P.,
                Dentovskaya, S., Detushev, K., Vagayskaya, A., Kartsev,
                N., Detusheva, E., Zeninskaya, N., Ivanov, S., Kartseva,
                A., Platonov, M., Hlyntseva, A., Khomyakov, A.,
                Chernysh, S., Krasilnikova, E., Ryabko, A., Solomentsev,
                V., Teymurazov, M., Bakhteeva, I., Borzilov, A.,
                Skryabin, Y., Kanashenko, M., Abaimova, A., Kolchanova,
                A., Novikova, T., Goncharova, J., Timofeev, V., Kuzina,
                E., Fursov, M., Zhumakaev, R., Romanenko, I., Marin, M.,
                Denisenko, E., Trunyakova, A. and Kuzin, V.
```

```
TITLE          Direct Submission
JOURNAL        Submitted (25-MAY-2020) Science Department, SRCAMB,
               Building 1, Obolensk, Moscow region 142279, Russia
COMMENT        ##Assembly-Data-START##
               Assembly Method       :: Unicycler v. v0.4.7
               Sequencing Technology :: BGISEQ-500
               ##Assembly-Data-END##
FEATURES             Location/Qualifiers
     source          1..29544
                     /organism="Severe acute respiratory syndrome
                     coronavirus 2"
                     /mol _type="genomic RNA"
                     /isolate="SARS-CoV-2/human/RUS/
                     SCPM-O-cDNA-01/2020"
                     /host="Homo sapiens"
                     /db _xref="taxon:2697049"
                     /country="Russia: Moscow region"
                     /collection _date="2020-03-20"


     CDS             21497..25318
                     /gene="S"
                     /codon _start=1
                     /product="surface glycoprotein"
                     /protein _id="QJY78005.1"

/translation="MFVFLVLLPLVSSQCVNLTTRTQLPPAYTNSFTRGVYYPDKVFR
SSVLHSTQDLFLPFFSNVTWFHAIHVSGTNGTKRFDNPVLPFNDGVYFASTEKSNIIR
GWIFGTTLDSKTQSLLIVNNATNVVIKVCEFQFCNDPFLGVYYHKNNKSWMESEFRVY
SSANNCTFEYVSQPFLMDLEGKQGNFKNLREFVFKNIDGYFKIYSKHTPINLVRDLPQ
GFSALEPLVDLPIGINITRFQTLLALHRSYLTPGDSSSGWTAGAAAYYVGYLQPRTFL
LKYNENGTITDAVDCALDPLSETKCTLKSFTVEKGIYQTSNFRVQPTESIVRFPNITN
LCPFGEVFNATRFASVYAWNRKRISNCVADYSVLYNSASFSTFKCYGVSPTKLNDLCF
TNVYADSFVIRGDEVRQIAPGQTGKIADYNYKLPDDFTGCVIAWNSNNLDSKVGGNYN
YLYRLFRKSNLKPFERDISTEIYQAGSTPCNGVEGFNCYFPLQSYGFQPTNGVGYQPY
RVVVLSFELLHAPATVCGPKKSTNLVKNKCVNFNFNGLTGTGVLTESNKKFLPFQQFG
RDIADTTDAVRDPQTLEILDITPCSFGGVSVITPGTNTSNQVAVLYQGVNCTEVPVAI
HADQLTPTWRVYSTGSNVFQTRAGCLIGAEHVNNSYECDIPIGAGICASYQTQTNSPR
RARSVASQSIIAYTMSLGAENSVAYSNNSIAIPTNFTISVTTEILPVSMTKTSVDCTM
YICGDSTECSNLLLQYGSFCTQLNRALTGIAVEQDKNTQEVFAQVKQIYKTPPIKDFG
GFNFSQILPDPSKPSKRSFIEDLLFNKVTLADAGFIKQYGDCLGDIAARDLICAQKFN
GLTVLPPLLTDEMIAQYTSALLAGTITSGWTFGAGAALQIPFAMQMAYRFNGIGVTQN
VLYENQKLIANQFNSAIGKIQDSLSSTASALGKLQDVVNQNAQALNTLVKQLSSNFGA
ISSVLNDILSRLDKVEAEVQIDRLITGRLQSLQTYVTQQLIRAAEIRASANLAATKMS
ECVLGQSKRVDFCGKGYHLMSFPQSAPHGVVFLHVTYVPAQEKNFTTAPAICHDGKAH
FPREGVFVSNGTHWFVTQRNFYEPQIITTDNTFVSGNCDVVIGIVNNTVYDPLQPELD
SFKEELDKYFKNHTSPDVDLGDISGINASVVNIQKEIDRLNEVAKNLNESLIDLQELG
KYEQYIKWPWYIWLGFIAGLIAIVMVTIMLCCMTSCCSCLKGCCSCGSCCKFDEDDSE
PVLKGVKLHYT"
```

Note: The letters which are shown to be struck through are not included in the final mRNA product.

21481 ~~aacaactaaa~~ ~~cgaaca~~atgt ttgtttttct tgttttattg ccactagtct ctagtcagtg
21541 tgttaatctt acaaccagaa ctcaattacc ccctgcatac actaattctt tcacacgtgg
21601 tgtttattac cctgacaaag ttttcagatc ctcagtttta cattcaactc aggacttgtt

21661 cttaccttc ttttccaatg ttacttggtt ccatgctata catgtctctg ggaccaatgg
21721 tactaagagg tttgataacc ctgtcctacc atttaatgat ggtgtttatt ttgcttccac
21781 tgagaagtct aacataataa gaggctggat ttttggtact actttagatt cgaagaccca
21841 gtccctactt attgttaata acgctactaa tgttgttatt aaagtctgtg aatttcaatt
21901 ttgtaatgat ccatttttgg gtgtttatta ccacaaaaac aacaaaagtt ggatggaaag
21961 tgagttcaga gtttattcta gtgcgaataa ttgcactttt gaatatgtct ctcagccttt
22021 tcttatggac cttgaaggaa aacagggtaa tttcaaaaat cttagggaat ttgtgtttaa
22081 gaatattgat ggttatttta aaatatattc taagcacacg cctattaatt tagtgcgtga
22141 tctccctcag ggtttttcgg ctttagaacc attggtagat ttgccaatag gtattaacat
22201 cactaggttt caaactttac ttgctttaca tagaagttat ttgactcctg gtgattcttc
22261 ttcaggttgg acagctggtg ctgcagctta ttatgtgggt tatcttcaac ctaggacttt
22321 tctattaaaa tataatgaaa atggaaccat tacagatgct gtagactgtg cacttgaccc
22381 tctctcagaa acaaagtgta cgttgaaatc cttcactgta gaaaaaggaa tctatcaaac
22441 ttctaacttt agagtccaac caacagaatc tattgttaga tttcctaata ttacaaactt
22501 gtgccctttt ggtgaagttt ttaacgccac cagatttgca tctgtttatg cttggaacag
22561 gaagagaatc agcaactgtg ttgctgatta ttctgtccta tataattccg catcattttc
22621 cacttttaag tgttatggag tgtctcctac taaattaaat gatctctgct ttactaatgt
22681 ctatgcagat tcatttgtaa ttagaggtga tgaagtcaga caaatcgctc cagggcaaac
22741 tggaaagatt gctgattata attataaatt accagatgat tttacaggct gcgttatagc
22801 ttggaattct aacaatcttg attctaaggt tggtggtaat tataattacc tgtatagatt
22861 gtttaggaag tctaatctca aaccttttga gagagatatt tcaactgaaa tctatcaggc
22921 cggtagcaca ccttgtaatg gtgttgaagg ttttaattgt tactttcctt tacaatcata
22981 tggtttccaa cccactaatg gtgttggtta ccaaccatac agagtagtag tactttcttt
23041 tgaacttcta catgcaccag caactgtttg tggacctaaa aagtctacta atttggttaa
23101 aaacaaatgt gtcaatttca acttcaatgg tttaacaggc acaggtgttc ttactgagtc
23161 taacaaaaag tttctgcctt tccaacaatt tggcagagac attgctgaca ctactgatgc
23221 tgtccgtgat ccacagacac ttgagattct tgacattaca ccatgttctt ttggtggtgt
23281 cagtgttata acaccaggaa caaatacttc taaccaggtt gctgttcttt atcagggtgt
23341 taactgcaca gaagtccctg ttgctattca tgcagatcaa cttactccta cttggcgtgt
23401 ttattctaca ggttctaatg tttttcaaac acgtgcaggc tgtttaatag ggctgaaca
23461 tgtcaacaac tcatatgagt gtgacatacc cattggtgca ggtatatgcg ctagttatca
23521 gactcagact aattctcctc ggcgggcacg tagtgtagct agtcaatcca tcattgccta
23581 cactatgtca cttggtgcag aaaattcagt tgcttactct aataactcta ttgccatacc
23641 cacaaatttt actattagtg ttaccacaga aattctacca gtgtctatga ccaagacatc
23701 agtagattgt acaatgtaca tttgtggtga ttcaactgaa tgcagcaatc ttttgttgca
23761 atatggcagt ttttgtacac aattaaaccg tgctttaact ggaatagctg ttgaacaaga
23821 caaaaacacc caagaagttt ttgcacaagt caaacaaatt tacaaaacac caccaattaa
23881 agattttggt ggttttaatt tttcacaaat attaccagat ccatcaaaac caagcaagag
23941 gtcatttatt gaagatctac ttttcaacaa agtgacactt gcagatgctg gcttcatcaa
24001 acaatatggt gattgccttg gtgatattgc tgctagagac ctcatttgtg cacaaaagtt
24061 taacggcctt actgttttgc cacctttgct cacagatgaa atgattgctc aatacacttc
24121 tgcactgtta gcgggtacaa tcacttctgg ttggaccttt ggtgcaggtg ctgcattaca
24181 aataccattt gctatgcaaa tggcttatag gtttaatggt attggagtta cacagaatgt
24241 tctctatgag aaccaaaaat tgattgccaa ccaatttaat agtgctattg gcaaaattca
24301 agactcactt tcttccacag caagtgcact tggaaaactt caagatgtgg tcaaccaaaa
24361 tgcacaagct ttaaacacgc ttgttaaaca acttagctcc aattttggtg caatttcaag
24421 tgttttaaat gatatccttt cacgtcttga caaagttgag gctgaagtgc aaattgatag
24481 gttgatcaca ggcagacttc aaagtttgca gacatatgtg actcaacaat taattagagc
24541 tgcagaaatc agagcttctg ctaatcttgc tgctactaaa atgtcagagt gtgtacttgg
24601 acaatcaaaa agagttgatt tttgtggaaa gggctatcat cttatgtcct tccctcagtc
24661 agcacctcat ggtgtagtct tcttgcatgt gacttatgtc cctgcacaag aaaagaactt
24721 cacaactgct cctgccattt gtcatgatgg aaaagcacac tttcctcgtg aaggtgtctt
24781 tgtttcaaat ggcacacact ggtttgtaac acaaaggaat tttatgaac cacaaatcat
24841 tactacagac aacacatttg tgtctggtaa ctgtgatgtt gtaataggaa ttgtcaacaa
24901 cacagtttat gatcctttgc aacctgaatt agactcattc aaggaggagt tagataaata
24961 ttttaagaat catacatcac cagatgttga tttaggtgac atctctggca ttaatgcttc
25021 agttgtaaac attcaaaaag aaattgaccg cctcaatgag gttgccaaga atttaaatga
25081 atctctcatc gatctccaag aacttggaaa gtatgagcag tatataaaat ggccatggta
25141 catttggcta ggttttatag ctggcttgat tgccatagta atggtgacaa ttatgctttg
25201 ctgtatgacc agttgctgta gttgtctcaa gggctgttgt tcttgtggat cctgctgcaa
25261 atttgatgaa gacgactctg agccagtgct caaaggagtc aaattacatt acaca**taa**

The CD8A cell surface receptor genome genetic information as described on the NCBI website.[23] Struck through sections of nucleotides are presented for clarity of position of nucleotides, but are not included in the final version of the mRNA.

In this text, the terms cell surface receptor (CSR) and cell surface glycoprotein have the same meaning.

CD8A Cell Surface Receptor Genome

```
LOCUS          NC_000002 23792 bp DNA linear CON 02-MAR-2020
DEFINITION     Homo sapiens chromosome 2, GRCh38.p13 Primary Assembly.
ACCESSION      NC_000002 REGION: complement(86784605..86808396)
VERSION        NC_000002.12
DBLINK         BioProject: PRJNA168
               Assembly: GCF_000001405.39
KEYWORDS       RefSeq.
SOURCE         Homo sapiens (human)
  ORGANISM     Homo sapiens
               Eukaryota; Metazoa; Chordata; Craniata; Vertebrata;
               Euteleostomi; Mammalia; Eutheria; Euarchontoglires;
               Primates; Haplorrhini; Catarrhini; Hominidae; Homo.
REFERENCE      1 (bases 1 to 23792)
AUTHORS        Hillier, L.W., Graves, T.A., Fulton, R.S., Fulton, L.A.,
               Pepin, K.H., Minx, P., Wagner-McPherson, C., Layman, D.,
               Wylie, K., Sekhon, M., Becker, M.C., Fewell, G.A., Delehaunty,
               K.D., Miner, T.L., Nash, W.E., Kremitzki, C., Oddy, L.,
               Du, H., Sun, H., Bradshaw-Cordum, H., Ali, J., Carter, J.,
               Cordes, M., Harris, A., Isak, A., van Brunt, A., Nguyen,
               C., Du, F., Courtney, L., Kalicki, J., Ozersky, P., Abbott,
               S., Armstrong, J., Belter, E.A., Caruso, L., Cedroni, M.,
               Cotton, M., Davidson, T., Desai, A., Elliott, G., Erb, T.,
               Fronick, C., Gaige, T., Haakenson, W., Haglund, K., Holmes,
               A., Harkins, R., Kim, K., Kruchowski, S.S., Strong, C.M.,
               Grewal, N., Goyea, E., Hou, S., Levy, A., Martinka, S., Mead,
               K., McLellan, M.D., Meyer, R., Randall-Maher, J., Tomlinson,
               C., Dauphin-Kohlberg, S., Kozlowicz-Reilly, A., Shah, N.,
               Swearengen-Shahid, S., Snider, J., Strong, J.T., Thompson, J.,
               Yoakum, M., Leonard, S., Pearman, C., Trani, L., Radionenko,
               M., Waligorski, J.E., Wang, C., Rock, S.M., Tin-Wollam, A.M.,
               Maupin, R., Latreille, P., Wendl, M.C., Yang, S.P., Pohl, C.,
               Wallis, J.W., Spieth, J., Bieri, T.A., Berkowicz, N., Nelson,
               J.O., Osborne, J., Ding, L., Meyer, R., Sabo, A., Shotland,
               Y., Sinha, P., Wohldmann, P.E., Cook, L.L., Hickenbotham,
               M.T., Eldred, J., Williams, D., Jones, T.A., She, X.,
               Ciccarelli, F.D., Izaurralde, E., Taylor, J., Schmutz, J.,
               Myers, R.M., Cox, D.R., Huang, X., McPherson, J.D., Mardis,
               E.R., Clifton, S.W., Warren, W.C., Chinwalla, A.T., Eddy, S.R.,
               Marra, M.A., Ovcharenko, I., Furey, T.S., Miller, W., Eichler,
               E.E., Bork, P., Suyama, M., Torrents, D., Waterston, R.H. and
               Wilson, R.K.
```

TITLE	Generation and annotation of the DNA sequences of human chromosomes 2 and 4
JOURNAL	Nature 434 (7034), 724-731 (2005)
PUBMED	15815621
REFERENCE	2 (bases 1 to 23792)
CONSRTM	International Human Genome Sequencing Consortium
TITLE	Finishing the euchromatic sequence of the human genome
JOURNAL	Nature 431 (7011), 931-945 (2004)
PUBMED	15496913
REFERENCE	3 (bases 1 to 23792)
AUTHORS	Lander, E.S., Linton, L.M., Birren, B., Nusbaum, C., Zody, M.C., Baldwin, J., Devon, K., Dewar, K., Doyle, M., FitzHugh, W., Funke, R., Gage, D., Harris, K., Heaford, A., Howland, J., Kann, L., Lehoczky, J., LeVine, R., McEwan, P., McKernan, K., Meldrim, J., Mesirov, J.P., Miranda, C., Morris, W., Naylor, J., Raymond, C., Rosetti, M., Santos, R., Sheridan, A., Sougnez, C., Stange-Thomann, N., Stojanovic, N., Subramanian, A., Wyman, D., Rogers, J., Sulston, J., Ainscough, R., Beck, S., Bentley, D., Burton, J., Clee, C., Carter, N., Coulson, A., Deadman, R., Deloukas, P., Dunham, A., Dunham, I., Durbin, R., French, L., Grafham, D., Gregory, S., Hubbard, T., Humphray, S., Hunt, A., Jones, M., Lloyd, C., McMurray, A., Matthews, L., Mercer, S., Milne, S., Mullikin, J.C., Mungall, A., Plumb, R., Ross, M., Shownkeen, R., Sims, S., Waterston, R.H., Wilson, R.K., Hillier, L.W., McPherson, J.D., Marra, M.A., Mardis, E.R., Fulton, L.A., Chinwalla, A.T., Pepin, K.H., Gish, W.R., Chissoe, S.L., Wendl, M.C., Delehaunty, K.D., Miner, T.L., Delehaunty, A., Kramer, J.B., Cook, L.L., Fulton, R.S., Johnson, D.L., Minx, P.J., Clifton, S.W., Hawkins, T., Branscomb, E., Predki, P., Richardson, P., Wenning, S., Slezak, T., Doggett, N., Cheng, J.F., Olsen, A., Lucas, S., Elkin, C., Uberbacher, E., Frazier, M., Gibbs, R.A., Muzny, D.M., Scherer, S.E., Bouck, J.B., Sodergren, E.J., Worley, K.C., Rives, C.M., Gorrell, J.H., Metzker, M.L., Naylor, S.L., Kucherlapati, R.S., Nelson, D.L., Weinstock, G.M., Sakaki, Y., Fujiyama, A., Hattori, M., Yada, T., Toyoda, A., Itoh, T., Kawagoe, C., Watanabe, H., Totoki, Y., Taylor, T., Weissenbach, J., Heilig, R., Saurin, W., Artiguenave, F., Brottier, P., Bruls, T., Pelletier, E., Robert, C., Wincker, P., Smith, D.R., Doucette-Stamm, L., Rubenfield, M., Weinstock, K., Lee, H.M., Dubois, J., Rosenthal, A., Platzer, M., Nyakatura, G., Taudien, S., Rump, A., Yang, H., Yu, J., Wang, J., Huang, G., Gu, J., Hood, L., Rowen, L., Madan, A., Qin, S., Davis, R.W., Federspiel, N.A., Abola, A.P., Proctor, M.J., Myers, R.M., Schmutz, J., Dickson, M., Grimwood, J., Cox, D.R., Olson, M.V., Kaul, R., Raymond, C., Shimizu, N., Kawasaki, K., Minoshima, S., Evans, G.A., Athanasiou, M.,Schultz, R., Roe, B.A., Chen, F., Pan, H., Ramser, J., Lehrach, H., Reinhardt, R., McCombie, W.R., de la Bastide, M., Dedhia, N.,Blocker, H., Hornischer, K., Nordsiek, G., Agarwala, R., Aravind, L., Bailey, J.A.,

```
            Bateman, A., Batzoglou, S., Birney, E., Bork, P., Brown,
            D.G., Burge, C.B., Cerutti, L., Chen, H.C., Church, D.,
            Clamp, M., Copley, R.R., Doerks, T., Eddy, S.R., Eichler,
            E.E., Furey, T.S., Galagan, J., Gilbert, J.G., Harmon, C.,
            Hayashizaki, Y., Haussler, D., Hermjakob, H., Hokamp, K.,
            Jang, W., Johnson, L.S., Jones, T.A., Kasif, S., Kaspryzk,
            A., Kennedy, S., Kent, W.J., Kitts, P., Koonin, E.V.,
            Korf, I., Kulp, D., Lancet, D., Lowe, T.M., McLysaght,
            A., Mikkelsen, T., Moran, J.V., Mulder, N., Pollara, V.J.,
            Ponting, C.P., Schuler, G., Schultz, J., Slater, G., Smit,
            A.F., Stupka, E., Szustakowski, J., Thierry-Mieg, D.,
            Thierry-Mieg, J., Wagner, L., Wallis, J., Wheeler, R.,
            Williams, A., Wolf, Y.I., Wolfe, K.H., Yang, S.P., Yeh,
            R.F., Collins, F., Guyer, M.S., Peterson, J., Felsenfeld,
            A., Wetterstrand, K.A., Patrinos, A., Morgan, M.J., de
            Jong, P., Catanese, J.J., Osoegawa, K., Shizuya, H., Choi,
            S. and Chen, Y.J.
CONSRTM     International Human Genome Sequencing Consortium
TITLE       Initial sequencing and analysis of the human genome
JOURNAL     Nature 409 (6822), 860-921 (2001)
PUBMED      11237011
REMARK      Erratum:[Nature 2001 Aug 2;412(6846):565]
COMMENT     REFSEQ INFORMATION: The reference sequence is identical
            to CM000664.2.
            On Feb 3, 2014 this sequence version replaced NC_000002.11.
            Assembly Name: GRCh38.p13 Primary Assembly
            The DNA sequence is composed of genomic sequence,
            primarily finished clones that were sequenced as part of
            the Human Genome Project. PCR products and WGS shotgun
            sequence have been added where necessary to fill gaps
            or correct errors. All such additions are manually
            curated by GRC staff. For more information see: https://
            genomereference.org.

            ##Genome-Annotation-Data-START##
            Annotation Provider         :: NCBI
            Annotation Status           :: Updated annotation
            Annotation Name             :: Homo sapiens Updated
                                           Annotation Release
                                           109.20200228
            Annotation Version          :: 109.20200228
            Annotation Pipeline         :: NCBI eukaryotic genome
                                           annotation pipeline
            Annotation Software Version :: 8.3
            Annotation Method           :: Best-placed RefSeq;
                                           propagated RefSeq model
            Features Annotated          :: Gene; mRNA; CDS; ncRNA
            ##Genome-Annotation-Data-END##
FEATURES             Location/Qualifiers
     source          1..23792
                     /organism="Homo sapiens"
                     /mol_type="genomic DNA"
                     /db_xref="taxon:9606"
                     /chromosome="2"
     gene            1..23792
```

/gene="CD8A"
/gene _synonym="CD8; Leu2; p32"
/note="CD8a molecule; Derived by automated computational
analysis using gene prediction method: BestRefSeq."
/db _xref="GeneID:925"
/db _xref="HGNC:HGNC:1706"
/db _xref="MIM:186910"

mRNA

join(1..278,615..950,6740..6886,17302..17620,17716..18069, 18647..18757,18964..19074,19837..19867,22426..23792)
/gene="CD8A"
/gene _synonym="CD8; Leu2; p32"
/product="CD8a molecule, transcript variant 3"
/note="Derived by automated computational analysis using
gene prediction method: BestRefSeq."
/transcript _id="NM_001145873.1"
/db _xref="GeneID:925"
/db _xref="HGNC:HGNC:1706"
/db _xref="MIM:186910"

CD8A CSR 5' Region:

Section 1: 1..278,

Section 2: 615..950,

Section 3: 6740..6886

Section 1:
1..278

Note: The letters which are shown to be struck through are not included in the final mRNA product.

ORIGIN

1 ctctgtaaaa taaatgcgct gggccggatc ttttctgagt tctcttctcc cctacgaatt
61 ctagatccct cctctgtcct ccctgcgcca gggaccttcg ggcgaccctt ccctgtaccc
121 ccaccccacc ctctctggac cccgtttctg cctcagtacg gcgcgctgag ctctgccccc
181 tgcccaggcc ctgacccccct caggagccgc ggtttcctgg ggtaacagtg ggaaacgtgt
241 cggccgtctc cgctcaggcg cttgctgtgt acagaaag~~gt~~ ~~gaattcatgg~~ ~~gaaaggtggc~~

Section 2:
615..950

601 ~~tccgtctcct~~ ~~ttag~~gctgat tcaggcacac cggctctcgt cgccttggtg gccctcccca
661 gccctcctcc gcgcctgctc cgggtggcgc tccgctgggc tcctcgtgcg cctgtccgcg
721 accgcaccca cctcatcctg gcacccccat cgtggcatca cgtgttccct catctgtcct
781 catggctggc gtgcccctct gcggtgagac ctgcagaaca ggaattggtg ccgggtcagc
841 agccggcgat gaagccggac gaagcctgca aaccccaccc atacgccagc ttcacatagc
901 tcctatccat tgcacagcag cgtggggaag caccgttctc taccctccaa ~~gtaagaagct~~

Section 3:
6740..6886

6721 ~~tcctttttttt ttcaaaaag~~a caaaagcatg aaccaggtgc agtggctcac gtctgtaatc
6781 ccagcatttt ggaggccaag gtggatggat ggattccttg agtccaggag ttcaagacca
6841 gcctgggcaa catggtgaac ccccatctct acaaaaattt agccag~~gtat gatggtgtgc~~

CD8A CSR 3' Region:

22478-23792

22441 ~~gggagacaag cccagccttt cggcgagata cgtctaa~~ccc tgtgcaacag ccactacatt
22501 acttcaaact gagatccttc cttttgaggg agcaagtcct tccctttcat tttttccagt
22561 cttcctccct gtgtattcat tctcatgatt attattttag tgggggcggg gtgggaaaga
22621 ttacttttc tttatgtgtt tgacgggaaa caaaactagg taaaatctac agtacaccac
22681 aagggtcaca atactgttgt gcgcacatcg cggtagggcg tggaaagggg caggccagag
22741 ctacccgcag agttctcaga atcatgctga gagagctgga ggcacccatg ccatctcaac
22801 ctcttccccg cccgttttac aaagggggag gctaaagccc agagacagct tgatcaaagg
22861 cacacagcaa gtcagggttg gagcagtagc tggagggacc ttgtctccca gctcagggct
22921 ctttcctcca caccattcag gtctttcttt ccgaggcccc tgtctcaggg tgaggtgctt
22981 gagtctccaa cggcaaggga acaagtactt cttgatacct gggatactgt gcccagagcc
23041 tcgaggaggt aatgaattaa agaagagaac tgcctttggc agagttctat aatgtaaaca
23101 atatcagact ttttttttt ataatcaagc ctaaaattgt atagacctaa aataaaatga
23161 agtggtgagc ttaaccctgg aaaatgaatc cctctatctc taaagaaaat ctctgtgaaa
23221 cccctatgtg gaggcggaat tgctctccca gcccttgcat tgcagagggg cccatgaaag
23281 aggacaggct accccttac aaatagaatt tgagcatcag tgaggttaaa ctaaggccct
23341 cttgaatctc tgaatttgag atacaaacat gttcctggga tcactgatga ctttttatac
23401 tttgtaaaga caattgttgg agagcccctc acacagccct ggcctctgct caactagcag
23461 atacagggat gaggcagacc tgactctctt aaggaggctg agagcccaaa ctgctgtccc
23521 aaacatgcac ttccttgctt aaggtatggt acaagcaatg cctgcccatt ggagagaaaa
23581 aacttaagta gataaggaaa taagaaccac tcataattct tcaccttagg aataatctcc
23641 tgttaatatg gtgtacattc ttcctgatta ttttctacac atacatgtaa aatatgtctt
23701 tctttttaa atagggttgt actatgctgt tatgagtggc tttaatgaat aaacatttgt
23761 agcatcctct ttaatgggta aacagcatcc ga **aaaaaaaaaaaaa** //

Consolidating CD8A 5' region and 3' region:

CD8A CSR 5' Region:

1 ctctgtaaaa taaatgcgct gggccggatc ttttctgagt tctcttctcc cctacgaatt
61 ctagatccct cctctgtcct ccctgcgcca gggaccttcg ggcgaccctt ccctgtaccc
121 ccaccccacc ctctctggac cccgtttctg cctcagtacg gcgcgctgag ctctgccccc
181 tgcccaggcc ctgacccct caggagccgc ggtttcctgg ggtaacagtg ggaaacgtgt
241 cggccgtctc cgctcaggcg cttgctgtgt acagaaag
615 gctgat tcaggcacac cggctctcgt cgccttggtg gccctcccca
661 gccctcctcc gcgcctgctc cgggtggcgc tccgctgggc tcctcgtgcg cctgtccgcg
721 accgcaccca cctcatcctg gcacccccat cgtggcatca cgtgttccct catctgtcct
781 catggctggc gtgcccctct gcggtgagac ctgcagaaca ggaattggtg ccgggtcagc
841 agccggcgat gaagccggac gaagcctgca aaccccaccc atacgccagc ttcacatagc
901 tcctatccat tgcacagcag cgtggggaag caccgttctc taccctccaa
6740 a caaaagcatg aaccaggtgc agtggctcac gtctgtaatc
6781 ccagcatttt ggaggccaag gtggatggat ggattccttg agtccaggag ttcaagacca
6841 gcctgggcaa catggtgaac ccccatctct acaaaaattt agccag

Insert between CD8A CSR 5' leader end and 3' terminal end the polypeptide nucleotide coding sequences for Wuhan-Hu-1 'S' protein probe, the 'uaa' (taa) codon, and the nucleotide coding sequence for the Moscow 'S' protein probe. Following the nucleotide coding sequence for the Moscow 'S' protein probe is a second 'uaa' (taa) codon, prior to the nucleotide code of the 3' terminal end.

Second STOP Code codon:

```
taa
```

Native Human CD8A CSR 3' Terminal End Region:

```
22478 ccc tgtgcaacag ccactacatt
22501 acttcaaact gagatccttc cttttgaggg agcaagtcct tccctttcat tttttccagt
22561 cttcctccct gtgtattcat tctcatgatt attattttag tgggggcggg gtgggaaaga
22621 ttactttttc tttatgtgtt tgacgggaaa caaaactagg taaaatctac agtacaccac
22681 aagggtcaca atactgttgt gcgcacatcg cggtagggcg tggaaagggg caggccagag
22741 ctacccgcag agttctcaga atcatgctga gagagctgga ggcacccatg ccatctcaac
22801 ctcttccccg cccgttttac aaagggggag gctaaagccc agagacagct tgatcaaagg
22861 cacacagcaa gtcagggttg gagcagtagc tggagggacc ttgtctccca gctcagggct
22921 ctttcctcca caccattcag gtctttcttt ccgaggcccc tgtctcaggg tgaggtgctt
22981 gagtctccaa cggcaaggga acaagtactt cttgatacct gggatactgt gcccagagcc
23041 tcgaggaggt aatgaattaa agaagagaac tgcctttggc agagttctat aatgtaaaca
23101 atatcagact tttttttttt ataatcaagc ctaaaattgt atagacctaa aataaaatga
23161 agtggtgagc ttaaccctgg aaaatgaatc cctctatctc taaagaaaat ctctgtgaaa
23221 cccctatgtg gaggcggaat tgctctccca gcccttgcat tgcagagggg cccatgaaag
23281 aggacaggct acccctttac aaatagaatt tgagcatcag tgaggttaaa ctaaggccct
23341 cttgaatctc tgaatttgag atacaaacat gttcctggga tcactgatga ctttttatac
23401 tttgtaaaga caattgttgg agagcccctc acacagccct ggcctctgct caactagcag
23461 atacagggat gaggcagacc tgactctctt aaggaggctg agagcccaaa ctgctgtccc
23521 aaacatgcac ttccttgctt aaggtatggt acaagcaatg cctgcccatt ggagagaaaa
23581 aacttaagta gataaggaaa taagaaccac tcataattct tcaccttagg aataatctcc
23641 tgttaatatg gtgtacattc ttcctgatta ttttctacac atacatgtaa aatatgtctt
23701 tctttttaa atagggttgt actatgctgt tatgagtggc tttaatgaat aaacatttgt
23761 agcatcctct ttaatgggta aacagcatcc ga aaaaaaaaaaaaaa    //
```

Note: letters which are struck through are not included in the mRNA coding.

CONSTRUCTING mRNA CD8A VACCINE to place COVID-19 virion surface probe both the Wuhan-Hu-1 version and the Moscow version on cell surface of human cell:

Consolidating CD8A 5' region and 3' region and adding the Coronavirus 'S' protein nucleic acid coding for both Wuhan-Hu-1 and Moscow:

Native Human CD8A CSR 5' Leader End Region:

```
  1 ctctgtaaaa taaatgcgct gggccggatc ttttctgagt tctcttctcc cctacgaatt
 61 ctagatccct cctctgtcct ccctgcgcca gggaccttcg ggcgaccctt ccctgtaccc
121 ccaccccacc ctctctggac cccgtttctg cctcagtacg gcgcgctgag ctctgccccc
181 tgcccaggcc ctgacccccct caggagccgc ggtttcctgg ggtaacagtg ggaaacgtgt
241 cggccgtctc cgctcaggcg cttgctgtgt acagaaag
279 gctgat tcaggcacac cggctctcgt cgccttggtg gccctcccca
325 gccctcctcc gcgcctgctc cgggtggcgc tccgctgggc tcctcgtgcg cctgtccgcg
385 accgcaccca cctcatcctg gcacccccat cgtggcatca cgtgttccct catctgtcct
445 catggctggc gtgcccctct gcggtgagac ctgcagaaca ggaattggtg ccgggtcagc
505 agccggcgat gaagccggac gaagcctgca aaccccaccc atacgccagc ttcacatagc
565 tcctatccat tgcacagcag cgtggggaag caccgttctc taccctccaa
615 a caaaagcatg aaccaggtgc agtggctcac gtctgtaatc
656 ccagcatttt ggaggccaag gtggatggat ggattccttg agtccaggag ttcaagacca
716 gcctgggcaa catggtgaac cccatctct acaaaaattt agccag
```

CORONAVIRUS Wuhan-Hu-1 'S' Protein Probe nucleic acid coding:

```
 762 atgtttgt ttttcttgtt ttattgccac tagtctctag
 800 tcagtgtgtt aatcttacaa ccagaactca attacccct gcatacacta attctttcac
 860 acgtggtgtt tattaccctg acaaagtttt cagatcctca gttttacatt caactcagga
 920 cttgttctta cctttctttt ccaatgttac ttggttccat gctatacatg tctctgggac
 980 caatggtact aagaggtttg ataaccctgt cctaccattt aatgatggtg tttattttgc
1040 ttccactgag aagtctaaca taataagagg ctggattttt ggtactactt tagattcgaa
1100 gacccagtcc ctacttattg ttaataacgc tactaatgtt gttattaaag tctgtgaatt
1160 tcaatttgt aatgatccat ttttgggtgt ttattaccac aaaaacaaca aaagttggat
1220 ggaaagtgag ttcagagttt attctagtgc gaataattgc actttgaat atgtctctca
1280 gcctttctt atggaccttg aaggaaaaca gggtaatttc aaaaatctta gggaatttgt
1340 gtttaagaat attgatggtt atttaaaat atattctaag cacacgccta ttaatttagt
1400 gcgtgatctc cctcagggtt tttcggcttt agaaccattg gtagatttgc caataggtat
1460 taacatcact aggtttcaaa ctttacttgc tttacataga agttatttga ctcctggtga
1520 ttcttcttca ggttggacag ctggtgctgc agcttattat gtgggttatc ttcaacctag
1580 gactttcta ttaaaatata atgaaaatgg aaccattaca gatgctgtag actgtgcact
1640 tgaccctctc tcagaaacaa agtgtacgtt gaaatccttc actgtagaaa aaggaatcta
1700 tcaaacttct aactttagag tccaaccaac agaatctatt gttagatttc ctaatattac
1760 aaacttgtgc ccttttggtg aagtttttaa cgccaccaga tttgcatctg tttatgcttg
1820 gaacaggaag agaatcagca actgtgttgc tgattattct gtcctatata attccgcatc
1880 attttccact tttaagtgtt atggagtgtc tcctactaaa ttaaatgatc tctgctttac
1940 taatgtctat gcagattcat ttgtaattag aggtgatgaa gtcagacaaa tcgctccagg
2000 gcaaactgga aagattgctg attataatta taaattacca gatgatttta caggctgcgt
2060 tatagcttgg aattctaaca atcttgattc taaggttggt ggtaattata attacctgta
2120 tagattgttt aggaagtcta atctcaaacc ttttgagaga gatatttcaa ctgaaatcta
2180 tcaggccggt agcacacctt gtaatggtgt tgaaggtttt aattgttact ttcctttaca
2240 atcatatggt ttccaaccca ctaatggtgt tggttaccaa ccatacagag tagtagtact
2300 ttcttttgaa cttctacatg caccagcaac tgtttgtgga cctaaaaagt ctactaattt
2360 ggttaaaaac aaatgtgtca atttcaactt caatggttta acaggcacag gtgttcttac
2420 tgagtctaac aaaaagtttc tgcctttcca acaatttggc agagacattg ctgacactac
2480 tgatgctgtc cgtgatccac agacacttga gattcttgac attacaccat gttcttttgg
2540 tggtgtcagt gttataacac caggaacaaa tacttctaac caggttgctg ttctttatca
2600 ggatgttaac tgcacagaag tccctgttgc tattcatgca gatcaactta ctcctacttg
2660 gcgtgtttat tctacaggtt ctaatgtttt tcaaacacgt gcaggctgtt taataggggc
2720 tgaacatgtc aacaactcat atgagtgtga catacccatt ggtgcaggta tatgcgctag
2780 ttatcagact cagactaatt ctcctcggcg ggcacgtagt gtagctagtc aatccatcat
2840 tgcctacact atgtcacttg gtgcagaaaa ttcagttgct tactctaata actctattgc
2900 catacccaca aattttacta ttagtgttac cacagaaatt ctaccagtgt ctatgaccaa
2960 gacatcagta gattgtacaa tgtacatttg tggtgattca actgaatgca gcaatctttt
3020 gttgcaatat ggcagttttt gtacacaatt aaaccgtgct ttaactggaa tagctgttga
```

```
3080 acaagacaaa aacacccaag aagtttttgc acaagtcaaa caaatttaca aaacaccacc
3140 aattaaagat tttggtggtt ttaatttttc acaaatatta ccagatccat caaaaccaag
3200 caagaggtca tttattgaag atctactttt caacaaagtg acacttgcag atgctggctt
3260 catcaaacaa tatggtgatt gccttggtga tattgctgct agagacctca tttgtgcaca
3320 aaagtttaac ggccttactg ttttgccacc tttgctcaca gatgaaatga ttgctcaata
3380 cacttctgca ctgttagcgg gtacaatcac ttctggttgg acctttggtg caggtgctgc
3440 attacaaata ccatttgcta tgcaaatggc ttataggttt aatggtattg gagttacaca
3500 gaatgttctc tatgagaacc aaaaattgat tgccaaccaa tttaatagtg ctattggcaa
3560 aattcaagac tcactttctt ccacagcaag tgcacttgga aaacttcaag atgtggtcaa
3620 ccaaaatgca caagctttaa acacgcttgt taaacaactt agctccaatt ttggtgcaat
3680 ttcaagtgtt ttaaatgata tcctttcacg tcttgacaaa gttgaggctg aagtgcaaat
3740 tgataggttg atcacaggca gacttcaaag tttgcagaca tatgtgactc aacaattaat
3800 tagagctgca gaaatcagag cttctgctaa tcttgctgct actaaaatgt cagagtgtgt
3860 acttggacaa tcaaaaagag ttgatttttg tggaaagggc tatcatctta tgtccttccc
3920 tcagtcagca cctcatggtg tagtcttctt gcatgtgact tatgtccctg cacaagaaaa
3980 gaacttcaca actgctcctg ccatttgtca tgatggaaaa gcacactttc ctcgtgaagg
4040 tgtctttgtt tcaaatggca cacactggtt tgtaacacaa aggaattttt atgaaccaca
4100 aatcattact acagacaaca catttgtgtc tggtaactgt gatgttgtaa taggaattgt
4160 caacaacaca gtttatgatc ctttgcaacc tgaattagac tcattcaagg aggagttaga
4220 taaatatttt aagaatcata catcaccaga tgttgattta ggtgacatct ctggcattaa
4280 tgcttcagtt gtaaacattc aaaaagaaat tgaccgcctc aatgaggttg ccaagaattt
4340 aaatgaatct ctcatcgatc tccaagaact tggaaagtat gagcagtata taaaatggcc
4400 atggtacatt tggctaggtt ttatagctgg cttgattgcc atagtaatgg tgacaattat
4460 gctttgctgt atgaccagtt gctgtagttg tctcaagggc tgttgttctt gtggatcctg
4520 ctgcaaattt gatgaagacg actctgagcc agtgctcaaa ggagtcaaat tacattacac
4580 a

4581 taa
```

Note: nucleotides 4581-4583 is 'taa' which is functioning as a STOP/AND codon.[14,15]

CORONAVIRUS Moscow 'S' Protein Probe nucleic acid coding:

```
4584 atgt       ttgtttttct tgttttattg ccactagtct ctagtcagtg
4628 tgttaatctt acaaccagaa ctcaattacc ccctgcatac actaattctt tcacacgtgg
4688 tgtttattac cctgacaaag ttttcagatc ctcagtttta cattcaactc aggacttgtt
4748 cttacctttc ttttccaatg ttacttggtt ccatgctata catgtctctg ggaccaatgg
4808 tactaagagg tttgataacc ctgtcctacc atttaatgat ggtgtttatt ttgcttccac
4868 tgagaagtct aacataataa gaggctggat ttttggtact actttagatt cgaagaccca
4928 gtccctactt attgttaata acgctactaa tgttgttatt aaagtctgtg aatttcaatt
4988 ttgtaatgat ccatttttgg gtgtttatta ccacaaaaac aacaaaagtt ggatggaaag
5048 tgagttcaga gtttattcta gtgcgaataa ttgcactttt gaatatgtct ctcagccttt
5108 tcttatggac cttgaaggaa aacagggtaa tttcaaaaat cttagggaat ttgtgtttaa
5168 gaatattgat ggttatttta aaatatattc taagcacacg cctattaatt tagtgcgtga
5228 tctccctcag ggtttttcgg ctttagaacc attggtagat ttgccaatag gtattaacat
5288 cactaggttt caaactttac ttgctttaca tagaagttat ttgactcctg gtgattcttc
5348 ttcaggttgg acagctggtg ctgcagctta ttatgtgggt tatcttcaac ctaggacttt
5408 tctattaaaa tataatgaaa atggaaccat tacagatgct gtagactgtg cacttgaccc
5468 tctctcagaa acaaagtgta cgttgaaatc cttcactgta gaaaaaggaa tctatcaaac
5528 ttctaacttt agagtccaac caacagaatc tattgttaga tttcctaata ttacaaactt
5588 gtgccctttt ggtgaagttt ttaacgccac cagatttgca tctgtttatg cttggaacag
5648 gaagagaatc agcaactgtg ttgctgatta ttctgtccta tataattccg catcattttc
5708 cacttttaag tgttatggag tgtctcctac taaattaaat gatctctgct ttactaatgt
5768 ctatgcagat tcatttgtaa ttagaggtga tgaagtcaga caaatcgctc cagggcaaac
5828 tggaaagatt gctgattata attataaatt accagatgat tttacaggct gcgttatagc
5888 ttggaattct aacaatcttg attctaaggt tggtggtaat tataattacc tgtatagatt
```

```
5948 gtttaggaag tctaatctca aacctttga gagagatatt tcaactgaaa tctatcaggc
6008 cggtagcaca ccttgtaatg gtgttgaagg ttttaattgt tactttcctt tacaatcata
6068 tggtttccaa cccactaatg gtgttggtta ccaaccatac agagtagtag tactttcttt
6128 tgaacttcta catgcaccag caactgtttg tggacctaaa aagtctacta atttggttaa
6188 aaacaaatgt gtcaatttca acttcaatgg tttaacaggc acaggtgttc ttactgagtc
6248 taacaaaaag tttctgcctt tccaacaatt tggcagagac attgctgaca ctactgatgc
6308 tgtccgtgat ccacagacac ttgagattct tgacattaca ccatgttctt ttggtggtgt
6368 cagtgttata acaccaggaa caaatacttc taaccaggtt gctgttcttt atcagggtgt
6428 taactgcaca gaagtccctg ttgctattca tgcagatcaa cttactccta cttggcgtgt
6488 ttattctaca ggttctaatg tttttcaaac acgtgcaggc tgtttaatag gggctgaaca
6548 tgtcaacaac tcatatgagt gtgacatacc cattggtgca ggtatatgcg ctagttatca
6608 gactcagact aattctcctc ggcgggcacg tagtgtagct agtcaatcca tcattgccta
6668 cactatgtca cttggtgcag aaaattcagt tgcttactct aataactcta ttgccatacc
6728 cacaaatttt actattagtg ttaccacaga aattctacca gtgtctatga ccaagacatc
6788 agtagattgt acaatgtaca tttgtggtga ttcaactgaa tgcagcaatc ttttgttgca
6848 atatggcagt ttttgtacac aattaaaccg tgctttaact ggaatagctg ttgaacaaga
6908 caaaaacacc caagaagttt ttgcacaagt caaacaaatt tacaaaacac caccaattaa
6968 agattttggt ggttttaatt tttcacaaat attaccagat ccatcaaaac caagcaagag
7028 gtcatttatt gaagatctac ttttcaacaa agtgacactt gcagatgctg gcttcatcaa
7088 acaatatggt gattgccttg gtgatattgc tgctagagac ctcatttgtg cacaaaagtt
7148 taacggcctt actgttttgc cacctttgct cacagatgaa atgattgctc aatacacttc
7208 tgcactgtta gcgggtacaa tcacttctgg ttggaccttt ggtgcaggtg ctgcattaca
7268 aataccattt gctatgcaaa tggcttatag gtttaatggt attggagtta cacagaatgt
7328 tctctatgag aaccaaaaat tgattgccaa ccaatttaat agtgctattg gcaaaattca
7388 agactcactt tcttccacag caagtgcact tggaaaactt caagatgtgg tcaaccaaaa
7448 tgcacaagct ttaaacacgc ttgttaaaca acttagctcc aattttggtg caatttcaag
7508 tgttttaaat gatatccttt cacgtcttga caaagttgag gctgaagtgc aaattgatag
7568 gttgatcaca ggcagacttc aaagtttgca gacatatgtg actcaacaat taattagagc
7628 tgcagaaatc agagcttctg ctaatcttgc tgctactaaa atgtcagagt gtgtacttgg
7688 acaatcaaaa agagttgatt tttgtggaaa gggctatcat cttatgtcct tccctcagtc
7748 agcacctcat ggtgtagtct tcttgcatgt gacttatgtc cctgcacaag aaaagaactt
7808 cacaactgct cctgccattt gtcatgatgg aaaagcacac tttcctcgtg aaggtgtctt
7868 tgtttcaaat ggcacacact ggtttgtaac acaaaggaat tttatgaac cacaaatcat
7928 tactacagac aacacatttg tgtctggtaa ctgtgatgtt gtaataggaa ttgtcaacaa
7988 cacagtttat gatcctttgc aacctgaatt agactcattc aaggaggagt tagataaata
8048 ttttaagaat catacatcac cagatgttga tttaggtgac atctctggca ttaatgcttc
8108 agttgtaaac attcaaaaag aaattgaccg cctcaatgag gttgccaaga atttaaatga
8168 atctctcatc gatctccaag aacttggaaa gtatgagcag tatataaaat ggccatggta
8228 catttggcta ggttttatag ctggcttgat tgccatagta atggtgacaa ttatgctttg
8288 ctgtatgacc agttgctgta gttgtctcaa gggctgttgt tcttgtggat cctgctgcaa
8348 atttgatgaa gacgactctg agccagtgct caaaggagtc aaattacatt acaca

8403 taa
```

Note nucleotides 8403-8405 is 'taa', which is a STOP codon.[14,15]

Native Human CD8A CSR 3' Terminal End Region:

```
8406 ccc        tgtgcaacag ccactacatt
8429 acttcaaact gagatccttc cttttgaggg agcaagtcct tccctttcat tttttccagt
8489 cttcctccct gtgtattcat tctcatgatt attattttag tgggggcggg gtgggaaaga
8549 ttactttttc tttatgtgtt tgacgggaaa caaaactagg taaaatctac agtacaccac
8609 aagggtcaca atactgttgt gcgcacatcg cggtagggcg tggaaagggg caggccagag
8669 ctacccgcag agttctcaga atcatgctga gagagctgga ggcacccatg ccatctcaac
8729 ctcttccccg cccgttttac aaagggggag gctaaagccc agagacagct tgatcaaagg
8789 cacacagcaa gtcagggttg gagcagtagc tggagggacc ttgtctccca gctcagggct
8849 ctttcctcca caccattcag gtctttcttt ccgaggcccc tgtctcaggg tgaggtgctt
```

```
8909 gagtctccaa cggcaaggga acaagtactt cttgatacct gggatactgt gcccagagcc
8969 tcgaggaggt aatgaattaa agaagagaac tgcctttggc agagttctat aatgtaaaca
9029 atatcagact tttttttttt ataatcaagc ctaaaattgt atagacctaa aataaaatga
9089 agtggtgagc ttaaccctgg aaaatgaatc cctctatctc taaagaaaat ctctgtgaaa
9149 cccctatgtg gaggcggaat tgctctccca gcccttgcat tgcagagggg cccatgaaag
9209 aggacaggct acccctttac aaatagaatt tgagcatcag tgaggttaaa ctaaggccct
9269 cttgaatctc tgaatttgag atacaaacat gttcctggga tcactgatga ctttttatac
9329 tttgtaaaga caattgttgg agagcccctc acacagccct ggcctctgct caactagcag
9389 atacagggat gaggcagacc tgactctctt aaggaggctg agagcccaaa ctgctgtccc
9449 aaacatgcac ttccttgctt aaggtatggt acaagcaatg cctgcccatt ggagagaaaa
9509 aacttaagta gataaggaaa taagaaccac tcataattct tcaccttagg aataatctcc
9569 tgttaatatg gtgtacattc ttcctgatta ttttctacac atacatgtaa aatatgtctt
9629 tcttttttaa atagggttgt actatgctgt tatgagtggc tttaatgaat aaacatttgt
9689 agcatcctct ttaatgggta aacagcatcc g
9720 aaaaaaaaaa aaaaaaaaaa aaaaaaaaaa aaaa    //
```

The modified mRNA containing two separate coronavirus probes, to function as a COVID-19 RNA vaccine is 9720 nucleotides long, though the final length depends upon the number of adenine nucleotides comprising the 3' tail of the mRNA. Above mRNA is shown with 33 adenine nucleotides comprising the tail, similar to the positive-sense coronavirus mRNA. Number of adenine nucleotides in the 3' tail is a function of the optimal performance of the mRNA inside a target cell.

To summarize, the construct of this mRNA coronavirus vaccine is comprised of: 5' leader nucleotide sequence of a native human mRNA for CD8A glycoprotein cell surface receptor, attached to the nucleotide coding sequence for coronavirus Wuhan-Hu-1 'S' probe, then is attached the 'taa' STOP/AND code codon, then is attached nucleotide coding sequence for coronavirus Moscow 'S' probe, then is attached a second 'taa' STOP code codon, then is attached the 3' terminal end nucleotide sequence of a native human mRNA coding for CD8A glycoprotein cell surface receptor, then is attached a sequence of adenine nucleotides comprising the tail of the molecule.

To code like a mRNA, the COVID-19 mRNA vaccine nucleotide coding with t's replaced by u's as by convention the construct of a messenger ribonucleic acid.

Native Human CD8A CSR 5' Leader End Region:

```
  1 cucuguaaaa uaaaugcgcu gggccggauc uuuucugagu ucucuucucc ccuacgaauu
 61 cuagaucccu ccucuguccu cccugcgcca gggaccuucg ggcgacccuu cccuguaccc
121 ccaccccacc cucucuggac cccguuucug ccucaguacg gcgcgcugag cucugccccc
181 ugcccaggcc cugacccccu caggagccgc gguuuccugg gguaacagug ggaaacgugu
241 cggccgucuc cgcucaggcg cuugcugugu acagaaag
```

```
279 gcugau ucaggcacac cggcucucgu cgccuuggug gcccucccca
325 gcccuccucc gcgccugcuc cggguggcgc uccgcugggc uccucgugcg ccuguccgcg
385 accgcaccca ccucauccug gcacccccau cguggcauca cguguucccu caucuguccu
445 cauggcuggc gugccccucu gcggugagac cugcagaaca ggaauuggug ccgggucagc
505 agccggcgau gaagccggac gaagccugca aaccccaccc auacgccagc uucacauagc
565 uccuauccau ugcacagcag cguggggaag caccguucuc uacccuccaa
615 a caaaagcaug aaccaggugc aguggcucac gucuguaauc
656 ccagcauuuu ggaggccaag guggauggau ggauuccuug aguccaggag uucaagacca
716 gccugggcaa cauggugaac ccccaucucu acaaaaauuu agccag
```

CORONAVIRUS Wuhan-Hu-1 'S' Protein Probe nucleic acid coding:

```
 762 auguuugu uuuucuuguu uuauugccac uagucucuag
 800 ucaguguguu aaucuuacaa ccagaacuca auuacccccu gcauacacua auucuuucac
 860 acgugguguu uauuacccug acaaaguuuu cagauccuca guuuuacauu caacucagga
 920 cuuguucuua ccuuucuuuu ccaauguuac uugguuccau gcuauacaug ucucugggac
 980 caaugguacu aagagguuug auaacccugu ccuaccauuu aaugauggug uuuauuuugc
1040 uuccacugag aagucuaaca uaauaagagg cuggauuuuu gguacuacuu uagauucgaa
1100 gacccagucc cuacuuauug uuaauaacgc uacuaauguu guuauuaaag ucugugaauu
1160 ucaauuuugu aaugauccau uuuugggugu uuauuaccac aaaaacaaca aaaguuggau
1220 ggaaagugag uucagaguuu auucuagugc gaauaauugc acuuuugaau augucucuca
1280 gccuuuucuu auggaccuug aaggaaaaca ggguaauuuc aaaaaucuua gggaauuugu
1340 guuuaagaau auugaugguu auuuuaaaau auauucuaag cacacgccua uuaauuuagu
1400 gcgugaucuc ccucaggguu uuucggcuuu agaaccauug guagauuugc caauagguau
1460 uaacaucacu agguuucaaa cuuuacuugc uuuacauaga aguuauuuga cuccugguga
1520 uucuucuuca gguuggacag cuggugcugc agcuuauuau gugguuauc uucaaccuag
1580 gacuuuucua uuaaaauaua augaaaaugg aaccauuaca gaugcuguag acugugcacu
1640 ugacccucuc ucagaaacaa aguguacguu gaaauccuuc acuguagaaa aaggaaucua
1700 ucaaacuucu aacuuuagag uccaaccaac agaaucuauu guuagauuuc cuaauauuac
1760 aaacuugugc ccuuuuggug aaguuuuuaa cgccaccaga uuugcaucug uuuaugcuug
1820 gaacaggaag agaaucagca acuguguugc ugauuauucu guccuauaua auuccgcauc
1880 auuuuccacu uuuaaguguu auggaguguc uccuacuaaa uuaaaugauc ucugcuuuac
1940 uaaugucuau gcagauucau uuguaauuag aggugaugaa gucagacaaa ucgcuccagg
2000 gcaaacugga aagauugcug auuauaauua uaaauuacca gaugauuuua caggcugcgu
2060 uauagcuugg aauucuaaca aucuugauuc uaagguuggu gguaauuaua auuaccugua
2120 uagauuguuu aggaagucua aucucaaacc uuuugagaga gauauuucaa cugaaaucua
2180 ucaggccggu agcacaccuu guaauggugu ugaagguuuu aauuguuacu uuccuuuaca
2240 aucauauggu uuccaaccca cuaauggugu ugguuaccaa ccauacagag uaguaguacu
2300 uucuuuugaa cuucuacaug caccagcaac uguuugugga ccuaaaaagu cuacuaauuu
2360 gguuaaaaac aaauguguca auuucaacuu caaugguuua acaggcacag guguucuuac
2420 ugagucuaac aaaaaguuuc ugccuuucca acaauuuggc agagacauug cugacacuac
2480 ugaugcuguc cgugauccac agacacuuga gauucuugac auuacaccau guucuuuugg
2540 uggugucagu guuauaacac caggaacaaa uacuucuaac cagguugcug uucuuuauca
2600 ggauguuaac ugcacagaag ucccuguugc uauucaugca gaucaacuua cuccuacuug
2660 gcguguuuau ucuacagguu cuaauguuuu ucaaacacgu gcaggcuguu uaauaggggc
2720 ugaacauguc aacaacucau augaguguga cauacccauu ggugcaggua uaugcgcuag
2780 uuaucagacu cagacuaauu cuccucggcg ggcacguagu guagcuaguc aauccaucau
2840 ugccuacacu augucacuug gugcagaaaa uucaguugcu uacucuaaua acucuauugc
2900 cauacccaca aauuuuacua uuaguguuac cacagaaauu cuaccagugu cuaugaccaa
2960 gacaucagua gauuguacaa uguacauuug uggugauuca acugaaugca gcaaucuuuu
3020 guugcaauau ggcaguuuuu guacacaauu aaaccgugcu uuaacuggaa uagcuguuga
3080 acaagacaaa aacacccaag aaguuuuugc acaagucaaa caaauuuaca aaacaccacc
3140 aauuaaagau uuuggugguu uuaauuuuuc acaaauauua ccagauccau caaaaccaag
3200 caagagguca uuuauugaag aucuacuuuu caacaaagug acacuugcag augcuggcuu
3260 caucaaacaa uauggugauu gccuugguga uauugcugcu agagaccuca uuugugcaca
3320 aaaguuuaac ggccuuacug uuuugccacc uuugcucaca gaugaaauga uugcucaaua
3380 cacuucugca cuguuagcgg guacaaucac uucugguugg accuuuggug caggugcugc
3440 auuacaaaua ccauuugcua ugcaaauggc uuauagguuu aaugguauug gaguuacaca
```

```
3500 gaauguucuc uaugagaacc aaaaauugau ugccaaccaa uuuaauagug cuauuggcaa
3560 aauucaagac ucacuuucuu ccacagcaag ugcacuugga aaacuucaag auguggucaa
3620 ccaaaaugca caagcuuuaa acacgcuugu uaaacaacuu agcuccaauu uuggugcaau
3680 uucaaguguu uuaaaugaua uccuuucacg ucuugacaaa guugaggcug aagugcaaau
3740 ugauagguug aucacaggca gacuucaaag uuugcagaca uaugugacuc aacaauuaau
3800 uagagcugca gaaaucagag cuucugcuaa ucuugcugcu acuaaaaugu cagagugugu
3860 acuuggacaa ucaaaaagag uugauuuuug uggaaagggc uaucaucuua uguccuuccc
3920 ucagucagca ccucauggug uagucuucuu gcaugugacu uauguccug cacaagaaaa
3980 gaacuucaca acugcuccug ccauuuguca ugauggaaaa gcacacuuuc cucgugaagg
4040 ugucuuuguu ucaaauggca cacacugguu uguaacacaa aggaauuuuu augaaccaca
4100 aaucauuacu acagacaaca cauuuguguc ugguaacugu gauguuguaa uaggaauugu
4160 caacaacaca guuuaugauc cuuugcaacc ugaauuagac ucauucaagg aggaguuaga
4220 uaaauauuuu aagaaucaua caucaccaga uguugauuua ggugacaucu cuggcauuaa
4280 ugcuucaguu guaaacauuc aaaaagaaau ugaccgccuc aaugagguug ccaagaauuu
4340 aaaugaaucu cucaucgauc uccaagaacu uggaaaguau gagcaguaua uaaaauggcc
4400 augguacauu uggcuagguu uuauagcugg cuugauugcc auaguaaugg ugacaauuau
4460 gcuuugcugu augaccaguu gcuguaguug ucucaagggc uguuguucuu guggauccug
4520 cugcaaauuu gaugaagacg acucugagcc agugcucaaa ggagucaaau uacauuacac
4580 a

4581 uaa
```

Note: nucleotides 4581-4583 is ‘uaa’, which is functioning as a STOP/AND codon.[14,15]

CORONAVIRUS Moscow ‘S’ Protein Probe nucleic acid coding:

```
4584 augu uuguuuuucu uguuuuauug ccacuagucu cuagucagug
4628 uguuaaucuu acaaccagaa cucaauuacc cccugcauac acuaauucuu ucacacgugg
4688 uguuuauuac ccugacaaag uuuucagauc cucaguuuua cauucaacuc aggacuuguu
4748 cuuaccuuuc uuuuccaaug uuacuugguu ccaugcuaua caugucucug ggaccaaugg
4808 uacuaagagg uuugauaacc cuguccuacc auuuaaugau gguguuuauu uugcuuccac
4868 ugagaagucu aacauaauaa gaggcuggau uuuugguacu acuuuagauu cgaagaccca
4928 gucccuacuu auuguuaaua acgcuacuaa uguuguuauu aaagucugug aauuucaauu
4988 uuguaaugau ccauuuuugg guguuuauua ccacaaaaac aacaaaaguu ggauggaaag
5048 ugaguucaga guuuauucua gugcgaauaa uugcacuuuu gaauaugucu cucagccuuu
5108 ucuuauggac cuugaaggaa aacaggguaa uuucaaaaau cuuagggaau uuguguuuaa
5168 gaauauugau gguuauuuua aaauauauuc uaagcacacg ccuauuaauu uagugcguga
5228 ucucccucag gguuuuucgg cuuuagaacc auugguagau uugccaauag guauuaacau
5288 cacuagguuu caaacuuuac uugcuuuaca uagaaguuau uugacuccug gugauucuuc
5348 uucagguugg acagcuggug cugcagcuua uuaugugggu uaucuucaac cuaggacuuu
5408 ucuauuaaaa uauaaugaaa auggaaccau uacagaugcu guagacugug cacuugaccc
5468 ucucucagaa acaaagugua cguugaaauc cuucacugua gaaaaaggaa ucuaucaaac
5528 uucuaacuuu agaguccaac caacagaauc uauuguuaga uuuccuaaua uuacaaacuu
5588 gugcccuuuu ggugaaguuu uuaacgccac cagauuugca ucuguuuaug cuuggaacag
5648 gaagagaauc agcaacugug uugcugauua uucuguccua uauaauuccg caucauuuuc
5708 cacuuuuaag uguuauggag ugucuccuac uaaauuaaau gaucucugcu uuacuaaugu
5768 cuaugcagau ucauuuguaa uuagagguga ugaagucaga caaaucgcuc cagggcaaac
5828 uggaaagauu gcugauuaua auuauaaauu accagaugau uuuacaggcu gcguuauagc
5888 uuggaauucu aacaaucuug auucuaaggu ugguggua au uauaauuacc uguauagauu
5948 guuuaggaag ucuaaucuca aaccuuuuga gagagauauu ucaacugaaa ucuaucaggc
6008 cgguagcaca ccuuguaaug guguugaagg uuuuaauugu uacuuuccuu uacaaucaua
6068 ugguuuccaa cccacuaaug guguugguua ccaaccauac agaguaguag uacuuucuuu
6128 ugaacuucua caugcaccag caacuguuug uggaccuaaa aagucuacua auuugguuaa
6188 aaacaaaugu gucaauuuca acuucaaugg uuuaacaggc acagguguuc uuacugaguc
6248 uaacaaaaag uuucugccuu uccaacaauu uggcagagac auugcugaca cuacugaugc
6308 uguccgugau ccacagacac uugagauucu ugacauuaca ccauguucuu uugguggugu
```

```
6368 caguguuaua acaccaggaa caaauacuuc uaaccagguu gcuguucuuu aucagggugu
6428 uaacugcaca gaagucccug uugcuauuca ugcagaucaa cuuacuccua cuuggcgugu
6488 uuauucuaca gguucuaaug uuuuucaaac acgugcaggc uguuuaauag gggcugaaca
6548 ugucaacaac ucauaugagu gugacauacc cauuggugca gguauaugcg cuaguuauca
6608 gacucagacu aauucuccuc ggcgggcacg uaguguagcu agucaaucca ucauugccua
6668 cacuauguca cuuggugcag aaaauucagu ugcuuacucu aauaacucua uugccauacc
6728 cacaaauuuu acuauuagug uuaccacaga aauucuacca gugucuauga ccaagacauc
6788 aguagauugu acaauguaca uuugugguga uucaacugaa ugcagcaauc uuuuguugca
6848 auauggcagu uuuuguacac aauuaaaccg ugcuuuaacu ggaauagcug uugaacaaga
6908 caaaaacacc caagaaguuu uugcacaagu caaacaaauu uacaaaacac caccaauuaa
6968 agauuuuggu gguuuuaauu uuucacaaau auuaccagau ccaucaaaac caagcaagag
7028 gucauuuauu gaagaucuac uuuucaacaa agugacacuu gcagaugcug gcuucaucaa
7088 acaauauggu gauugccuug gugauauugc ugcuagagac cucauuugug cacaaaaguu
7148 uaacggccuu acuguuuugc caccuuugcu cacagaugaa augauugcuc aauacacuuc
7208 ugcacuguua gcggguacaa ucacuucugg uuggaccuuu ggugcaggug cugcauuaca
7268 aauaccauuu gcuaugcaaa uggcuuauag guuuaauggu auuggaguua cacagaaugu
7328 ucucuaugag aaccaaaaau ugauugccaa ccaauuuaau agugcuauug gcaaaauuca
7388 agacucacuu ucuuccacag caagugcacu uggaaaacuu caagaugugg ucaaccaaaa
7448 ugcacaagcu uuaaacacgc uuguuaaaca acuuagcucc aauuuuggug caauuucaag
7508 uguuuuaaau gauauccuuu cacgucuuga caaaguugag gcugaagugc aaauugauag
7568 guugaucaca ggcagacuuc aaaguuugca gacauaugug acucaacaau uaauuagagc
7628 ugcagaaauc agagcuucug cuaaucuugc ugcuacuaaa augucagagu guguacuugg
7688 acaaucaaaa agaguugauu uuuguggaaa gggcuaucau cuuauguccu ucccucaguc
7748 agcaccucau gguguagucu ucuugcaugu gacuuauguc ccugcacaag aaaagaacuu
7808 cacaacugcu ccugccauuu gucaugaugg aaaagcacac uuuccucgug aaggugucuu
7868 uguuucaaau ggcacacacu gguuuguaac acaaaggaau uuuuaugaac cacaaaucau
7928 uacuacagac aacacauuug ugucugguaa cugugauguu guaauaggaa uugucaacaa
7988 cacaguuuau gauccuuugc aaccugaauu agacucauuc aaggaggagu uagauaaaua
8048 uuuuaagaau cauacaucac cagauguuga uuuaggugac aucucuggca uuaaugcuuc
8108 aguuguaaac auucaaaaag aaauugaccg ccucaaugag guugccaaga auuuaaauga
8168 aucucucauc gaucuccaag aacuuggaaa guaugagcag uauauaaaau ggccauggua
8228 cauuuggcua gguuuuauag cuggcuugau ugccauagua auggugacaa uuaugcuuug
8288 cuguaugacc aguugcugua guugucucaa gggcuguugu ucuuguggau ccugcugcaa
8348 auuugaugaa gacgacucug agccagugcu caaaggaguc aaauuacauu acaca

8403 uaa
```

Note nucleotides 8403-8405 is 'uaa', which is a STOP codon.[14,15]

Native Human CD8A CSR 3' Terminal End Region:

```
8406 ccc ugugcaacag ccacuacauu
8429 acuucaaacu gagauccuuc cuuuugaggg agcaaguccu ucccuuucau uuuuuccagu
8489 cuuccucccu guguauucau ucucaugauu auuauuuuag ugggggcggg gugggaaaga
8549 uuacuuuuuc uuuauguguu ugacgggaaa caaaacuagg uaaaaucuac aguacaccac
8609 aagggucaca auacuguugu gcgcacaucg cgguagggcg uggaaagggg caggccagag
8669 cuacccgcag aguucucaga aucaugcuga gagagcugga ggcacccaug ccaucucaac
8729 cucuuccccg cccguuuuac aaaggggggag gcuaaagccc agagacagcu ugaucaaagg
8789 cacacagcaa gucaggguug gagcaguagc uggagggacc uugucuccca gcucagggcu
8849 cuuuccucca caccauucag gucuuucuuu ccgaggcccc ugucucaggg ugaggugcuu
8909 gagucuccaa cggcaaggga acaaguacuu cuugauaccu gggauacugu gcccagagcc
8969 ucgaggaggu aaugaauuaa agaagagaac ugccuuuggc agaguucuau aauguaaaca
9029 auaucagacu uuuuuuuuuu auaaucaagc cuaaaauugu auagaccuaa aauaaaauga
9089 aguggugagc uuaacccugg aaaaugaauc ccucuaucuc uaaagaaaau cucugugaaa
9149 ccccuaugug gaggcggaau ugcucuccca gcccuugcau ugcagagggg cccaugaaag
9209 aggacaggcu accccuuuac aaauagaauu ugagcaucag ugagguuaaa cuaaggcccu
9269 cuugaaucuc ugaauuugag auacaaacau guuccuggga ucacugauga cuuuuuauac
```

9329 uuuguaaaga caauuguugg agagccccuc acacagcccu ggccucugcu caacuagcag
9389 auacagggau gaggcagacc ugacucucuu aaggaggcug agagcccaaa cugcuguccc
9449 aaacaugcac uuccuugcuu aagguauggu acaagcaaug ccugcccauu ggagagaaaa
9509 aacuuaagua gauaaggaaa uaagaaccac ucauaauucu ucaccuuagg aauaaucucc
9569 uguuaauaug guguacauuc uuccugauua uuuucuacac auacauguaa aauaugucuu
9629 ucuuuuuuaa auaggguugu acuaugcugu uaugaguggc uuuaaugaau aaacauuugu
9689 agcauccucu uuaaugggua aacagcaucc g
9720 a**aaaaaaaaa aaaaaaaaaa aaaaaaaaaa aaaa** //

The modified mRNA is **9720** nucleotides long, though the final length depends upon the number of adenine nucleotides comprising the 3' tail of the mRNA. As shown above, the adenine tail is comprised of thirty-three 'a's'; the length of the adenine tail.

When an artificial mRNA is constructed for the purposes of a medical treatment, and one or more polypeptides are intended to be the product of the translation of the said artificial mRNA, then the use of a 'UAA' STOP codon is deliberate and a necessary part of the construction of the said mRNA. The 'UAA' STOP codon would be required to be present between the nucleotide sequencing coding for one or more polypeptides and the 3' terminal end of the mRNA. The use of the 'UAA' STOP codon between nucleotide sequences is required for a mRNA to be translated and properly produce one, two or more polypeptides during a single translation event cycle of the said mRNA, that is a for an mRNA to be translated once and produce one, two or more polypeptides, the 'UAA' STOP code codon is required to be present between two polypeptide generating nucleotide sequences and between a polypeptide generating nucleotide sequence and the 3' terminal end of the mRNA.

A single mRNA can produce more than one polypeptide by being translated more than one time, that is, undergoing more than one translation event cycle connected to a ribosome, with the number of translation event cycles being dictated by the number of adenine nucleotides attached to the 3' terminal end of the mRNA, also called the Poly (A) tail. Each adenine nucleotide comprising the Poly (A) tail dictates a repeat of the translation event cycle of the said mRNA to create a polypeptide. The invention described in this provisional patent application describes how with the use of the 'UAA' STOP codon code inserted between two nucleotide coding sequences, that when the mRNA is translated each of the nucleotide coding sequences will generate a separate polypeptide during a single translation event cycle of the said mRNA. Thus, with the use of the specific 'UAA' STOP codon code, rather than the other two STOP codon codes, more than one polypeptide can be generated by an artificial mRNA during a single translation event cycle of the said mRNA. See Figure 29.

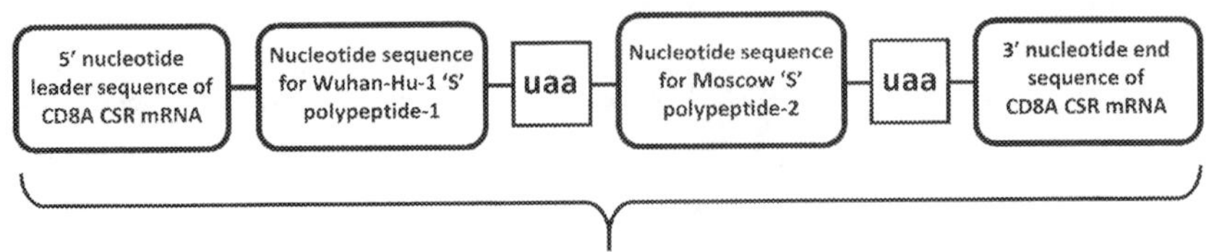

mRNA coded to generate 'S' protein for both Wuhan-Hu- 1 and Moscow strains of coronavirus with 'uaa' present between polypeptide coding segments and between last coding segment and the 3' end of the mRNA

Figure 29
Added UAA segment necessary between coding for second polypeptide and 3'end.

Likely to properly construct an mRNA to function as a multi-polypeptide coding sequence, not only do the differing nucleotide sequences coding for the polypeptides be separated by a UAA codon code, but also the last polypeptide coding sequences needs a UAA separating it from the 3' terminal end of the mRNA. Without the UAA codon coding code between the last polypeptide and the 3' end of the mRNA, the last polypeptide likely will not be released from the mRNA and the proximal (front) end of the mRNA will only be decoded once by the reading ribosome complex, rather than possibly multiple times as dictated by the length of the adenine tail. Likely the 3' end of the mRNA contains instructions regarding the protein being generated, which need to be decoded and acted upon. The UAA codon instructs the decoder to continue reading the mRNA and seek out the functional instructions

SUMMARY

The human race cannot allow a misguided scrap of malignant bio-programming code to ravage the world's population without being heatedly contested by our best efforts at innovation and invention. We must capitalize on the advancements in the knowledge of how the DNA is decoded, the construct of transcription factors and how mRNAs are translated. A single modified mRNA could generate, through the process of cellular translation, one, two or more polypeptides during the same translation process. In the case of coronavirus, two differing RNA vaccines could be coded into one mRNA molecule. The codon code 'UAA' or 'uaa' or 'TAA', or 'taa', is recognized generally as a STOP code codon, but actually acts as an 'AND' or continue function to facilitate the proper translation of the genetic code carried by the mRNA. With proper use of the 'UAA' STOP code codon, one artificial mRNA could carry the genetic instructions to mount two differing 'S' probes on the cell surface of the same human cell. The use of the 'UAA' STOP codon between nucleotide sequences is required for a mRNA to be translated and properly produce one, two or more polypeptides during a single translation event cycle of the said mRNA, that is a for an mRNA to be translated once and produce one, two or more polypeptides, the 'UAA' STOP code codon is required to be present between two polypeptide generating nucleotide sequences and between a polypeptide generating nucleotide sequence and the 3' terminal end of the mRNA.

CHAPTER FOURTEEN

METHODS OF MAKING AND DELIVERING mRNA THERAPIES

METHODS OF MAKING COMPOSITIONS OF THE INVENTION

Methods for making soluble molecules in general are well established in references such as A. Traunecker et al. "Bispecific single chain molecules (Janusins) target cytotoxic lymphocytes on HIV infected cells, EMBO Journal 10(12):3655-3659; Neuberger et al., Biotechniques. 4 (3):214-21 (1986); Ernst Winnacker, "From Genes to Clones: Introduction to Gene Technology" Chapter 7, 1987 at pages 239-317.[26.27.28]

The starting material can be a cDNA clone of TFIIIA gene. Using methods known in the art a restriction site can be positioned close to a start codon. The next step can be a digestion step which should cut DNA fragments asymmetrically. The mixture of DNA fragments obtained is then cloned into a vector, e.g., a pUC vector. Of course, a cleavage site must be present within the polylinker of a chosen vector. Since a wide spectrum of vectors are available, it should not be difficult to find a suitable vector containing the desired cleavage site. Once a suitable clone is identified, the cleavage site can be used for the insertion of the gene of interest, which can be obtained from the original cDNA clone. Messenger RNAs can be harvested from the cloned DNA.

METHODS FOR DELIVERING MESSENGER RNAS

Introducing the modified mRNA coded to produce the intended modified TFIIIA therapeutic polypeptides into host cells infected by the coronavirus may be accomplished by a number of practical means.[15,29] Once introduced into the body, modified mRNA is to cross the membrane of cells. Likely lung cells will be the primary target given COVID-19 is primarily a respiratory virus. Upon the mRNA diffusing across a cell membrane the mRNA will be engaged by a cell's ribosomes and translated as if the mRNA had been produced by the cell's nucleus. Once translated, said modified mRNA will generate said modified TFIIIA polypeptides as if it were a natural mRNA. Upon being generated per the cell's mRNA translation process, the modified TFIIIA polypeptide will seek out the uracil tail of the negative-sense coronavirus genome and bind to the COVID-19 genome. The number of modified TFIIIA polypeptides produced by one said mRNA is dictated by the adenine tail constructed in the said mRNA molecule. Optimal number of adenine nucleotides comprising the tail will be determined per clinical trials.

To introduce, the therapeutic modified mRNA coded to produce a modified TFIIIA polypeptide, into a cell, may be accomplished by packing the said mRNA in a polyethylene glycol (PEG)-polyamino acid block copolymer-based polyplex nanomicelles. Nanomicelles infused with the modified mRNA have been shown to be successfully injected into joints.[30] Such a device may be modified to be injected into plasma.

Other means are being actively explored to introduce mRNA directly to the lung tissues. Delivery mechanisms such as polyethylenimine (PEI) for delivering inhalable DNA to the lungs has been studied.[31] PEI fails to break down easily, and thus with repeated doses the polymer could accumulate in the lung tissues and result in side effects. An alternative to PEI is hyperbranched poly (beta amino esters). Hyperbranched poly (beta amino esters) are being developed to carry mRNAs, which could be inhaled by a patient in order to deliver the said modified mRNAs to the patient's lung cells without accumulation of toxic effects. [32]

Additional delivery method being developed include work on mRNA pulmonary delivery by dry powder formulation of PEGylated synthetic KL4 peptide.[33] Again a modified mRNA could be aerosolized. As an aerosol, delivered in a dry powder formulation of PEGylated synthetic KL4 peptide or similar construct, the modified mRNA could be delivered to the lung tissues to deliver modified mRNA to lung cells. See Figure 30.

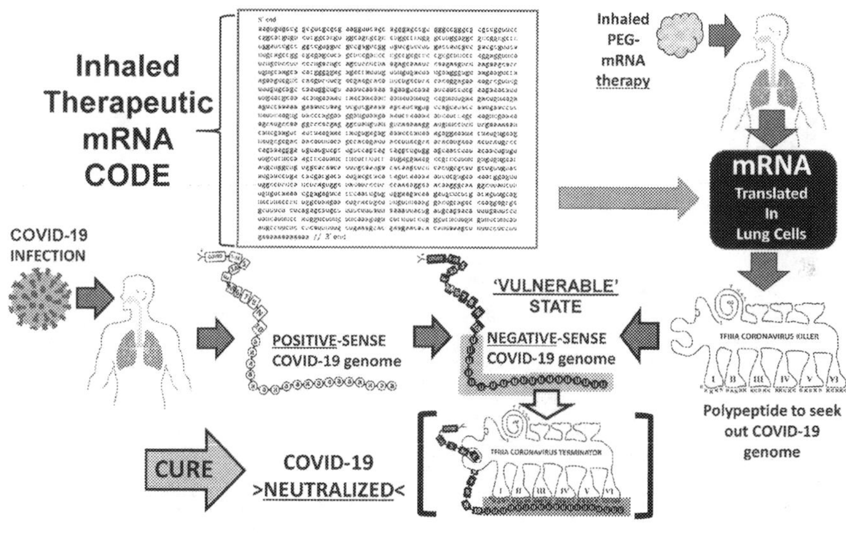

Figure 30
Delivery of mRNA therapies to the lungs to manage coronavirus.

An interesting approach would be editing COVID-19's own genome, extruding unnecessary viral elements, while embedding programming code sufficient to construct the modified mRNA to produce the modified TFIIIA molecule. Coronavirus virion's spike probe seeks out and binds to the ACE2 cell surface receptor present on a number of different human cells. Paradoxically, the bio-programming comprising the coronavirus's genome could be rewritten to generate COVID-19 virions which would deliver therapeutic mRNAs to be translated in a cell's cytoplasm to produce and mount coronavirus spike proteins on the surface of the same human cells the virus targets.[15]

CHAPTER FIFTEEN

NEXT CATASTROPHIC THREAT, A 'RESPIRATORY TRANSMITTED' EBOLA PANDEMIC

Zaire Ebolavirus Genome (EBOV)
Genus Ebolavirus
Family Filoviridae

Single stranded RNA virus (-)

≈19,000 bps

7 Primary Genes
7 encoded viral proteins and
3'leader and 5'trailer sequences

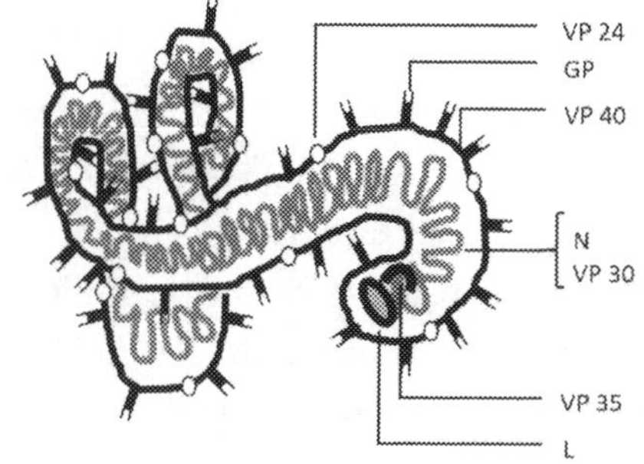

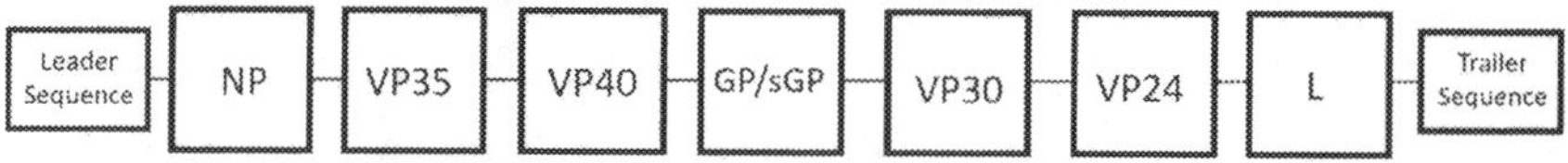

Seven Primary Genes:

NP = Predominant nucleocapsid protein.
VP35 = Cofactor in polymerase complex; Type I IFN antagonist.
VP40 = Matrix protein: Coalesce nucleocapsid and cell membrane.
GP = GP_1 Receptor binding gp120, GP_2 Receptor binding to gp41.
sGP = Soluble secreted protein to impede extracellular viral response.
VP30 = Encapsidation of viral genome.
VP 24 = Prevents intracellular viral response; Virion assembly; Matrix protein.
L = Transcription viral genome; Replication of viral genome.

Figure 31
The nucleotide coding segments comprising Ebolavirus.

Introduction to the next horrific viral threat

Ebola strikes fear in the heart of many whom hear the name. Over the years, the media has portrayed this virus as a vicious monster lurking in the jungles of Africa. Periodically, this virus is described as erupting as a pandemic striking those whom become infected with a horrific death. The mortality rate of this virus has been rather high compared to other viruses.

There are five distinct species of the Genus Ebolavirus. The WHO data suggests the species Zaire Ebola virus, first strain detected in 1976 and is the strain of virus responsible for the 2014 Ebola outbreak.[34,35] Fruit bats of the *Pteropodidae* family are considered to be the natural host of the Ebola virus. The Zaire strain has appeared 15 times since first detected along the Ebola river in 1976. The cycling of the virus suggests random contact of humans with the virus's natural reservoir or it possibly suggests the virus periodically slips into a dormant state only to reemerge with deadly consequences.

Ebola, like other viruses, is an intracellular pathogen. Replication of the virus occurs inside cells. The only trace of the virus in blood and body fluids is detectable when the virus virion is extracellular and antibodies generated as a response to the virus's presence.

There are a number of ways to classify viruses. Viruses can be classified by type of nucleic acids that comprise their genome, the method of replication, the host cell used for replication, the host organism that the virus utilizes for replication purposes, the type of disease the virus causes, the characteristics of the external shell that carries the virus. The two recognized authorities for viral classification include the International Committee on Taxonomy of Viruses (ICTV)[36] and the Baltimore classification system[37,38,39].

ICTV Classification

The ICTV is charged by the International Union of Microbiological Societies with establishing, refining, and maintaining virus taxonomy. Viral classification starts with features of the classification of cellular organisms including: Order (virales), Family (viridae), Subfamily (virinae), Genus (virus) and Species (generally the name of the disease). There are 7 Orders, 96 Families, 22 Sub Families, 450 Genera and 2618 Species of viruses defined by ICTV. The seven orders include: Caudovirales, Herpesvirales, Ligamenvirales, Mononegavirales, Nidovirales, Picornoavirales and Tymovirales. Caudovirales are tailed dsDNA bacteriophages. Herpesvirales are large eukaryotic dsDNA viruses. Ligamenvirales are linear acrhaean dsDNA viruses. Monogegavirales negative strand ssRNA plant and animal viruses. Nidovirales are positive strand ssRNA vertebrate host viruses. Picornavirales are positive strand ssRNA viruses that infect plane, insect and animal hosts. Tymovirales are monopartite positive ssRNA viruses that infect plants.

Baltimore Classification of Viruses

The Baltimore classification of viruses is based on separating the viruses regarding method of viral mRNA synthesis. The Baltimore classification was first introduced in 1971. There are three major types of mRNA viral genomes, which include DNA genome, RNA genome and reverse transcribing genomes. The Baltimore classification more completely divides viruses into seven categories. The seven classification categories includes: (I) dsDNA viruses, (II) ssDNA viruses, (III) dsRNA viruses, (IV) positive sense ssRNA viruses, (V) negative sense ssRNA viruses, (VI) ssRNA-RT, positive sense RNA with DNA intermediate (i.e. retroviruses), and (VII) dsDNA-RT viruses. Table 6 presents common viruses per the Baltimore classification.[37,38,39] Note: ssRNA refers to single stranded RNA versus dsRNA refers to double stranded RNA; +sense refers to positive-sense of the viral genome and -sense refers to negative-sense of the viral genome.

Nucleotide type	Group	Type of genome	Family	Virion	Common names
DNA	I	dsDNA	Adenoviridae	Nkd	Adenovirus, Canine hepatitis virus

Nucleotide type	Group	Type of genome	Family	Virion	Common names
DNA	I	dsDNA	Papovaridae	Nkd	Papillomavirus, Polyomaviridae, Simian vacuolating virus
DNA	I	dsDNA	Herpesviridae	Env	Herpes simplex virus, Varicella-zoster virus, Cytomegalovirus, Epstein-Barr virus
DNA	I	dsDNA	Poxviridae	Com	Smallpox virus, cow pox virus, sheep pox virus, monkey pox virus
DNA	II	ssDNA	Parvoviridae	Nkd	Parvovirus B19, Canine parvovirus
DNA	II	ssDNA	Anelloviridae	Nkd	Torque teno virus
RNA	III	dsRNA	Reoviridae	Nkd	Reovirus, Rotovirus,
RNA	IV	+sense ssRNA	Picornaviridae	Nkd	Enterovirus, Rhinovirus, Hepatovirus, Cardiovirus, Aphthovirus, Poliovirus, Parechovirus, Erbovirus, Kovbuvirus, Teschovirus, Coxsakie
RNA	IV	+sense ssRNA	Caliciviridae	Nkd	Norwalk virus
RNA	IV	+sense ssRNA	Togaviridae	Env	Rubella virus, Alphavirus
RNA	IV	+sense ssRNA	Flaviviridae	Env	Dengue virus, Hepatitis C, Yellow Fever virus
RNA	IV	+sense ssRNA	Coronaviridae	Env	Corona virus, Middle East respiratory syndrome (MERS-CoV) SARS COVID-19

Nucleotide type	Group	Type of genome	Family	Virion	Common names
RNA	IV	+sense ssRNA	Astroviridae	Nkd	Astrovirus
RNA	IV	+sense ssRNA	Arteriviridae	Env	Arterivirus, Equine arteritis virus
RNA	IV	+sense ssRNA	Hepeviridae	Nkd	Hepatitis E virus
RNA	V	-sense ssRNA	Arenaviridae	Env	Lymphocytic choriomeningitis virus
RNA	V	-sense ssRNA	Orthomyxoviridae	Env	Influenza A, Influenza B, Influenza C, Isavirus, Thogotovirus
RNA	V	-sense ssRNA	Paramyxoviridae	Env	Measles virus, Mumps virus, Respiratory syncytial virus, Rinderpest virus, Canine distemper virus
RNA	V	-sense ssRNA	Bunyaviridae	Env	California encephalitis, Hantavirus
RNA	V	-sense ssRNA	Rhabdoviridae	Env	Rabies virus
RNA	V	-sense ssRNA	Filoviridae	Env	Ebola virus Marburg virus
RNA	V	-sense ssRNA	Bornaviridae	Env	Borna disease virus
Reverse Transcribe RNA	VI	ssRNA	Retroviridae	Env	HIV
Reverse Transcribe DNA	VII	dsDNA	Hepadenaviridae	Env	Hepatitis B

Com = Complex
Env = Envelope
Nkd = Naked

Table 6

Classification of Viruses per Baltimore classification method.

By understanding the classification of viruses, especially the Baltimore classification, establishes how the virus generates mRNA for replication purposes. Knowing how a virus produces mRNA in order to replicate identifies possible means to silence a virus by exploiting areas of vulnerabilities. Obstructing transcription of viral DNA or obstructing translation of viral mRNA results in silencing the targeted viral genome, which arrests the viral disease.

Genus Ebolavirus is 1 of 3 members of the *Filoviridae* family (filovirus), along with genus Marburgvirus and genus Cuevavirus.[40] Genus Ebolavirus comprises 5 distinct species:

- Bundibugyo ebolavirus (BDBV)
- Zaire ebolavirus (EBOV)
- Reston ebolavirus (RESTV)
- Sudan ebolavirus (SUDV)
- Taï Forest ebolavirus (TAFV).

BDBV, EBOV, and SUDV have been associated with large EVD outbreaks in Africa, whereas RESTV and TAFV have not. The RESTV species, found in Philippines and the People's Republic of China, can infect humans, but no illness or death in humans from this species has been reported to date.

Zaire Ebolavirus History

There are five distinct species of the Genus Ebolavirus. The WHO data from www.who.int/mediacentre/factsheets/fs103/en/, suggests the species Zaire ebolavirus was the first species detected along the Ebola river in 1976.[41] The outbreaks of the Zaire ebolavirus YEAR (number infected) include: 1976 (318), 1977(1), 1994(52), 1995(315), 1996 (31), 1996(60), 2001-2002(65), 2001-2002(59), 2003(143), 2003(35), 2005(12), 2007(264), 2008(32), 2014(in progress); overall mortality rate from 1976-2008 is 79%. The appearance of the virus suggests either random contact of humans with the virus's natural reservoir as the population of humans becomes increasingly dense in the region where the reservoir resides, or this possibly suggests a cycling phenomenon where the virus exhibits a dormant state.

Ebola represents an intricately sophisticated bio computer program. Replication of the virus occurs inside the host cell. The only representation of the virus in blood and body fluids is detectable when (a) the virus virion is extracellular, (b) antibodies are generated as a response to the virus's presence or (c) if fragments of the virus are detectable when an infected host cell is being broken down and the contents of the infected cell are exposed. From 1976 through 2013 there have been 290 survivors of the 1,387 recorded to have been infected with the Zaire ebolavirus, which suggests there is limited knowledge regarding the virus's long-term effects in the human body.

EBOLA VIRUS: Eloquent example of a simple but, deadly biologic program

Ebola virus is a negative sense RNA virus. The virus's virion enters an endothelial cell, mononuclear phagocyte or a hepatic cell utilizing exterior probes that seek out such cell types. Once the virion has intercepted a potential host cell the nucleocapsid is injected into the cytoplasm of the

cell. The genome of the Ebola virus bypasses the nucleus of the cell and performs all of its life-cycle functions in the cytoplasm of the host cell.

Once in the cytoplasm of the cell, the Ebola virus is transcribed by an RNA-dependent RNA polymerase molecule the Ebola virion carries with it to the host cell. Transcription of the negative sense RNA changes the viral genome to a positive sense mRNA. Once the viral genome is in the form of a positive sense mRNA the genes can be translated by the cell's ribosomes.

Ebola's genome consists of seven proteins.[42,43,44] The seven proteins include 3'-NP- VP35-VP40-GP-VP30-VP24-L-5'. Once transcribed, the positive mRNA is sequenced in the opposite direction. As the genes of the Ebola genome are transcribed various proteins are generated. RNA-dependent RNA polymerase (L), polymerase cofactor protein VP35 and transcription activator protein VP30 accompany the viral genome. The viral polymerase uncoats the nucleocapsid. The viral polymerase then transforms the Ebola virus genome into a positive sense mRNA. The positive sense RNA is then translated to produce structural and nonstructural proteins. The L protein then switches from translation to viral genome replication. The L protein produces negative sense copies of the Ebola genome. The virus self assembles in the host cell. As the Ebola virion buds from the host cell, the transport vehicle acquires the exterior envelop from the cellular membrane of the host cell.

The Ebola virion carries the negative sense RNA genome. Some of Ebola's viral proteins exhibit multiple functions. The proteins generated by translating the Ebola genome include:

1. SEVgp4 (GP1) binds to receptors of target host cell.
2. SEVgp7 (L) polymerase uncoats the nucleocapsid.
3. SEVgp7 (L) + SEVgp2 (VP35) + SEVgp5 (VP30) transcribe the viral genome.
4. Translation mechanisms translate the viral mRNAs.
5. Translation of SEVgp4 mRNA generates secretable glycoprotein GP1,2.
6. Translation of SEVgp6 mRNA generates VP24.
7. Translation of SEVgp1 mRNA generates the nucleoprotein, predominant component of the nucleocapsid. Translation SEVgp5 mRNA of produces VP 30 minor nucleoprotein.
8. Translation of GP1,2 produces the virion probes.
9. SEVgp7 (L) polymerase replicates the viral mRNA producing a negative sense RNA genome.
10. VP24 assists with virion assembly.
11. Translation of the SEVgp3 mRNA produces VP40 coalesce nucleocapsids and cell membrane in virion assembly and budding.

The construct of the Ebola virus genome is presented in Table 7.

RNA Gene	mRNA	SUDV Protein id	Name	Function
----	---	---	Leader sequence	Noncoding; contains replication signal
SEVgp1	NP	YP 138521.1	Nucleoprotein	Predominant component of nucleocapsid; Encapsulation of genomic RNA
SEVgp2	VP35	YP 138522.1		Cofactor in polymerase complex; type I IFN antagonist
SEVgp3	VP40	YP 138523.1	Matrix Protein	Coalesce nucleocapsids and cell membranes in virion assembly (budding)
SEVgp4	GP	YP 138524.1	Glycoprotein	Nonstructural, soluble, secreted glycoprotein Forms dimmers liked by disulfide bonds; processed by furin to yield SGP and delta peptide
SEVgp5	VP30	YP 138525.1	Minor Nucleoprotein	Encapsidation of genomic RNA
SEVgp6	VP24	YP 138526.1	Membrane Associated Structural Protein	Prevents intracellular establishment of viral state by blocking; Virion assembly; Matrix protein
7	L	YP 138527.1	Polymerase Complex Protein	Transcription of viral genome; Replication of viral genome
----	---	----	Trailer sequence	Noncoding, contains replication signal

Table 7

Construct of the SUDV Ebola viral genome.

Ebola virus is representative of a biologic computer program consisting of both mechanisms of protein production and instruction. The Ebola virus program accomplishes the means to translate its genome, defeat host defenses against its existence, copy its genome, assemble its transport vessel (virion), and bud from the host cell. The virus's biologic computer programming is rather compact and very elegant.

The quaternary Biologic Programming steps exhibited by Ebola include:

1. Seeks out and intercepts target host cell.
2. Uncoat the nucleocapsid.
3. Transcribe the genome from negative sense to positive sense.
4. Translate the positive sense viral mRNA.
5. Generate secreted glycoproteins to decrease endothelial barrier function, down-modulated host cell surface molecules responsible for immune surveillance and cell adhesion.
6. Produce VP24 to down-regulate the cell's anti-viral response.
7. Produce copies of the nucleocapsid protein.
8. Produce copies of the exterior virion probes.
9. Replicate the viral genome.
10. Assemble the parts of the virion.
11. Bud the virion through the cell membrane encapsulating with envelope.

Ebola outbreaks occur when one comes in contact with the blood or body fluids of an infected animal and spreads the virus to a local community. Monkeys, pigs, bush game, fruit bats carry the virus. Manifestations of the virus begin with abrupt onset of influenza-like symptoms. The respiratory tract and central nervous system are attacked by the virus. Later stages, the body suffers from multiple organ failures, disseminated intravascular coagulation and focal tissue necrosis.

The Ebola virus is a pathogen which appears very capable of terminating its host. The virus boldly exhibits several decisive actions in order to evade the human surveillance system.

Ebola virus's VP24 protein acts to prevent the infected cell from responding to the presence of the virus. Generally, if a cell has been targeted by a virus, a human cell can alert the immune system that it is hosting a pathogen and cause the cells of the human immune system to kill the infected cell to prevent spread of the virus. VP24 protein interacts with STAT-1 binding of the alpha-1/KPNA1 protein, which prevents activated STAT1 from activating the transcription of IFN-induced genes. By blocking the intracellular interferon alpha/beta (IFN-alpha/beta) and interferon gamma (IFN-gamma) signaling pathways the infected cell is unable to properly signal the body's immune system that it is harboring a lethal pathogen.

By disrupting cell to cell signaling, the Ebola virus delays the immune response against the presence of the virus. Infected mononuclear phagocytes which gobble up the virus, but then carry the pathogen throughout the body including to the lymph nodes, spleen, liver and lungs. Viral particles spread into human tissues activates cytokines, to include TNF-alpha, IL-6 and IL-8, which result in fever and inflammation. The cytopathic effects of the stimulation of signaling molecules results in loss of vascular integrity. Damage occurs to the liver, which leads to coagulopathy. Organ failure, coagulopathy and tissue necrosis leads to Ebola's high mortality.

CHAPTER SIXTEEN

MODIFYING TFIIIA INTO A HUNTER-KILLER PROTEIN TO COMBAT THE THREAT OF EBOLA

In homo sapiens the HIV, HSV, VZV and smallpox virus genomes exist in a DNA form to create the mRNA required to copy the viral genome. Ebola virus presents a different challenge with the fact that in humans the viral genome is a negative sense single stranded RNA virus. The genomes of HIV, HSV, VZV and smallpox can be targeted in the nucleus while the viral genome is embedded in the host nuclear DNA. The genome of the Ebola virus must be targeted in the cytoplasm as it exists as a negative sense RNA strand or a positive sense RNA strand since there is no DNA phase.

The design of the modified TFIIIA molecule utilized to silence the genomes of HIV, HSV, VZV, and smallpox virus may be carried over to silencing the RNA genomes of the Ebola virus. The TFIIIA molecule is generated in the cytoplasm of the cell. Introducing a therapeutic TFIIIA molecule modified to bind to the Ebola RNA genome into the cytoplasm of a cell is natural site for such a molecule to be located. Amino acids attach to thymine and uracil in a similar manner. If the TFIIIA molecule is encoded to target the unique identifier of a critical gene in the Ebola RNA genome then whether the Ebola genome is negative sense ssRNA or positive sense ssRNA, the modified TFIIIA molecule should silence the RNA molecule and arrest the infection. Alternately, modified rRNA molecules/ribosome proteins may be investigated as silencers of viral RNA genomes.

There are multiple versions of the Ebola viral genome. Table 8 lists several strains of Ebola virus. The nucleoprotein gene (NP) starts at nucleotide 54 to 56.

Ebola virus	Date	NCBI Number	Nucltd 30-33	Nucleotides 34-53	Nucltd 54-63
EBOV	06-Feb-2004 Zaire 1995	AY354458	agga agga	Tcttttgtgtgcgaataact Ucuuuugugcgaauaacu	Atgaggaaga Auaggaaga
SUDV	12-Feb-2009 Isolated 2000	NC_ 006432.1	tata uaua	Cttttgtgtgcgaataact Cuuuuugugugcgaauaact	Atgaggaga Augaggaaga
SUDV	14-Mar-2013 Collect 1979	KC242783	aaga aaga	Cttttgtgtgcgaataact cuuuuugugugcgaauaacu	Atgaggaaga Augaggaaga
RESTV	08-Sep-2002	NC_ 004161.1	aaga aaga	Cttttgtgtgcgagtaact cuuuuugugugcgaguaacu	Atgaggaaga Augaggaaga
BUBV	09-Aug-2010 Collect 2007	NC_ 014373.1	aatc aaua	Tttattgtgtgcgagtaact uuuauugugugcgaguaacu	Acgaggaaga Acgaggaaga
CIEBOV	08-Sep-2012 Collect 1994	NC_ 014372.1	gatc gauc	Tttattgtgtgcgaataact uuuauugugugcgaauaacu	Atgaggaaga Augaggaaga

*Note: as presented in the NCBI genome database.
**Nucltd: nucleotide.

Table 8
Multiple versions of Ebola genome regarding nucleotides 30-63.

The Sudan strains of Ebola virus share the genetic unique identifier 5'-ctttttgtgtgcgaataact atgaggaaga-3'; Sudan Ebola strains NC_ 006432.1 and KC242783.2. The Zaire Ebola strain GenBank: AY354458.1, has unique identifier 5'-tcttttgtgtgcgaataact atgaggaaga-3'. Note the difference is the 'c' and 't' at the beginning of the unique identifier are transposed between the Sudan and Zaire strains. The data in Table 8 suggests that a universal TFIIIA molecule could be configured to target the viral genome to include the nucleotides: 'ctttttgtgtgcgaataact atgaggaaga' (cuuuuugugugcgaauaacu augaggaaga). This sequence would appear to cover the two Sudan Ebola strains that are listed. The unique identifiers are similar enough, this configuration may possibly be sufficient to also silence the genomes of Zaire (EBOV), Reston ebolavirus (RESTV), CÔte d'Ivoier ebolavirus (TAFV), and Bundibugyo ebolavirus (BDBV). If not specific enough, molecules can be devised to target each individual Ebola strain as needed and as the Ebola virus may further evolve altering its genome. BLAST query of the human genome identifies 19/19 at 100% (tttttgtgtgcgaataact) of the 30 nucleotides comprising the above unique identifier. BLAST is Basic Local Alignment Search Tool finds regions of proteins or nucleotide sequences in the data base and calculates statistical significance of the matches; located ncbi.nlm.nih.gov/BLAST/. NCBI: National Center for Biotechnology Information.

Table 9 provides the original and modified amino acid sequence to silence the Sudan strains of the Ebola virus, by demonstrating the amino acid binding for the TFIIIA molecule to target the nucleotide sequence from nucleotide 34 to 63. Since Ebola is an RNA virus with no DNA phase, there is no reliable presence of a TATA box in an RNA genome.

Number	Loop	Original Amino Acid Sequence	Modified Amino Acid Sequence
1	Alpha	SANYSKAWKLDA	ESSKKSSKSSKK
2	Beta	GKAFIRDYHLSR	RSSKRSSKSSRE
3	Gamma	DQKFNTKSNLKK	RSSNNSSKSSNN
4	Delta	KKTFKKHQQLKI	ESSKNSSKSSRN
5	Epsilon	GKHFASPSKLKR	RSSRNSSNSSRN
6	Zeta	SFVAKTWTELLK	SFVASTWTELLS
7	Eta	RKTFKRKDYLKQ	SKTFKSKDYLKQ
8	Theta	GRTYTTVFNLGS	GSTYTTVFSLGS
9	Iota	GKTFAMKQSLTR	GSTFAMKQSLTS

Table 9

The modified amino acid sequences for the nine loops of TFIIIA.

Taking the modifications presented in Table 9 and applying them to the TFIIIA molecule results in the molecule presented in Figure 32. Alternately, the 25 nucleotide sequence 5'-ttttgtgtgcgaataactatgagga-3' is shared between the Zaire and Sudan strains and might be used as a universal unique identifier.

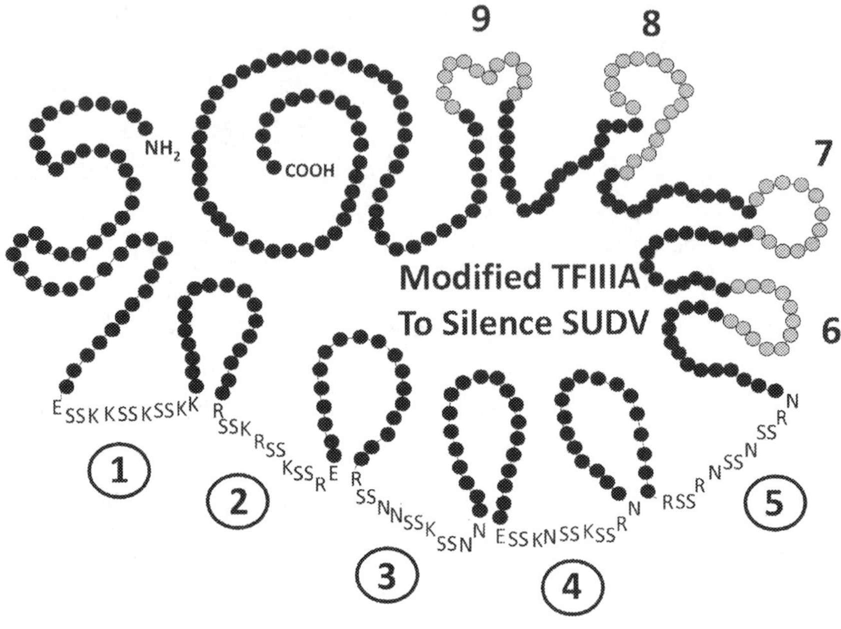

Figure 32
Modified Transcription Factor IIIA molecule to silence Ebola genome.

The TFIIIA molecule is a nuclear signaling protein and functions as a transport protein. The TFIIIA molecule migrates into the nucleus of the cell. Part of the construct of the TFIIIA molecule acts as a signal to usher the molecule into the nucleus. To silence DNA embedded viruses, it is an advantage to have the TFIIIA molecule naturally migrate into the nucleus. Given the Ebola virus bypasses the nucleus and functions solely in the cytoplasm of the cell, it is necessary to try to maintain the TFIIIA molecule in the cytoplasm rather than having the therapeutic TFIIIA molecule migrate into the nucleus of the cell.

Our intent is to additionally modify the TFIIIA molecule for Ebola virus to cause the TFIIIA molecule to remain in the cell's cytoplasm to optimize its opportunity to intercept the Ebola mRNA and silence transcription and/or translation of the Ebola genome. The 3' (COOH) end of the TFIIIA molecule offers the cell signaling means to restrict the modified TFIIIA molecule to the scope of the cytosol. As seen with the modified version of the TFIIIA polypeptide described to combat coronavirus, the 3' tail end of the protein can be altered to confine the modified version of the TFIIIA protein in the cytoplasm.

Polypeptides destined to enter the nucleus are labeled with a particular sequence of amino acids termed the nuclear location sequence (NLS). The gateways through the nuclear membrane separating the cytoplasm from the inner chamber of the nucleus recognize the NLS coded into the structure of the polypeptide and grant access to polypeptides which possess the proper NLS.

The amino acid sequence 'PDKKKMKLK' present in the 3' tail of the native TFIIIA polypeptide (TI9606) from amino acid 303 to 311 acts as the nuclear location sequence, giving the molecule access to the translocate from the cell's cytoplasm to the nucleus of the cell.[18] It is desirable to maintain the modified TFIIIA in the cytoplasm and prevent the polypeptide from entering into the nucleus. In order to trap the modified TFIIIA polypeptide in the cytoplasm of a cell to optimize the molecule's effectiveness, the lysine amino acids of the native NSL are changed to threonine. The modified TFIIIA polypeptide is to possess the modified amino acid sequence of amino acids 303 to 311 as described as 'PDTTTMTLT'.

As a point of discussion, the Ebolavirus's genome, like coronavirus, morphs between a negative-sense version and a positive-sense version. It is likely, that if the modified version of the TFIIIA polypeptide designed to seek out and bind to the uracil tail of the negative-sense version of the coronavirus evolved to be an effective therapy against coronavirus, then this same molecule would likely have a beneficial effect in combating ebolavirus infections. The advantage described herein is that there may be at least two different versions of TFIIIA protein which can be pursued to directly combat an Ebolavirus pandemic.

CHAPTER SEVENTEEN

THE FUTURE: MULTI-FUNCTION mRNA PHARMACEUTICAL AGENTS UTILIZING THE -UAA- 'AND' COMMAND

The use of UAA (TAA) codon as a joiner between two nucleotide coding sequences in artificial mRNAs will facilitate the opportunity to create two or more simultaneous actions inside a cell, given the administration of a single drug. This will lead to a new class of drugs, referred to as 'intelligent programable' pharmaceuticals. By using the UAA codon code, a nucleotide sequence for the production of a protein to include an enzyme, a cell surface receptor, a transcription factor can be activated inside a cell in synchrony with another or multiple enzymes, cell surface receptors, transcription factors or other polypeptides.

The option of being able to use an AND command between two nucleotide coding sequences allows for more than one coding sequence to be translated. Two, three, four or more coding sequences could be translated. The number of translated sequences comprising an artificial mRNA is limited only to the total number of nucleotides which can fit into one transport vehicle which will carry the artificial mRNA to the target cell.

The nucleotide sequences comprising an artificial mRNA can code for the same polypeptide or the nucleotide sequences can code for dissimilar polypeptides. If an artificial mRNA can carry two, three or four nucleotide coding sequences, then the mRNA could produce two, three or four of the same polypeptides respectfully; or two, three, or four dissimilar polypeptides respectfully. See Figure 33.

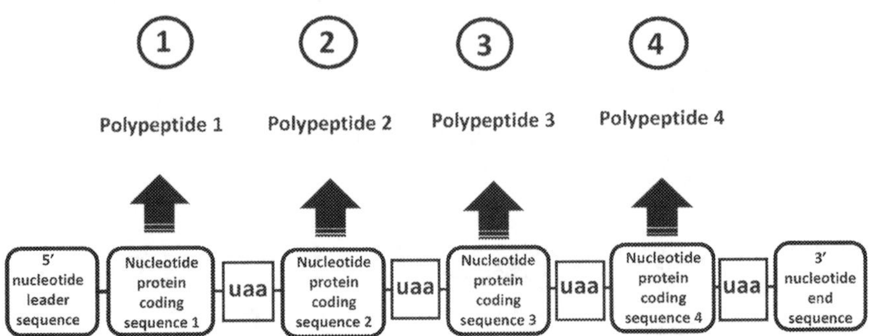

Figure 33
One mRNA could code for four different polypeptides.

Amplification of the therapeutic process. Instead of a target cell being given one therapeutic agent, multiple copies of the therapeutic agent can be delivered to a target cell. See Figure 34.

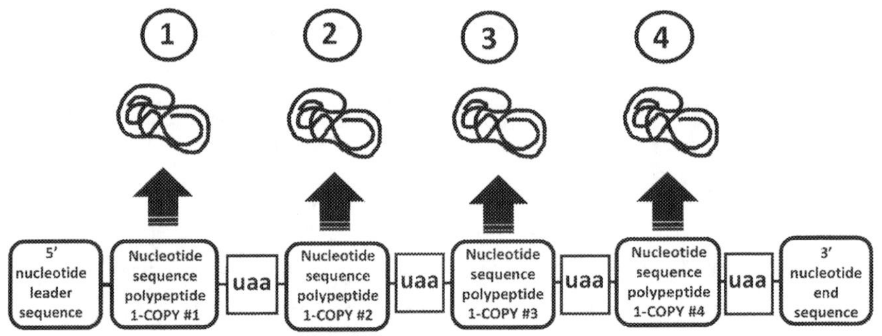

Figure 34
Multiple copies of the same polypeptide can be coded into a single mRNA.

Such an mRNA would amplify the therapy. If such an mRNA could code for four of the same proteins, and if this same mRNA had 30 adenine nucleotides comprising its tail, then 4 x 30 could generate 120 like therapeutic proteins with one mRNA.

There is a necessity to be able to assemble more than one functionally translatable nucleotide sequence in an artificial mRNA. Many cell surface receptors are comprised of alpha and beta components, thus in such a case two differing polypeptides are required to replicate such a cell surface receptor. Some molecules, such as hemoglobin are comprised of multiple proteins, thus there is a need for the capacity to generate at least four polypeptides in synchronicity if one were to attempt to generate complex intracellular molecules. See Figure 35.

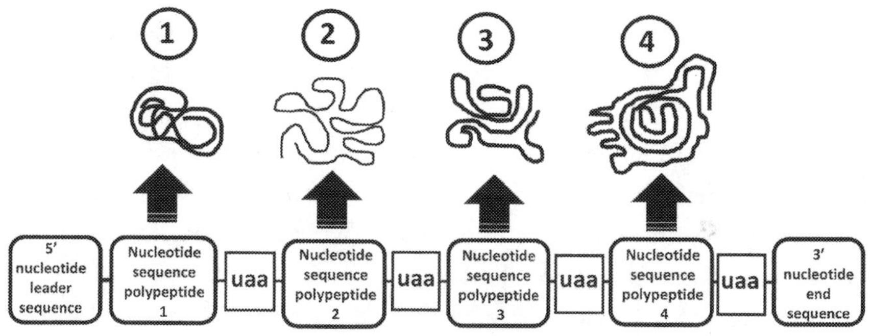

Figure 35
Different polypeptides can be coded into a single mRNA.

The ability to create several different proteins by selectively coding the nucleotide sequencing of one mRNA, paves the way to developing an entirely new and revolutionary branch of pharmaceuticals. The ability to create two different proteins by prompting the cellular ribosomes to decode a single mRNA, which is constructed with the nucleotide sequencing for two or more proteins, makes it possible to have two separate therapeutic effects being conducted inside a target cell simultaneously. This is different than treating a patient with two different drugs and hoping that the effects of both reach the same cell. Coding a mRNA to generate two different proteins, ensures that a cell being targeted for a specific therapy benefits from two different medically therapeutic effects at the same time.

An immediate use of the -UAA- AND application could be seen with the COVID-19 vaccine therapy. Certain proteins may be utilized to enhance the effectiveness of the coronavirus spike protein cell surface receptor. The ability to design an mRNA which carried both the coding for an effective coronavirus spike protein cell surface receptor and a booster protein to enhance the action of the spike protein cell surface receptor would optimize such a vaccine. Having the coding for both proteins written into the same mRNA would mean that it was guaranteed both proteins would be generated in the same target cell, and would ensure that the booster protein was actually physically present in the same cell as the coronavirus spike protein cell surface receptor.

Cell surface receptors are often comprised of two differing proteins. Having the means to design mRNAs to code for two different proteins makes it possible to mount artificial cell surface receptors on the exterior of the membrane of target cells. An incredibly diverse range of medically therapeutic possibilities comes into existence if medical science is able to mount artificial cell surface receptors on target cells. Several of the categories of pharmacologic intervention would include: (1) enhancing the recognition of threats by the immune system by alerting the immune system to pathologic cell surface receptors; (2) using artificial cell surface receptors to tag cancer cells or other pathologic cells for elimination; (3) utilizing artificial cell surface receptors to deliver large-size therapeutic molecules to target cells (diabetes, caused by faulty insulin cell surface receptors may be a promising therapeutic effort).

An entirely different and exciting use of the -UAA- 'AND' command would be to invoke an 'IF-THEN' pharmacologic treatment strategy. Abstract 'IF THEN' statements can be constructed using an artificial mRNA carrying nucleotide coding for two or more proteins. The actions of one polypeptide generated by an artificial mRNA may be dependent upon the conditions found in the target cell receiving the said mRNA or dependent upon the actions of the other polypeptides generated by the same mRNA. Intelligent pharmaceuticals using artificial mRNAs to deliver more than one polypeptide at a time to a target cell, may be able to positively react in a programmed fashion to the environment found inside a target cell to deliver a calculated medical therapeutic response.

Programmed intelligent responses can be contrived to occur in target cells. Such intelligent mRNA pharmaceuticals can be constructed to kill cancer cells, to combat viral infections, to destroy invading bacteria or parasites, to fix structural problems such as heart disease. Drugs which are capable of making decisions based on the environment existing inside a target cell is the intelligent pharmaceutical technology of the future, but could be realizable in the matter of just a few years.

CHAPTER EIGHTEEN

THE GAME CHANGER: 'IF-THEN' STATEGY TO CREATE INTELLIGENT mRNA PHARMACEUTICAL AGENTS

This recoding of the nucleotide sequencing of the messenger RNA technology to generate modified transcription factors as described herein, can be used to treat various medical disease processes in addition to viral diseases. Recoding of the nucleotide sequencing of the messenger RNA of TFIIIA supplies the means to generate other medically useful TFIIIA polypeptides that would be capable of intercepting and binding to other medically significant targets. The messenger RNA used to code for other transcription factors could also be recoded to generate transcription factors that would intercept and modulate additional medically therapeutic targets. Modifying mRNAs to generate through translation modified transcription factors would facilitate treatments for various viral diseases, bacterial diseases, parasitic infections, inflammatory arthritis, osteoarthritis, connective tissue diseases, myopathies, endocrinopathies, and many forms of cancer.

The development of new drugs will no longer be a 'hit-and-miss' venture which has plagued pharmaceutical research for centuries. The creation of mRNA therapies will be much more directed and specific, time from conception of a drug to marketing of a product will be dramatically shortened compared to current R&D science. This new approach to drug research and development will require a much more abstract approach to thinking about pharmaceuticals. Those pursuing such development will need to see the mRNAs as sophisticated computer programs.

The software of the IF-THEN intelligent mRNA pharmaceutical is dependent upon understanding that the three codon code of 'UAA' (TAA) causes a discontinuation of the translation process of a nucleotide coding sequence, but in addition represents the signal to continue reading the mRNA in search of another action to be taken; where three codon code of 'UAG' (TAG) specifies that the ribosome reader is to release the emerging polypeptide and disassemble. Thus 'UAA' exhibits an 'AND' function in the RNA and DNA coding schemes, while 'UAG' acts as a true 'STOP' code for purposes of the actions of the ribosome reading unit. There are thus at least three commands AUG which represents START, AUG which represents STOP, and UAA which represents AND.

With three commands to work with, abstract 'intelligent' pharmaceutical agents can be constructed. Intelligent mRNA pharmaceuticals provide the capacity to generate two or more polypeptides in cells simultaneously. Intelligent mRNA pharmaceuticals then can theoretically produce two or more actions inside of a cell at one time. Pharmaceutical agents to date are monoaction molecules. A single drug is intended to generate one medically therapeutic action. Unfortunately, one drug may lead to a wide variety of side effects in differing people.

Nature repeatedly demonstrates the use of the same polypeptide to generate different responses depending upon the cell type the polypeptide is created in or is interacting with in the human body. Adrenaline, is one example of a molecule which produces a wide variety of responses depending upon the cells the molecule interacts with throughout the body. Nature uses molecules of the same design and construct to accomplish differing actions, and in this manner efficiently conserves precious resources. Estrogen and testosterone both generate numerous actions throughout the human body, which are the key hormones responsible for the differing sexual features of the female and male bodies respectfully.

Having START, STOP and AND command functions to work with to construct mRNAs makes it possible to generate smart pharmaceutical mRNA agents which are capable of responding to the intracellular environment. The AND command allows for the mRNA to be constructed with one, two or more nucleotide segments which each are coded for and capable of generating a different polypeptide. Being able to generate more than one polypeptide using a single agent means multiple actions can be made to occur within a cell at the same time.

If a intelligent pharmaceutical mRNA is designed to generate two polypeptides, then two separate actions may occur as a result of two medically therapeutic proteins being produced through translation of the single mRNA. The IF-THEN statement would be exemplified by the intelligent pharmaceutical mRNA being translated and generating two different polypeptides. The first polypeptide generated by translating the intelligent-mRNA transits the cell in search of a target protein. If the first polypeptide encounters the target protein and binds to the target protein, then a conformational change occurs in the first polypeptide. The now altered tertiary structure of the first polypeptide interacts with the second polypeptide generated by the translation of the intelligent-mRNA. The binding of the first and second polypeptides generated by translation of the intelligent-mRNA causes a conformation change in the three-dimensional structure of the second polypeptide which activates the second polypeptide to take action inside the cell. Such actions may include the second polypeptide becoming an active enzyme, or the second polypeptide becoming an active transcription factor, or the second polypeptide becoming an intracellular or extracellular protein such as a hormone. See Figure 36.

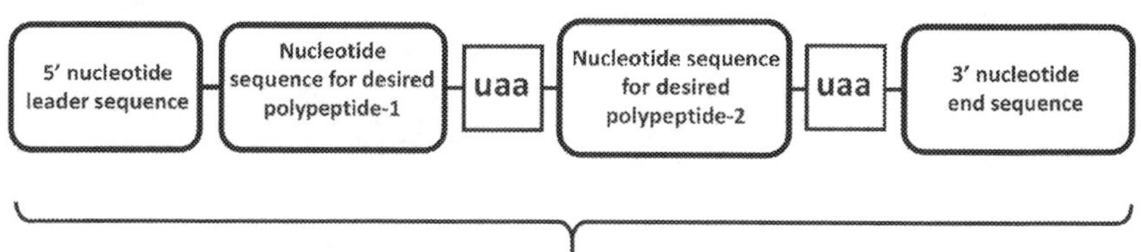

Figure 36
A medically therapeutic mRNA may contain nucleotide coding sequences for two polypeptides.

The two nucleotide coding sequences would produce two different polypeptides. See Figure 37.

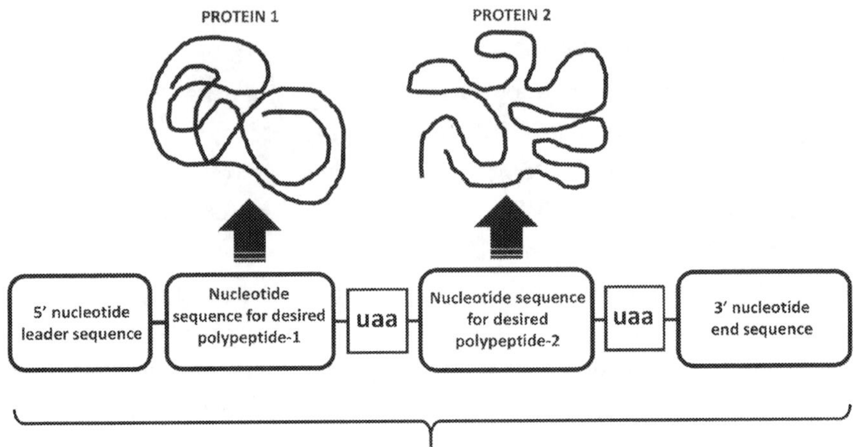

Figure 37
A medically therapeutic mRNA may contain nucleotide coding sequences for two polypeptides which would generate two different proteins.

Once generated by the ribosome decoding the mRNA, the two proteins would be released into the cytoplasm of the cell. See Figure 38.

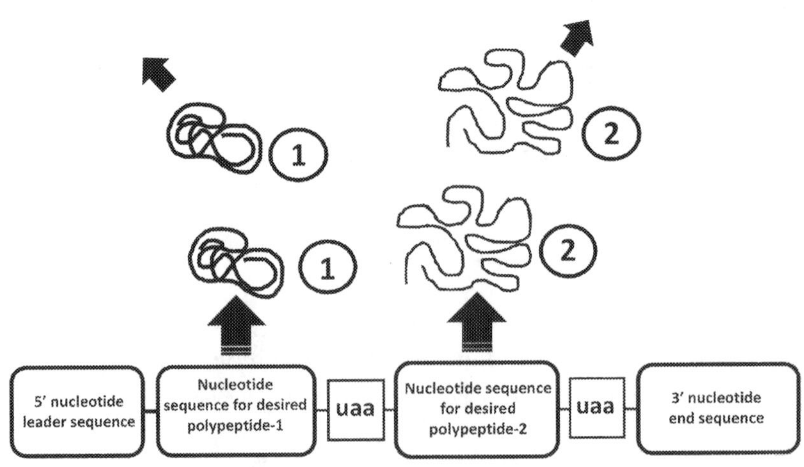

Figure 38
A medically therapeutic mRNA may contain nucleotide coding sequences for two polypeptides which would generate two different proteins which are then released into the cytoplasm.

In Figure 38, following translation of nucleotide sequence 1, polypeptide 1 is generated. If no target protein is encountered in the cell cytoplasm, then no further action takes place. Nucleotide sequence 2 of the artificial mRNA is translated, and polypeptide 2 is created, but polypeptide 2 in its current state is unable to bind with any intracellular molecules.

Scenario #2: Following translation of nucleotide sequence 1, polypeptide 1 is generated and polypeptide 1 does locate and makes contact with the intracellular target protein. The intracellular target protein could include such molecules as a viral protein or a protein produced by a cancerous cell or a protein produced by a bacterium or a protein produced by a genetic mutation. Upon binding to the intracellular target protein, polypeptide 1's three-dimensional structure is altered such that polypeptide 1 is now capable of binding to polypeptide 2. See Figure 39.

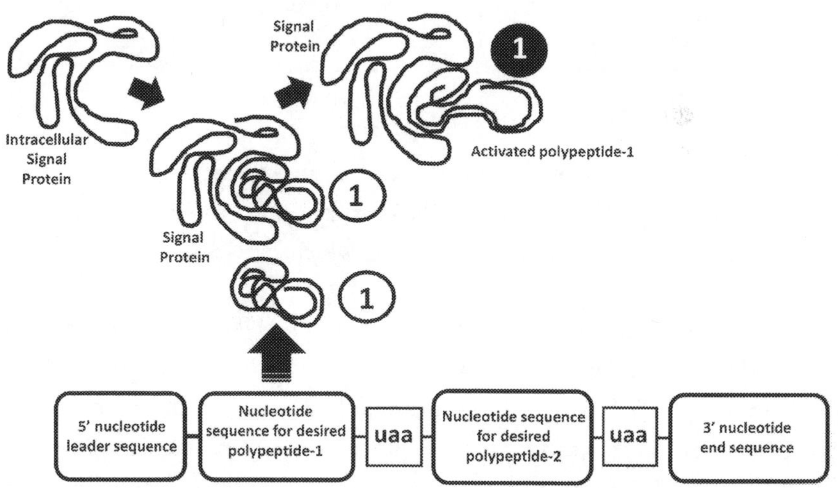

Figure 39

Protein #1 interacts with target proteins, undergoes a conformational change, which makes protein #1 capable of binding with protein #2.

Once the complex formed by the target protein and polypeptide 1 binds to polypeptide 2, the three-dimensional shape of polypeptide 2 is altered. With polypeptide 2 bonded to polypeptide 1, which is bonded to the target protein, polypeptide 2's shape is altered such that a portion of the molecule is transformed into one or more active binding sites. See Figure 40. The altered polypeptide 2 is capable of acting as a receptor or an enzyme or transcription factor. The altered polypeptide 2 can become an effective medical therapy given the proper circumstances inside the target cell which translated the artificial mRNA.

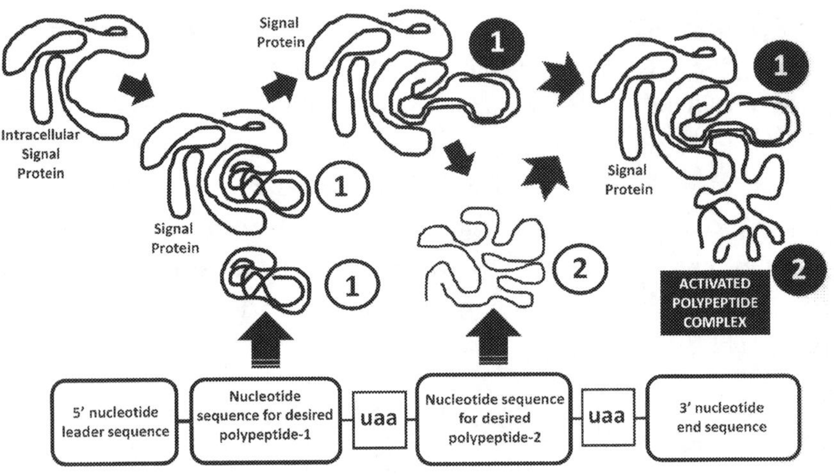

Figure 40
Protein #1 interacts with target proteins, undergoes a conformational change, binds with protein #2, which causes a conformation change in protein #2, which activates protein #2.

Understanding the role of the UAA as an AND command opens up the construct of intelligent-mRNAs to an almost infinite array of medically therapeutic possibilities. Such a therapeutic strategy could be enlisted to preferentially kill targeted cancer cells, or viral infected cells, or modify the behavior of genetically altered cells or change the course of cells suffering from an abnormal protein metabolism related to disease or due to aging.

CHAPTER NINETEEN

ESTABLISHING A mRNA RESEARCH & DEVELOPMENT TEAM

INTELLIGENT pharmaceuticals will demand much more abstract and spatial thinking than prior drug development has necessitated. Not only will future pharmaceutical research require the biomedical knowledge of the medical problem requiring treatment, but it will be necessary for researcher to understand how three-dimensional molecules interact with each other in the unique realm created by the cytoplasm of the human cell.

Future drug research will require the participants to understand not only the structure of molecules as they exist in space, but will necessitate that if the building blocks of such structures are changed in an attempt to improve the therapeutic value of the drug, how this will alter the three-dimensional shape of the molecule. Being intimately knowledgeable of the three-dimensional structure of proteins is a necessity in using proteins as therapeutic molecules. Proteins interact with other structures by means of their construct and resultant shape.

Pharmaceutical researchers will not only be required to understand how therapeutic proteins work as drugs, and how the shape of the polypeptide contributes to the therapeutic mission of the protein, but also they will be required to know how to code for the design of such therapeutic molecules utilizing nucleotide sequencing in order to construct medically therapeutic mRNA molecules.

The construct of medically therapeutic mRNA molecules will require teams of experts to accomplish such tasks. Engineers will play a vital role in designing and constructing such molecules. The inefficient, often disastrous prior 'Try and See' method of research will fall to the much more intense and target specific engineered means of drug development. The old means of making as many as 10,000 attempts at development of a drug before finding a suitable agent, will rapidly evolve into drug development where in essence novel pharmaceuticals will be generated with a high degree of reliability and functionality on the first try at drug testing.

The key to new drug development will be a team of integrated experts from differing science and engineering backgrounds designing new drugs and the use of dynamic 3D computer models of the interior environment of human cells to test the behavior of new drugs prior to animal or human testing.

Much more abstract thinking which will create much more specific therapy. Typically, you do not want to go to a doctor who wants to try a different method of medical management every time you go see him or her, but on the other hand, when confronted with a new threat of gigantic proportion such as the COVID-19 global pandemic, the population needs new ideas to combat such an emergency.

Members of a Messenger RNA Development Team should include:

Electrical Engineers (programmable coding expertise)
Mechanical Engineers (three-dimensional molecular structuring, fluid mechanics)
Chemical Engineers (thermodynamics, chemical bonding and repelling)
Molecular Biologists (amino acid-nucleotide bonding)
Biomedical Engineers (packaging and delivery expertise)
Infectious Disease Specialists (bacterial, viral, parasite threats)
Intensive Care Physicians (clinical expertise)
Virologists (Specific characteristics of a threatening virus)
Pharmaceutical Manufacturing (assembly, production, distribution of product)

Engineers and physicians traditionally do not 'think' the same. Core engineers such as electrical engineers, mechanical engineers and chemical engineers do not approach a problem in the same manner as a physician would attempt to solve a problem. Due to differences in fundamental thinking and training, the two disciplines tend to clash when placed in the same room to discuss matters of science and engineering.

The underlying reason behind the inability for core engineers to have a meaningful discussion with medical scientists is the two disciplines use differing portions of their brains and each discipline has been taught to approach a problem with a different set of protocols. Engineers tend to use the posterior aspect of their brain while physicians use the anterior portion of the brain. See Figure 41. Engineers utilize mathematical tools and known constants to approach solving a problem, were as physicians use memorized facts and learned algorithms to solve problems. The two approaches are as different, as a physician might comment, 'why don't you know that?', while an engineer might comment 'why can't you figure that out?'.

In general, a physician's deductive reasoning tends to organize observed facts into bundled information, and check such groupings of data against learned algorithms searching for a match. A physician's brain functions like a high-speed network router linked to a memory system. An engineer's brain enters a deep scanning mode in order to sift through fine details of a project in order to look for patterns not previously recognized or appreciated. Physicians often times take what appear to be a grouping of abstract facts and assimilate such data into medical diagnoses, in part because in some cases there is just not a clear concrete means, per physical exam or testing, to make a diagnosis. Engineers tend to almost always rely and build upon known constants and proven mathematical formulas to arrive at conclusions. The challenge is that many aspects of the human body remain poorly understood, testing often times produces limited information, more than one organic system may fail at any given time, and the body is dynamic, invariably changing the parameters of the medical condition. Both modes of approaching a problem bring to the research table differing, but important strengths.

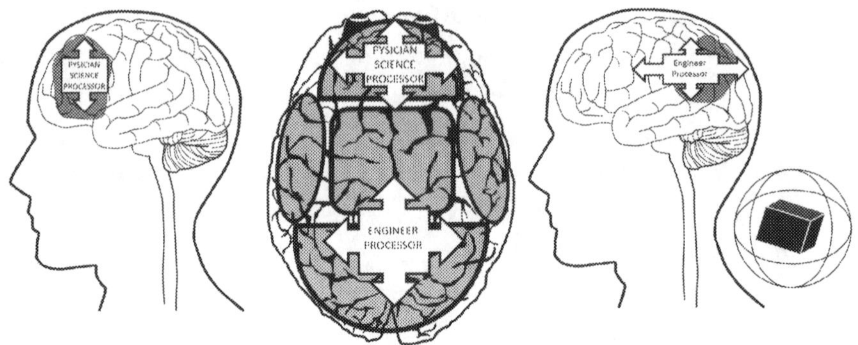

Figure 41

A physician/scientist uses anterior brain function, while and engineer's brain utilizes posterior spatial processing.

Still, both disciplines, engineering and medicine, need to find a common ground and work intellectually together to arrive at a means to generate effective mRNA therapies. The unique talents of both disciplines will yield far more success combining forces together, than either struggling without the other. It is important each discipline recognize the inherent strength the other discipline brings to the research and capitalize on the use of such talent.

Both engineers and physicians need to become comfortable with using computer modeling of a cell to predict the outcomes of introducing drugs into the human body. Physicians tend to be more comfortable with the outcomes of mouse, rat, ape and human experiments. Engineers tend to utilize mathematical models to build bridges, erect buildings, construct roads, design ground vehicles, tanker ships and aircraft. Computer models will become important with understanding and predicting how mRNAs and polypeptides will interact with in the intracellular environment.

CHAPTER TWENTY

VIRTUAL LABORATORY TO CREATE 3D INTELLIGENT PHARMACEUTICALS

Computer modeling will become vitally important when exploring the designs of proposed three-dimensional polypeptides. Medically therapeutic polypeptides created to interact with native molecules in the cell will require understanding of how differing three-dimensional amino acid structures fit together in space. But it is not only how the amino acids physically occupy space, but the electrical charges the amino acids carry, which dictate the success of a proposed medically therapeutic polypeptide.

Aberrant intracellular molecules existing as the result of a malignancy or a virus or a bacteria or other inflammatory conditions will complicate the research and development process above that of designing therapeutic polypeptides to interact with native molecules. Aberrant molecules refer to proteins which are generated inside a cell due to a cancerous condition or an infectious or inflammatory condition. Aberrant molecules are structurally different than native molecules and will need to be computer modeled as their own class of simulation with adjustments made to incorporate their own unique properties and behaviors in the intracellular environment.

The next level of complexity of the design of therapeutic intracellular polypeptides 'requires' computer simulation and engineering design skill. Designing a therapeutic polypeptide to interact with either a 'native' molecule or an 'aberrant' molecule in order to create a change in the therapeutic polypeptide's structure, enough such that the therapeutic polypeptide will now successfully bind to a second therapeutic polypeptide and evoke change in the structure of the second therapeutic polypeptide to cause the second therapeutic polypeptide to perform an action, would be impossible without computer modeling. Again, all of this modeling will need to be representative of the intracellular environment to include all of the organelles (to include the nuclear envelope, endoplasmic reticulum, Golgi apparatus, mitochondria, vacuoles) and the milieu of proteins occupying the cytoplasm. The computer modeling will need to account for the 3D physical presence of all of these structures as well as the electrical surface charges exerted by these organelles and proteins.

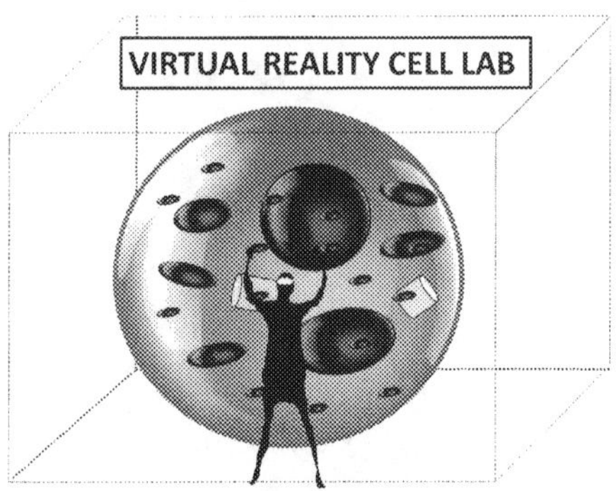

Figure 42
Virtual laboratory to facilitate animated real-time 3D modeling of the interior of a human cell.

Such computer modeling of the inner workings of the human cell and therapeutic polypeptides will result in the construct of dynamic intelligent drugs which will be capable of reacting to the environment found inside a target cell. Actions taken by such therapeutic mRNAs will be based just on not the mRNA finding its way into a cell, but based on factors the resultant polypeptides find inside the cell. Such drug development utilizing a multi-discipline approach and computer modeling will lead to cures for the most challenging cancers, the most virulent infections, the most devastating inflammatory and genetic medical conditions.

The virtual model of a human cell would be an essential tool to assist in the investigation of the actions of medically therapeutic proteins once introduced into target cells. Such a tool would be helpful in understanding how molecules navigate through the cytoplasm of the cell and how they would interact with the various internal structures of the cell. The virtual model of a cell would not only be able to assist in the study of how a proposed medically therapeutic protein would function inside a cell, but such modeling would help predict potential adverse side effects which might occur if such a protein were administered to human subjects.

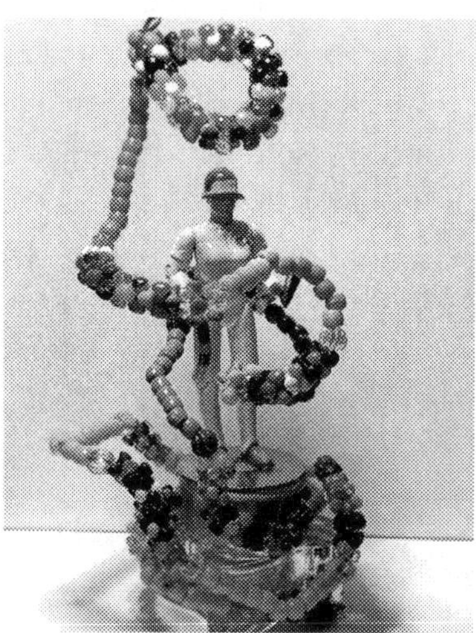

Figure 43
Virtual laboratory to dynamically change the construct of therapeutic molecules.

In the case of the ebolavirus, the real wild type ebolavirus can be broken down to a computer-generated model of the virus. Such a model could be introduced into the 3D model of a human cell to study how the virus functions inside the cell. Such modeling would be useful in analyzing strategies to neutralize the replication of the virus and halt the infectivity of the virus.

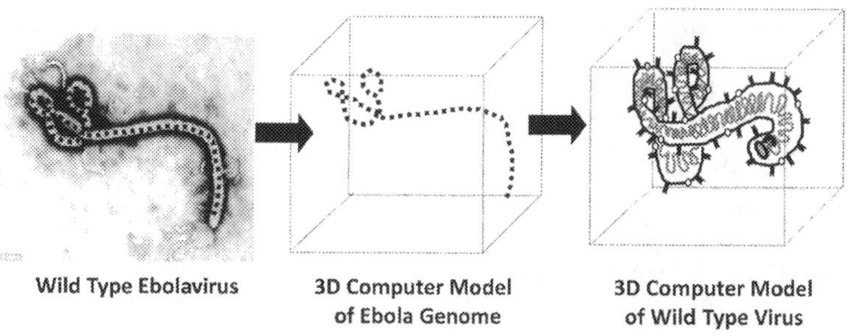

Figure 44
3D modeling of pathogens such as Ebola to better understand how they invade and take over human cells.

Such computer graphics modeling software would be able to generate 3D imagery of the Transcription Factor IIIA (TFIIIA) polypeptide. Such computer modeling would help analyze the structural changes of altering one or more amino acids comprising the protein, in order to predict what would happen to the overall shape of the protein and how this affect the bonding characteristics of the altered protein. Change of the three-dimensional structure of the protein may improve the therapeutic function of the molecule, while some changes in the structure of the protein may diminish the effectiveness of the protein as a pharmaceutical agent. The optimal design of a protein could be worked out in a virtual lab prior to animal or human testing.

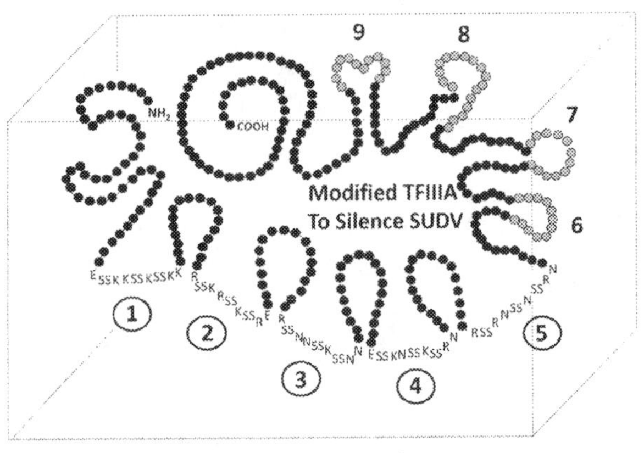

3D Computer Model of TFIIIA

Figure 45

Computer modeling of the 3D structure of the TFIIIA molecule to optimize design therapeutic agents to combat infectious agents.

Thus, molecules such as mRNAs which code for medically therapeutic TFIIIA polypeptides could be devised. A software version of the mRNA could be inserted into a computer model of the cell. Analysis of how effective the virtual mRNA would interact with the cell's ribosomes could be studied. The translation of the mRNA could be modeled and the resultant medically therapeutic TFIIIA polypeptide could be generated in the virtual cell. Once the mRNA is transcribed and the TFIIIA protein is released by the ribosome which constructed the polypeptide, the actions of the TFIIIA could be viewed in the virtual world of the cytoplasm of the cell. See Figure 46. How well the computer software generated version of the TFIIIA intercepts and binds to the intended therapeutic target can be studied. The TFIIIA can be modified in real time to enhance the performance of the medically therapeutic polypeptide.

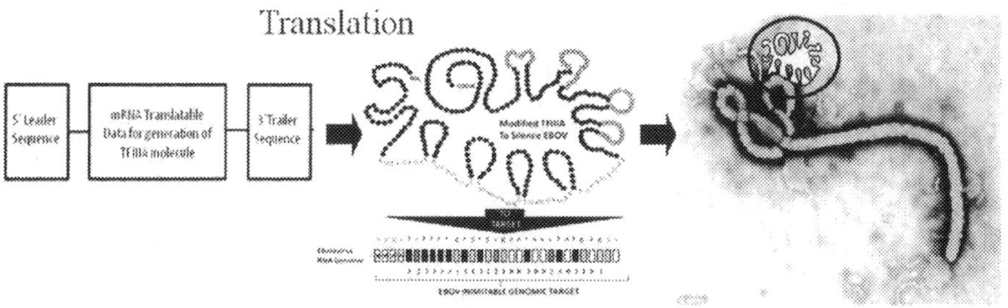

TFIIIA Messenger RNA TFIIIA To Silence Ebola TFIIIA Engaging Ebola

Figure 46
Computer modeling of the TFIIIA molecule binding to coronavirus genome to neutralize the virus.

A virtual lab modeling the details of the intracellular environment, would be able to take a therapeutic molecule and run through virtual scenarios to see if the artificial study molecule binds to or otherwise interacts with unintended native proteins or RNAs in the cell. A virtual lab could change cell type. There are approximately 220 differing cell types comprising the construct of the tissues of the human body. A virtual lab could alter the intracellular environment to match the therapeutic molecule with the proper cell type that the therapeutic molecule is to target. The potential side effects of intelligent pharmaceuticals could be predicted and possibly significantly diminished by optimizing the design of such intelligent therapeutic molecules.

CHAPTER TWENTY-ONE

PROPER STEWARDS OF THE PLANET

-Pollutants and Global Warming provide the perfect maelstrom for the incubation of increasingly malignant viruses-

Humans are the responsible stewards of planet Earth. COVID-19 has humanity realizing that a virus, a mere strip of genetic code comprised of a little over 29,900 bits of biocomputer information, is capable of infecting and killing a significant number of people, wreaking havoc on society and devastating the world economy.

The number of virus-like particles inhabiting our planet is thought to be somewhere in the order of 10^{31}, compared to humans, which is estimated to be approximately 7.8 billion inhabitants.[45,46,47,48] Viruses are thought to be the most numerous genetic coded entities on the planet.

So, to try to grasp how large of a number 10^{31} actually is, one might consider this would be equal to 1 trillion (10^{12}) x 1 trillion (10^{12}) x 1 billion (10^{6}) x 10. Another way to look at it, would be to count the number of stars in the universe. There are an estimated 100-200 billion stars in our galaxy.[49] There are an estimated 200 billion galaxies comprising the universe.[50] Thus, the high estimate of the total number of stars in the universe would equal 200 billion multiplied by 200 billion, which equals 4 x 10^{22}. So, even with a generous estimate, there are far less stars in the known universe, than virus particles inhabiting Earth. This suggests there is an abundance of genetic material carried by viruses, which is constantly entering and replicating in side hosts cells, and likely genetic material is being shared with host cells, all across the planet.

Typically, a select grouping of viruses, in general, will infect only a certain type of animal or plant life form, with infrequent transinfectivity of closely related species. As mentioned earlier, there are approximately

219 differing viruses which tend to infect humans. Viruses which infect humans, may be generated by other species. We have seen on news reports in the last few decades, viruses occasionally being transmitted to humans from bird species or higher order mammals.

Viruses are unable to replicate without a host cell. Viruses either carry their own replication machinery, such as coronavirus, or viruses depend upon the biologic machinery of the host cell which it invades, in order to generate copies of the viral genome and virion. Even if the virus brings with its genome the coding to construct its own ribosomal replication protein, all viruses still depend upon the host cell in order to utilize the resources and energy of the cell to generate copies of itself.

Viruses interacting with host cells is likely one of the driving forces of evolution. Viruses may work at all levels of life to change the DNA of species, which has led to the changes that have seen in life over the eons. Eight to ten percent of human DNA is thought to be comprised of segments of viral DNA.[51,52] This would suggest that humans are much more intimately connected to lower life forms than what we would generally like to realize.

As humanity has expanded across the face of the Earth and the presence of humans has polluted the planet, we may be adversely affecting the lower levels of the ecosystem, which we all depend upon. The plastics, polymers, toxins we continually introduce into the ground, water and atmosphere as we industrialize and dominate the planet for profit, may be influencing and altering the genetic code of viruses. Viruses infecting the lower life forms consisting of bacteria, insects, plants, reptiles, amphibians and lower level mammals may be a breeding increasingly aggressive and violent viral configurations. The changes in the viral coding become more virulent, as the destructive genetic code rises through the ecosystem to humans.

As the planet heats up due to the effects of progressive industrialization and burning of fossil fuels, any addition of heat to a biologic process generally causes increased activity of the biologic process. It is estimated that 200,000 species of virus live in the oceans and waterways spanning the globe.[53,54] As humans indiscriminately introduce pollutants into the general environment across the planet, the effects of these toxins may have deleterious consequences regarding alterations to the genomes of viruses and the many lower order lifeforms. The actions of humans may be directly affecting the mutation rates of malicious viruses throughout the ecosystem.

We may see and we may become victim of more aggressive viral infections at a rate faster than what would generally be expected, due to the combined effects of heating of the planet and widespread pollution of our air, land and oceans. Humans are the responsible custodians of the world we live in. Our race needs to act vigorously to protect the one and only planet we depend upon, for the health and welfare of our generation and for the sake of all of the future generations to come. We are the stewards of the planet, and the cultivators of our future offspring.

REFERENCES

1. M Woolhouse, F Scott, Z Hudson, R Howey, M Chase-Topping, Human viruses: discovery and emergence, Philos Trans R Soc Lond B Biol Sci. 2012 Oct 19; 367(1604): 2864–2871.

2. A M Hemenstine, The 5 kinds of nucleotides, ThoughtCo.com, 10 December 2019.

3. L C Brody, Nucleotide, National Human Genome Research Institute, genome.gov, accessed 14 Jun 2020.

4. Uridine, Wikipedia, en.m.wikipedia.org, last accessed 14 Jun 2020.

5. Amino acid, Wikipedia, en.m.wikipedia.org, last accessed 14 Jun 2020.

6. K Arms, P S Camp, Biology, Holt, Rinehart and Winston, W. B. Saunders Company, New York, 1979.

7. J K Pal, S S Ghaskadbi, Fundamentals of Molecular Biology, Oxford University Press, New York, 2009.

8. L Mousavizadeh, S Ghasemi, Genotype and phenotype of COVID-19: Their roles in pathogenesis, Journal of Microbiology, Immunology and Infection, 22 March 2020, https://doi.org/10.1016/j.jmii.

9. Y Chen, Q Liu, D Guo, Emerging coronaviruses: Genome structure, replication, and pathogenesis, J Med Virol, 2020;92:418–423, https://doi.org/10.1002/jmv.25681.

10. NCBI Website: Wuhan-Hu-1, https://www.ncbi.nlm.nih.gov/nuccore/MN908947, last accessed 7 Jun 2020.

11. A R Fehr, S Perlman, Coronaviruses: An Overview of Their Replication and Pathogenesis, Chapter 1, H J Maier et al. (eds.), Coronaviruses: Methods and Protocols, Methods in Molecular Biology, vol. 1282, DOI 10.1007/978-1-4939-2438-7_1, Springer Science+Business Media New York 2015.

12. M A Shereen, S Khan, A Kazmi, N Bashir, R Siddique, COVID-19 infection: Origin, transmission, and characteristics of human coronaviruses, Journal of Advanced Research 24 (2020) 91–98.

13. LOCUS NC_000013, 114364328 bp, DNA, linear, CON 29-MAY-2020
BioProject: PRJNA168, Homo sapiens chromosome 13, GRCh38.p13 Primary
Assembly, NCBI Reference Sequence: NC_000013.11,
https://www.ncbi.nlm.nih.gov/nuccore/ NC_000013.11,
report=gbwithparts&log$=seqview
Assembly: GCF_000001405.39 (Updated version).

14. L B Scheiber II, L B Scheiber, DNA Vaccines, Courier Gene Technology, Volume 5, iUniverse, NY, 2017.

15. L B Scheiber II, L B Scheiber, Fourth Generation Biologics: Molecular Virus Killers, Volume 4, iUniverse, NY, 2014.

16. UniProtKB - Q92664 (TF3A_HUMAN), https://www.uniprot.org/uniprot/Q92664.

17. Homo sapiens general transcription factor IIIA (GTF3A), mRNA, NCBI Reference Sequence: NM_002097.3, 16 Jun 2020 (updated), https://www.ncbi.nlm.nih.gov/nuccore/1519315333.

18. M Hodel, A Corbett, A Hodel, Dissection of a Nuclear Localization Signal, J Bio Chem, Vol. 276, No. 2, Issue of 12 Jan 2001, 1317–1325.

19. B J Bosch, R van der Zee, C A M de Haan, et al., The Coronavirus Spike Protein Is a Class I Virus Fusion Protein: Structural and Functional

Characterization of the Fusion Core Complex, J of Virology, DOI: 10.1128/JVI.77.16.8801-8811.2003.

20. J Shang, Y Wan, C Luo, et al., Cell entry mechanisms of SARS-CoV-2, PNAS May 26, 2020 117 (21) 11727-11734.

21. J A Owens, J Punt, S A Stranford, PP Jones, Kuby Immunology, W. H. Freeman and Company, New York, 2013.

22. B Alberts, A Johnson, J Lewis, et al., Molecular Biology of the Cell, 4th Edition, Garland Science, New York, 2002. https://www.ncbi.nlm.nih.gov/books/NBK26926/.

23. CD8A Genbank, National Center for Biotechnology Information (NCBI), https://www.ncbi.nlm.nigh.gov/nuccore/NC_000002.12?report=genbank&from=86784605&to=86808396&strand=true, last accessed 14 Jun 2020.

24. L H Hartwell, M L Goldberg, J A Fischer, et al., Genetics: From Genes to Genomes, Fifth Edition, McGraw-Hill Education, New York, 2015.

25. NCBI Website: https://www.ncbi.nlm.nih.gov/nuccore/MT510643.1, last accessed 7 June 2020.

26. A Traunecker, et al., Bispecific single chain molecules (Janusins) target cytotoxic lymphocytes on HIV infected cells, EMBO Journal 10(12): 1991, 3655-3659.

27. Neuberger et al., Biotechniques. 4 (3): 1986, 214-21.

28. Ernst Winnacker, From Genes to Clones: Introduction to Gene Technology, Chapter 7, 1987, 239-317.

29. L B Scheiber II, L B Scheiber, Medical Vector Therapy, Changing the Global Approach to Medicine, Volume 2, iUniverse, NY, 2011.

30. H Aini, K Itaka, A Fujisawa, et al., Messenger RNA delivery of a cartilage-anabolic transcription factor as a disease-modifying strategy for osteoarthritis treatment, Scientific Reports, 6:18743; 05 Jan 2016.

31. A Trafton, Engineers create an inhalable form of messenger RNA, Patients with lung disease could find relief by breathing in messenger RNA molecules, MIT News Office 4 Jan 2019.

32. A Patel, J Kaczmarek, S Bose, Inhaled nanoformulated mRNA polyplexes for protein production in lung epithelium, Advanced Materials, 31(8), 22 Feb 2019.

33. Q Yingshan, R Man, Q Liao, et al., Effective mRNA pulmonary delivery by dry powder formulation of PEGylated synthetic KL4 peptide, J Controlled Release, ScienceDirect, 314, 28 Nov 2019, 102-115.

34. History of Ebola Virus Disease, Emergence of Ebola in Humans, https://www.cdc.gov/vhf/ebola/history/summaries.html.

35. L Baseler, D Chertow, et al., The Pathogenesis of Ebola Virus Disease. *Annu. Rev. Pathol. Mech. Dis.* 2017. 12:387–418.

36. International Committee on Taxonomy of Viruses (ICTV): Taxonomy, https://talk.ictvonline.org/taxonomy/.

37. D Baltimore, Expression of Animal Virus Genomes, Bacteriological Reviews, Vol. 35, No. 3., p. 235-241, Sep 1971.

38. G Mahmoudabadi, R Phillips, A comprehensive and quantitative exploration of thousands of viral genomes, eLife 2018;7: e 31955 https://www.ncbi.nlm.nih.gov/pmc/articles/PMC5908442/pdf/elife-31955.pdf.

39. Virus Classification, https://en.wikipedia.org/wiki/Virus_classification.

40. R Reece, M A Smit, T P Flanigan, Ebola Virus, Encyclopedia of Immunobiology, Volume 4, Pages 355-362, 2016.

41. World Health Organization website: Ebola virus disease, 10 Feb 2020, https://www.who.int/news-room/fact-sheets/detail/ebola-virus-disease.

42. S Watanabe, T Noda, Y Kawaoka, Functional Mapping of the Nucleoprotein of Ebola Virus, J Virol.; 80(8): 3743–3751, Apr 2006.

43. D Goodsell, Molecule of the Month, Ebola Virus Proteins, Protein Data Bank-101, Oct 2014, https://pdb101.rcsb.org/motm/178.

44. R A Hammou, Y Kasmi, K Khataby, et al., Roles of VP35, VP40 and VP24 Proteins of Ebola Virus in Pathogenic and Replication Mechanisms, Ebola, Crtomir Podlipnik, IntechOpen, 10 August 2016, https://www.intechopen.com/books/ebola/roles-of-vp35-vp40-and-vp24-proteins-of-ebola-virus-in-pathogenic-and-replication-mechanisms.

45. C A Suttle, Viruses in the sea. Nature 437(7057):356-361, 2005.

46. C H Wigington, D Sonderegger, C P Brussaard, et al., Re-examination of the relationship between marine virus and microbial cell abundances. Nature microbiology 1:15024, 2016.

47. V Racaniello, How many viruses on Earth?, 6 Sep 2013, HTTPS://WWW.VIROLOGY.WS/2013/09/06/HOW-MANY-VIRUSES-ON-EARTH/.

48. https://www.worldometers.info/world-population/.

49. E Howell, How Many Stars are in the Galaxy?, Space.com, 18 May 2017.

50. E Howell, How Many Galaxies Are There?, Space.com, 20 Mar 2018.

51. F P Ryan, Human endogenous retroviruses in health and disease: a symbiotic perspective, JR Soc Med, 97(12) 560-565,Dec 2004

52. Our complicated relationship with viruses, National Institute of General Medical Sciences, 28 Nov 2016, ScienceDaily.com.

53. A C Gregory, A A Zayed, N Conceição-Neto, et al., Marine DNA viral macro- and microdiversity from pole to pole, Cell, Volume 177, Issue 5, 16 May 2019, Pages 1109-1123.

54. E I Garcia de Jesus, Hundreds of thousands of marine viruses discovered in the world's oceans, nature, 25 Apr 2019, natue.com.

55. R White, How Computers Work Millennium Edition, Illustrated by T E Downs, Que, A Division of Macmillan Computer Publishing, Indianapolis, 1999.

56. C W Keenam, J H Wood, D C Kleinfelter, General College Chemistry, Fifth Edition, Harper & Ron Publishers, New York, 1976.

57. H Lodish, A Berk, C A Kaiser, et al., Molecular Cell Biology, Seventh Edition, W. H. Freeman and Company, New York, 2013.

APPENDIX ONE

ANALYSIS OF NUCLEOTIDE-AMINO ACID BONDING CHARACTERISTICS

Basic Binding Processes

With the DNA target site defined, the next step is to define an amino acid sequence that will bind to it. This requires some knowledge of how the binding process works. For example, which amino acids bind to which nucleic acids and how does the binding process take place? Further, a protein is made of a string of amino acids. As it is being made, its form changes. What are the possible forms and how do they impact the possible binding capability of the resulting molecule? We will cover these aspects in the next few parts of this section. Once the basics are in place, we will be in a position to begin the design of the DNA binding molecule.

a) How do Amino Acids Bind to Nucleic Acids?

There are two main binding processes that occur between these two sets of acids: the sharing of electrons, generally referred to as hydrogen bonds, and van der Waals (a sort of mutual attraction). In the following we will have a close look at these. We start with the hydrogen bonding process and what the binding process has to work with in both the nucleic acids and the amino acids.

Nucleic Acids

Figure 47 shows the types of hydrogen bonds associated with each type of nucleic acid for both the major and minor groves of the DNA. An inward pointing arrow indicates the ability to accept an electron to be shared while an outward pointing arrow indicate the availability of an electron to be shared. Thus, for example, the oxygen atom at the 4 position in the major grove of Thymine (t) can accept an electron while the hydrogen atom in the 4 position of Cytosine (c) can provide or donate one. Table 10 shows the complete set of hydrogen bond possibilities with which the binding process has to work with. The dash symbol indicates no elements are available.

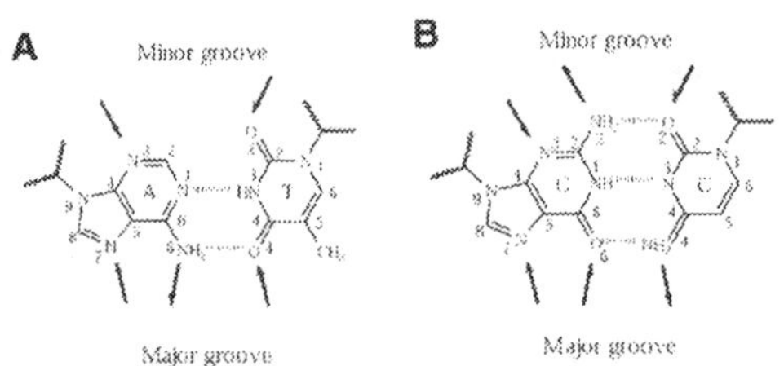

Figure 47[1]
Electron Acceptors and Donators.

The letter 'a' represents adenine, 'c' represents cytosine, 'g' represents guanine, and t represents thymine. Right away we can see the possibility of selectivity. That is in the major groove, 'a' can both provide and accept electrons, 't' can accept one, 'c' can donate one and 'g' can accept two. In the next section we will see how these characteristics marry up with the capabilities of the amino acids.

Nucleic Acid	Accept/Donate	Major Grove		Minor Grove	
		Number	Elements	Number	Elements
A	A	1	N	1	N
	D	1	NH_2	-	
T	A	1	O	1	O
	D	-		-	
C	A	-		1	O
	D	1	NH_2	-	
G	A	2	N & O	1	N
	D	-		1	NH_2

Table 10
Hydrogen bonding possibilities.

[1] This type of diagram appears in many places. We direct your attention to the following as it also contains additional explanatory material that we will draw your attention to later in this document: Nicholas M. Luscombe, Et Al, Amino acid-base interactions: a three-dimensional analysis of protein-DNA interactions at an atomic level.

b) Which Amino Acids Bind to Which Nucleic Acids and other elements of the DNA?

The 20 amino acids used in the construction of proteins have a number of characteristics that a designer needs to understand. These characteristics include the number of electrons that each can accept or donate, the type of amino acid e.g., polar, the charge that is on it and its reaction to water to name a few. First, we investigate the electron sharing capability and match it to the corresponding capability of the nucleic acids.

We note that Arg (R) has a strong affinity for 'g' while Asn (N) has a strong affinity for 'a'. Further, Lys (K) has an affinity for 't' and Glu (E) for 'c'. While there are other possibilities, to keep the discussion as clear as possible we will take these to be our primary amino acids, the ones that we will use in the design to bind to specific nucleic acids.

We also note that Ser (S) does not have an affinity for any of the nucleic acids, but binds very well with the DNA backbone or rail. We will use it as our spacer/stabilizing amino acid. These selections are summarized in Table 11.

Bonds To Basis		
Amino Acid	**Base**	**Bond Type**
Arg R	G	Multiple Donor
Asn N	A	Accepter + Donor
Lys K	T	Single Hydrogen Bond
Glu E	C	Single Hydrogen Bond
Bonds To Backbone		
Ser S		Van der Waals attractions generally appear to be used for stability and Serine has a large attraction for the phosphate elements in the DNA backbone[2].

Table 11

Bonds to Basis and Backbone.

2 See for example Table 6 in Nichoias M. Luscombe, Et Al, Amino acid-base interactions: a three-dimensional analysis of protein-DNA interactions at an atomic level.

c) *Basic Protein Structures*

In this section we look at the configuration sequences that amino acids go through as they transitions from the manufacturing process, as a string, to a DNA binding protein configuration. We first look at the basic protein structures and then how some of those structures facilitate the binding of the amino acids they consist of to the elements of the DNA.

Proteins have many different shapes. When they are first manufactured they are just a one dimensional string of amino acids, which is called the primary structure. It is also the backbone of the protein. However, in this form it actually consists of amino acid residues as opposed to amino acids because as the amino acids are connected together a water molecule is lost at the point where the connection occurs.

As an illustration[3], let's suppose that we are going to connect an alanine amino acid to a glycine amino acid. Figure 48a and 48b show the equations for glycine and alanine, respectively, while Figure 48c shows the equation when they are connected together. As can be seen in the figures, the water molecule at the site of the connection is lost. What remains of the amino acid is called the residue and it is the string of residues that make up the backbone of the protein. Although not quite evident yet, the backbone consists of a repeating sequence of the elements **CH-C-N**. Note: C = carbon atom, H = hydrogen atom, and N = nitrogen atom. This will become important in the following.

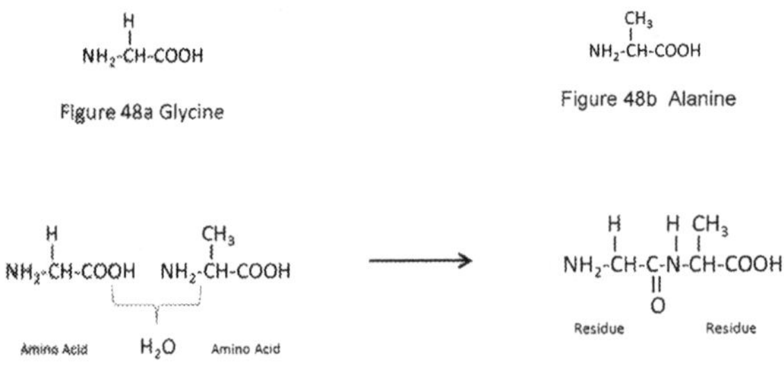

Figure 48
Creation of protein backbone.

[3] For a more detailed discussion see Chemguide's 'The Structure of Proteins' at http://www.chemguide.co.uk/organicprops/aminoacids/proteinstruct.html.

Although this string is indeed a molecule, it is not a functional protein. For it to become a functional protein the string must have starting and ending sequences and the entire sequence must be folded into a three-dimensional shape. Three steps are used to describe the process of folding. Level is sometimes used in place of step. Level 1 is the string as it is manufactured. Level 2 is a two-dimensional view of the first fold. Level 3 is the three-dimensional configuration.

At the second level most proteins, or parts thereof, fold into one of two shapes called alpha helix (α-helix) and beta sheet (β sheet). The α-helix form tends to fit into the major and minor grooves of the DNA, while the β sheet tends to attach to the DNA's backbone. Thus, herein we will describe the alpha helix form since we are designing a protein to bind to DNA bases as opposed to its backbone.

We will use conventional biological symbols and abbreviations. For example, when discussing the backbone we will use the letter R in place of the amino acids side chain when the makeup of the side chain has no impact on the discussion[4]. Thus, glycine would be shown as:

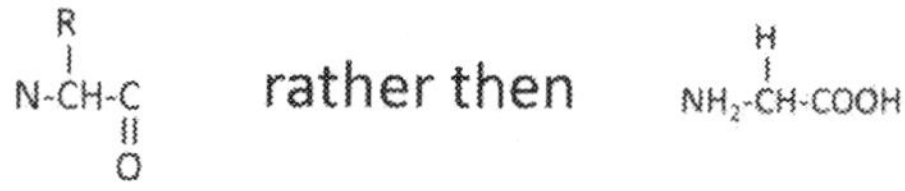

```
  R                          H
  |                          |
N-CH-C     rather then   NH2-CH-COOH
     ||
     O
```

Figure 49

Or for a string of residues making up a portion of a protein we might simply write what is presented as:

$\underline{N_H\text{-}C_R\text{-}C_O}\text{-}\underline{N_H\text{-}C_R\text{-}C_O}\text{-}\underline{N_H\text{-}C_R\text{-}C_O}\text{-}\underline{N_H\text{-}C_R\text{-}C_O}\text{-}\underline{N_H\text{-}C_R\text{-}C_O}\text{-}\underline{N_H\text{-}C_R\text{-}C_O}$

1 2 3 4 5 6 7 8 9 10 11 12 13 14 15 16 17 18

Figure 50

Where N_H is the NH complex, C_R is the CH with the side chain attached, C_O is the Carbon with the Oxygen attached and $\underline{N_H\text{-}C_R\text{-}C_O}$

[4] The amino acid proline is an exception as in it the hydrogen on the nitrogen nearest the "R" group is missing, and the "R" group loops around and is attached to that nitrogen as well as to the carbon atom in the chain.

represents the residue of a single amino acid. In the literature this is often written as NCO and, from time to time when the context makes it clear, we may use that form as well.

d) The Alpha Helix Structure - *Overview*

In an alpha helix amino acid residue string there is a slight right hand twist at the point where one amino acid residue attaches to the next. This leads to the alpha helix having a shape like a coiled spring. The right hand twist causes the sequence of atoms to be coiled in the clockwise direction when looking in the direction of the protein build[5]. Each loop consists of exactly 11 atoms[6] – the C_R combo with the side chain attached is counted as one atom. Thus, each turn has 3 complete amino acid residues and two atoms from the next residue. That means that the residues in each turn are offset from the ones above and below by two atoms. How this fits together can be seen in Figure 51.

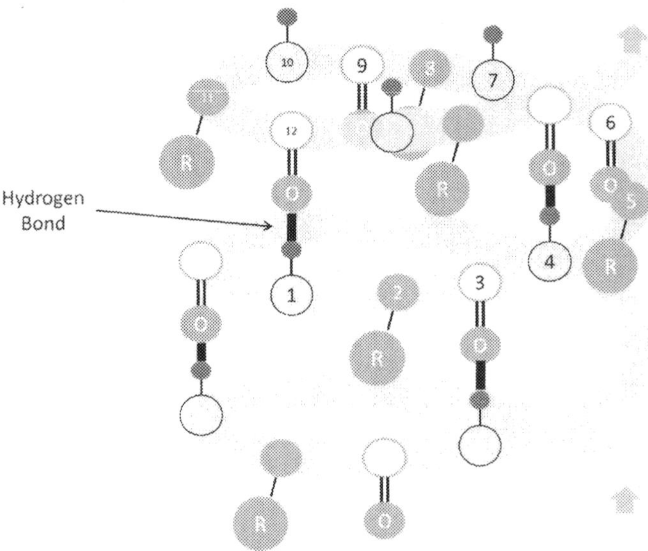

Figure 51
Alpha helix structure.

[5] That is, an α-helix is right-handed. It turns in the direction that the fingers of a right hand curl when its thumb points in the direction that the helix rises.

[6] See numbers in Figure 51.

This diagram shows several important features of the alpha helix structure. First, the N_H elements[7], with their hydrogen atoms pointing up, occur just before the carbon atoms to which the side chains are attached and the C_O elements, with their oxygen atoms pointing down, occur just after the carbon atoms. Since it is the hydrogen bonds between the N_H and C_O elements that hold the alpha helix in its coiled configuration, these elements need to be brought into alignment. The two extra atoms in a coil bring these elements into the proper orientation so the hydrogen bonds can take place. A solid line is used to show that the hydrogen atom in the N_H element points in the up direction. The dashed line shows that if it pointed in the down direction there could not be 11 amino acids in each coil. The positions of N_H and C_O in the coil results in a strong hydrogen bond between them that has the nearly optimum N to O distance of 2.8 Å[8,9].

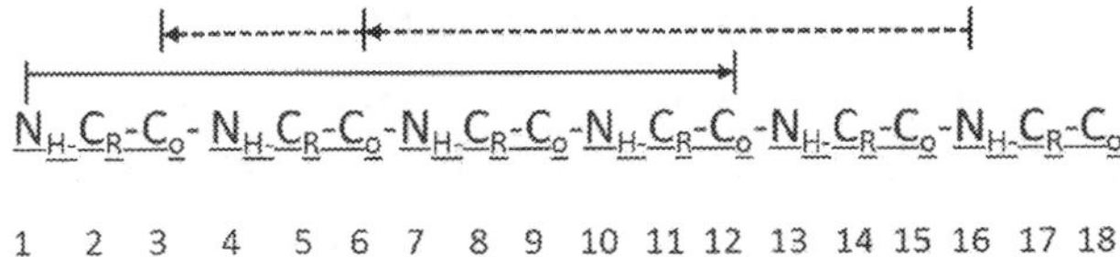

Figure 52

Hydrogen atom points in the up direction.

This shows, if one looks along the left side for example, that the alignment of the atoms in the vertical direction is such that C_O is always above N_H while C_R is always below it. What this is telling us is that if a residue's side chain is pointing in a particular direction that three coils above or below it is another residue which may have its side chain pointing in the same direction. Since residues are all of the way around each coil, we need to determine the direction of each as some, it would seem, will be in a better position to bind to bases than others. Thus, the angular position of the amino acids around the coil must be considered as one of the design constraints. Further, the amino acid side chains

---

[7] N_H elements are light gray, C_O elements are dotted with double lines to oxygen, hydrogen bonds are black, and Carbons are solid with attached side chains marked R.

[8] Å = 0.1 nm

[9] See for example Proteins: Three-Dimensional Structure at http://biochem118.stanford.edu/Papers/Protein%20Papers/Voet%26Voet%20chapter6.pdf.

project outward and downward from the helix thereby avoiding steric interference with the polypeptide backbone and with each other. If the side chains did not stick out away from the internal structure of the alpha helix they would not be able to bind to the nucleotides as the core of the helix is tightly packed; that is, its atoms are in van der Waals contact[10]. Why they stick out is discussed below.

In addition to the α-helix having 3.6 residues per turn, it has a pitch (the distance the helix rises along its axis per turn) of 5.4 Å. The α-helices of proteins have an average length of 12 residues, which corresponds to over three helical turns, and a height of 18 Å.

1. Design of a α-Helix DNA-Binding Protein

Proteins are very complex molecules. Before a molecular architect attempts to design one, the design parameters and constraints need to be well in mind. While we will introduce the major parameters, resources do not permit all of them to be covered in detail. Thus, in this section we will first cover the parameters associated with the protein and then those associated with the DNA. We include those introduced above for completeness. This will be followed by a discussion of how these two sets of parameters interact, e.g., generate constraints.

A. Design Parameters and Constraints

1) Associated with the Binding Structure of the Protein

a) *Amino Acids*

Amino acid characteristics which need to be considered in the design of a protein include:

- Type – Polar, charge, etc[11].

---

[10] See for example Proteins: Three-Dimensional Structure.

[11] To address the question as to "What causes polypeptide chains to fold into functional protein?" one notes that the amino acids in proteins can be divided into four groups: acidic, basic, polar and non-polar. Based on these classifications, the amino acids have varying

- Length of side chain.
- DNA elements to which they tend to bind.
- Types of binding – Hydrogen and van der Waals (vdW)
- Interaction with other amino acids. For example, in α-helixes the amino acid side chains project outward and downward from the helix thereby avoiding space interference with the polypeptide backbone and with each other.
- Function – e.g., C and H binding to zinc ion in zinc fingers.

b) *Alpha Helixes*

In designing a α-helix protein characteristics that need to be taken into account including:

- Alpha helixes are right-handed; that is, they turn in the direction that the fingers of a right hand curl when its thumb points in the direction that the helix rises.
- An α-helix has 3.6 (more precisely 3.67) residues per turn and rises about 5.4 Å along its axis per turn (called pitch).

When the backbone of a protein is generated there are angles formed at the N_H-C_R and C_R-C_O junctions called torsion or dihedral angles. The magnitudes of the angles are 57.8 degrees at the N_H-C_R junction and 47.0 degrees at the C_R-C_O junction[12]. The total is 104.8 degrees which is a bit more than a quarter of a turn (90 degrees). Thus, the change in direction of the protrusions of the side chains from the α-helix, from one side chain to the next, is about 105 degrees.

2) Associated with the DNA Structure

The DNA helix can assume one of three slightly different geometries, of which the "B" form described by James D. Watson and Francis Crick

---

affinities to bond with other amino acids. The specific tertiary structure is the result of such bonding between amino acids. For example, two polar amino acids may create hydrogen bonds, while an acid and a base may bond based on electron charges. Polar amino acids are those with side-chains that prefer to reside in a water environment. For this reason, one generally finds these amino acids exposed on the surface of a protein.

[12] See for example Figure 6-4 in Proteins: Three-Dimensional Structure.

is believed to predominate in cells. It is 20 Å wide and extends 34 Å per 10 bp of sequence (rises 3.4 Å from the center of one nucleic acid to the next).

The B form of the DNA helix twists 360° per 10.6 bp in the absence of strain. But many molecular biological processes can induce strain. A DNA segment with excess or insufficient helical twisting is referred to, respectively, as positively or negatively 'supercoiled'.

B. Design Aspects

1) General

Aspects that might make the molecule being designed fold further than the α-helix form are intentionally avoided. For example, cysteine amino acids are not used as they make the disulfide bonds which result in molecules folding to the third level.

Certain amino acids are specified as primary because they are known to bind to nucleic acids. However, others do as well and could be used instead of those used herein.

It may not be necessary to have an amino acid attached to each and every nucleic acid. That is, having some of the primary positions (those facing the DNA) filled with non-nucleic acid binding amino acids may not matter so long as the binding attraction of the protein sequence is sufficient to cause the protein to bind permanently to the HIV binding site.

2) Twist of the DNA

In an unstressed state, the DNA twists along its central axis at the rate of one complete turn about every 10.4 nucleotides or 34.46 degrees between each nucleic acid. This is referred to as twist ω[13]. As the α-helix is pulled into the major groove of the DNA by the amino acid to nucleotide attraction (binding), there may be some distortion. This distortion may occur in the DNA twist, other parts of the DNA structure,

[13] The twist is in the same direction as that of an α-helix (which is right-handed). That is, it turns in the direction that the fingers of a right hand curl when its thumb points in the direction that the DNA strand rises.

in the structure of the α-helix or in all of the above. While we make note of these possibilities, in the following analyses and design we assume that the α-helix structure remains unchanged and that the DNA twist is unchanged ($\omega = 34.46$ per nucleotide).

3) Rotational Position of the Primary Amino Acids

The α-helix fits into the major groove of the DNA. The direction of the α-helix at its closest point to the center of the major groove is taken to be zero degrees. To provide for the maximum potential binding between the targeted nucleic acids and the amino acids side chain direction, as measured around the α-helix, we will restrict it to $\pm$ 90 degrees which might sometimes be referred to a 0 to 90 degrees and 270 to 360 (or 0) degrees.

5) Stabilizing the Structure

Given that some of the amino acids will be beyond $\pm$ 90 degrees described above as our imposed angular condition for an amino acid to attach to a nucleic acid, one might chose amino acids for those positions that tend to bind to the rails of the DNA structure, either the sugar or the phosphate elements, which would provide stability for the binding process.

C. The Design Process

The design of a DNA binding molecule is a problem involving the simultaneous optimization of a number of parameters such as selecting the targets for the amino acids, matching the height of the amino acids with their targeted nucleosides along the DNA helix, and positioning the amino acids such that their side chains point in the direction of their intended targets. In this section we describe our approach to this multidimensional problem. From the above the nucleotides are already known as are the amino acids that we expect to bind to them.

In this initial design we will consider a single α-helix. However, if need be, it could be broken up into a number of connected α-helixes.

1) Matching the Heights

Along the DNA helix the nucleotides rise 3.4 Å from the center of one nucleic acid to the next while the amino acids in the α-helix rise at rate of 0.49 Å from one atom to the next.

As a first step we layout the protein backbone in a linear fashion. This is done by making a table listing the atoms in the backbone of the α-helix structure using the sequence NCO with the C, representing the atom with the side chain.

The list is made sufficiently long to include the expected number of amino acids in the α-helix. The heights of the atoms are added in the α-helix. In the general case, zero height is taken to be the position where the first amino acid's side chain is directly in line with the center of the first target nucleotide. However, the zero position could be defined as occurring in other places including the middle of the target sequence or at its end.

An angle is added to each atom. The angle of interest is its rotation about the zero point of the α-helix. The reason for this will become apparent later.

Using the height of the atoms, we then note on this list the height of each nucleotide along the DNA. The twist of the DNA at the position of each of the nucleotides is added. We refer to this list as the Protein Design Template an example of which is shown in Table 12.

2) Add the Names of the Nucleic Acids in the Target Sequence

Since we know the names of the nucleic acids in the target nucleotide sequence these are added to the list.

3) Identifying the Amino Acids

In a DNA binding protein the amino acid side chains have two different purposes: bind to the target nucleotide sequence and bind to the DNA backbone to enhance stability of the attachment of the α-helix to the DNA helix. In designing an efficient layout of the α-helix structure it is necessary to position the amino acid side chains around the curve of the α-helix such that they point, as near as possible, in the direction of their intended targets. Our current guiding rule for this is that a side chain intended to bind to a selected nucleotide should not exceed ± 90 degrees from the perpendicular direction to the nucleotide and should not be above or below it by more than 1 Å.

Thus, the position of each C atom is examined in relationship to the nearest nucleotide to see if it meets the above angular and height rules. If it meets these two criteria, the appropriate binding amino acid for the nucleotide is entered from Table 10. If it does not, we enter the stability amino acid from the table. Table 12 is used to show the results of the analysis.

Atom No	Atom Sym	Residual Side Chain	Coil Number	Side Chain Angle Deg	Residual Atom Height in Å	Amino Acid	Nucleotide Height in Å	DNA Twist ω	Nucleo-tide Name
1	N		1	-35					
2	C	1		0	0		1 @ 0	0	
3	O			35	0.49				
4	N			70	0.98				
5	C	2		105	1.47				
6	O			140	1.96				
7	N			175	2.45				
8	C	3		210	2.94				
9	O			245	3.43		2 @ 3.4	34.46	
10	N			280	3.92				
11	C	4		315	4.41				
12	O		2	350	4.9				
13	N			25	5.39				
14	C	5		60	5.88				
15	O			95	6.37				
16	N			130	6.86		3 @ 6.8	68.92	
17	C	6		165	7.35				
18	O			200	7.84				

Table 12

Example of a Protein Design Template.

The first nucleotide is noted in the target sequence is A (adenine). Since there is an amino acid with a side chain angle of zero and it is at the same height as the nucleotide[14], there is a binding opportunity. From Table 11 we see that Asn is the amino acid that we have selected to bind to A. We enter Asn into our results table, Table 13, for the amino acid. We also color that row light gray to provide an indication as to where binding strategies have been setup.

[14] Both deltas are zero since we selected this as our starting condition. Each of the remainder alignments we will have to check.

The C atom is investigated for the second amino acid and it is found to fail the height test for the second (G) nucleotides: 1.47 Å vs. 3.4 Å for G. We enter the stabilizing amino acid (Ser S) from Table 11 in its cell in the amino acid column. We also mark its row with dots, to indicate that the amino acid provides stabilization, and its cell in the Residual Atom Height column we make dark gray with white letters to indicate height is the reason it is not binding to a nucleotide. Since it would meet the angle test for G (105 vs. 34.64 for a delta of 70.36 degrees) we leave the marking of its Side Change Angle cell unchanged.

The third amino acid's side chain is more than 90 degrees displaced from the second nucleotide (210 vs. 34.64 degrees). It is treated the same as the second amino acid with the exception that we mark its Side Chain Angle cell to indicate that it fails the angle requirement. Its height is within 1 Å of the G nucleotide so we leave its height cell unchanged.

Atom No	Atom Sym	Residual Side Chain	Coil Number	Side Chain Angle Deg	Residual Atom Height in Å	Amino Acid	Nucleotide Height in Å	DNA Twist ω	Nucleotide Name
1	N		1	-35					
2	C	1		0	0	ASN N	1 @ 0	0	A
3	O			35	0.49				
4	N			70	0.98				
5	C	2		105	1.47	Ser S			
6	O			140	1.96				
7	N			175	2.45				
8	C	3		210	2.94	Ser S			
9	O			245	3.43		2 @ 3.4	34.64	G
10	N			280	3.92				
11	C	4		315	4.41	ARG R	ΔH = 1 Å	Δω=79.64	
12	O		2	350	4.9				
13	N			25	5.39				
14	C	5		60	5.88	GLU E	ΔH = 1 Å	Δω=9.28	
15	O			95	6.37				
16	N			130	6.86		3 @ 6.8	69.28	C
17	C	6		165	7.35	Ser S			
18	O			200	7.84				

Table 13

Initial Portion of the Design of a DNA Binding Molecule for HIV Killer Protein.

The fourth amino acid meets both the height and the angle conditions, ΔH = 1Å and Δω = 79.64 degrees respectively. From Table 11 we see that Arg binds to G. We enter it into our results table along with the delta values and then color the appropriate cells gray.

The remaining amino acid/nucleotide/stability combinations for our DNA binding molecule are established in the same manor. The binding molecule has 56 amino acids. The alignment of the amino acids with the nucleotides they are designed to bind to is shown below. The small letters in the figure indicate nucleotides to which the molecule is unable to bind.

```
N S S R E S S N S S R E S S K S S R S S E K S S K S S K
a     g c     a     g c     t     g     c t     t     t

K S K S S R S E S E S S K S R S K S S N S E S K S S R R
t   t     g   c   c     t   g   t     a   c   t     g g
```

HIV binding molecule.

4) Observations on the Design of the HIV Binding Molecule

An examination of the data shown above for the HIV binding molecule provides the following points about the design:

- 56 amino acids are needed to cover the nucleotide sequence of about 82 Å.
- Amino acids are positioned to bind with 21 of the 25 nucleotides.
- Of the 4 nucleotides which are not bound to amino acids none are adjacent.
- 35 of the amino acids bind to the DNA backbone.

We might get a somewhat different amino acid sequence if we chose a different amino acid/nucleotide combination as the starting point. In fact, we might be able to select a starting point that provides an optimum amino acid sequence. One approach is to use the center of the amino acid binding sequence and the center of the DNA binding target as the starting point. We call this technique 'Centering'.

5) Examination of Variations of the Design Parameter Constraints

As part of this engineering analysis, one always examines variations in the design parameters used to determine their impact on the results. Here we report two results.

- First, we look at increasing the Height Limit of 1 Å.
  - Three additional amino acids would bind with their target nucleotides if the vertical distance limit was raised from 1 to 1.5 Å.
  - Increasing it 2 Å permits all of the amino acids to reach a nucleotide.
- Next, we examine to see if there is an advantage of the protein binding to the DNA before or after the current design position. Since there are only three amino acids per residue in the protein's backbone, we look one amino acid (0.5 Ås) in each direction.

  The data derived in the analysis indicates that there is no significant difference among the three positions.

6) Multi Section Options for Alpha Helix Approach

There may be situations where a large binding section (for example, 56 amino acids in the discussion above) exceeds the physical limits of DNA binding protein to DNA binding site process. To accommodate these limitations, we describe several alternatives to the single alpha helix design. We refer to them as Sectioning, Sectioning with Centering, Sectioning with Gaps, and Sectioning with Change of Direction.

a) Sectioning
   Sectioning simply refers to breaking the string of amino acids constituting a single alpha helix into a set of amino acids, each constituting an alpha helix of its own. For example, one might want to use a zinc finger approach and spread the binding molecule across several of its fingers.

b) Sectioning with Centering
   Sectioning an alpha helix binding molecule provides the potential to slightly modify its binding arrangements, especially in the sequence of the amino acids. One way to do this is to treat each section as a separate alpha helix and use centering as described above.

c) Sectioning with Gaps
Sectioning an alpha helix binding molecule provides the potential to alter the sequence of nucleotides that are bound to. For example, if the binding becomes constrained by insufficient space, the space between fingers could be used to inject gaps. That is, by adjusting the number of binding amino acids placed in each finger and the positions within the fingers as to where the binding starts and ends.

d) Sectioning with Change of Direction
Sectioning an alpha helix binding molecule provides the potential to reverse the sequence of nucleotides that are intended to bind to a specific DNA binding site. This might occur, for example, if the binding becomes constrained by insufficient space for the linking molecules. One solution is to turn one or more of the sections around to give the linkers more room. If a section is intended to be turned around, then its sequence might have to be reversed.

e) Combinations of the above
Most of the above can be used in combination to optimize the intended binding.

2. Designing the HIV Killer Protein – Level 1

Having a molecule that can bind to a particular nucleotide sequence is necessary but insufficient in the development of our protein to kill HIV. Once the molecule gets into the cell's cytoplasm it must be able to get into the nucleus so that it can get to the HIV's genome. That is, it needs a transport mechanism that is acceptable to the cell, otherwise the cell may just disassemble it and reuse the amino acids elsewhere. This transport mechanism is referred to as the Intracellular Transporter.

This transporter must have several aspects to carry out its mission. First, it must appear to the cell to belong in the cell. Second, it must have the characteristic of a molecule that the cell normally transports to its nucleus. Third, it must be able to carry the binding molecule in such a way that the binding molecule's amino acids can locate and attach to the intended nucleotides. Finally, the transporter must in itself support the mission of stopping the transcription of the HIV genome.

Other aspects of the overall design mentioned in the Approach include the intercellular transporter and the manufacturing process. The intercellular transporter is the mechanism that transports the killer protein from the outside world to the cytoplasm of the cell. That is, it is available in some form like a pill or injectable fluid such that it can be placed in the body in such a way that it enters the blood stream and that the blood stream carries it to the intended cell type, the T-Helper cell. Once finding a T-Helper cell, the transporter must attach to it in such a way that the killer protein it is carrying is injected into the cytoplasm of the cell.

The design must also consider how the killer protein and its transporters are to be manufactured. Generally, one would consider each of the steps necessary in the manufacturing process. For example:

- The building the killer protein with the binding molecule
- The building of the transporter
    - Including the killer protein in the transporter
    - Affixing the appropriate molecules to the surface of the transporter which will allow the transporter to insert the protein into the cell

Summary of Amino Acid Characteristics and Bindings to Nucleic Acids

In designing a protein, one selects the amino acids that make up the protein to cause the protein to carry out specific tasks. The specific task at hand is to design a specific area of a protein to bind to a specific area of the DNA which is defined by a specific nucleotide sequence. The DNA is made up of nucleic acids. Thus, as a first step, we examine the binding of amino acids to nucleic acids of which there are, in general, three types; hydrogen bonds, van der Waals contacts and water-mediated bonds. We note that in the design of a protein, at least those associated with binding, to prevent transcription the objective is to select the amino acids which make strong bonds with specific nucleic acids. Thus, van der Waals contacts and water-mediated bonds, both of which are generally not specific in their bindings, are of less interest than hydrogen bonds. That is, hydrogen bonds are much stronger that either van der Waals contacts or water-mediated bonds. Thus, in the following we shall emphases hydrogen bonds[15].

From the literature, points that might be worth keeping in mind from a 'trying to understand the bonding process' point of view include:

- Greater specificity is more likely to occur in major grooves than minor grooves.
- Protein-DNA interactions are at the atomic level.
- Some amino acids can bind using multiple donor or accepter plus donor configurations. Amino acids binding with two sites show more specificity for specific bases.
- Single hydrogen bonds are usually not indicators of specificity, more in the role of stabilization of the structure.
- On protein side, polar and charged residues play a central role in hydrogen bonds.
- Arginine and lysine hydrogen bonding strongly favor guanine while hydrogen bonds of asparagine and glutamine favor adenine.
- Where hydrogen bonds are considered, amino acids with short side chains, like serine and threonine, have limited access to bases and therefore generally contribute to stability rather than specificity.
- Cys, Met & Trp have no base contact.
- Some amino acids such as A, C, F, I, L, M and V are hydrophobic and tend to move away from water. Others like E, G, H, K, N, Q, R, S and T are hydrophilic and tend to move toward water. Others are neutral about water. In developing a protein that binds to the DNA one observes that the side chains of the hydrophobic amino acids tend to force their way inside the three-dimensional protein which is fine for developing the correct structure, but of

[15] For more on this see for example Nicholas M. Luscombe, Et Al, Amino acid-base interactions: a three-dimensional analysis of protein-DNA interactions at an atomic level.

no value in actually binding to the DNA. The side chains of the amino acids that are used to bind to the DNA need to stick out of the protein. Thus, they need to be hydrophilic or at least neutral.

Hydrogen bonds result when a hydrogen atom shares electrons with another atom, usually nitrogen or oxygen. The acid containing the hydrogen atom is referred to as the donor and the molecule it bonds to is referred to as the acceptor.

Examining the data in the literature[16] we see the following:

- Amino Acids
  - Only Asn, Gln and His have both acceptors and donors
  - Arg, Lys, Ser, Thr and Tyr only have donors
  - Glu and Asp have only acceptors
  - None of the rest have acceptors or donors
- Nucleic Acids
  - Adenine has both a donor and an acceptor
  - Cytosine only has an donor
  - Guanine has two acceptors and no donors
  - Thymine has only an acceptor

Next we make the following selections of amino acids to bind to specific nucleic acids.

- Asn (N) will be used to bind to Adenine (a)
  - Gln (Q) is one link longer than Asn and the literature indicates it does not bind to Adenine as well as Asn. It is a possible alternative.
  - His (H) is one of the atoms that create the zinc fingers. Thus, we hesitate to use it in case fingers become involved even though nature does to some degree.
- Glu (E) will be used to bind to Cytosine (c)
  - No nucleotides have two donors that can bind to Glu's two acceptors. Further, no normal paring of nucleotides (a-t

[16] See for example Luscombe.

or g-c) have major grove donors that can bind to these acceptors.

- Asp (D) seems similar to but shorter than Glu, but maybe an alternate.

- Arg (R) will be used to bind to Guanine (g)
  - Only amino acid with two donors to bind to G's two acceptors.
- Lys (K) will be used to bind to Thymine (t)
  - Thr (T) has shorter side chain, seems to bind well with rails.
  - Tyr (Y) has complex side chain.
- Ser (S) will be used in positions on the backside of the alpha helix to add stability
  - It has short side chains.
  - The literature indicates it attaches very well to the rails.
  - Thr (T) is similar, but with more baggage – 2nd CH_3.

These selections and additional information on the other amino acids is provided in Table 14.

Nucleic Acids →				**A**denine		**T**hymine		**G**uanine			**C**ytosine	
Donate/Accept →				A	D	A	D	A_1	A_2	D	A	D
Amino Acid		Donate/Accept		N	NH_2	O	-	N	O	-	-	NH_2
N	Asn	D	NH_2	x								
		A	O		X							
K	Lys	D	NH_3^+			X						
		A	-									
R	Arg	D_1	NH_2^+					X				
		D_2	NH_2						x			
		A	-									
E	Glu	D	-									
		A	O	No nucleotides have two donors that can bind to Glu's two acceptors. But it seems to bind well to cytosine.								X
		A	O^-									
S	Ser	D	OH	Short side chain (2 elements). Binds well with DNA rails.								
		A	-									

T	Thr	D	OH	Short side chain (2 elements). Binds well with DNA rails. Seems equivalent to Ser, but has second CH_3. Possible alternative.
		A	-	
Q	Gln	D	NH_2	One link longer than Asn. Reference 12 indicates it does not bind to A as well as Asn. Possible alternative.
		A	O	
Y	Tyr	D	OH	The hydrogen it has available for bonding is off its 6 carbon molecule, a more difficult side chain to work with.
		A	-	
D	Asp	D	-	Similar to Glu. Note that no nucleotides have two donors that can bind to Asp's two acceptors. Further, no normal paring of nucleotides (A-T or G-C) have major grove donors that can bind to these acceptors.
		A_1	O	
		A_2	O^-	
H	His	D	NH^+	Second part of Zinc connecter.
		A	NH	
P	Pro	D	-	Nonpolar side chains. No As or Ds to share.
		A	-	
L	Leu	D	-	Nonpolar side chains. No As or Ds to share.
		A	-	
M	Met	D	-	Nonpolar side chains. No As or Ds to share.
		A	-	
V	Val	D	-	Nonpolar side chains. No As or Ds to share.
		A	-	
I	Ile	D	-	Nonpolar side chains. No As or Ds to share.
		A	-	
C	Cys	D	-	Nonpolar side chains. No As or Ds to share.
		A	-	
W	Trp	D	-	Nonpolar side chains. No As or Ds to share.
		A	-	
F	Phe	D	-	Nonpolar side chains. No As or Ds to share.
		A	-	
G	Gly	D	-	Nonpolar side chains. No As or Ds to share.
		A	-	
A	Ala	D	-	Nonpolar side chains. No As or Ds to share.
		A	-	

Table 14

Rational for Selecting Amino Acids to Bind to Nucleotides and DNA Rails.

APPENDIX TWO

UNIQUE FUNCTIONS OF EACH 'STOP' CODON IN THE GENETIC CODE

Summary

The fact that the genetic code contains three stop codons, but only one start codon has troubled researchers ever since the code was uncovered. Many seem to proceed as if there is no difference in their function. However, the results of this study, which examined stop codon usage in prokaryotic, eukaryotic and viral genomes, indicate that each stop codon, in addition to its command to release the emerging protein, has one or more additional functions that are both necessary and unique. Thus, the stop codons are not interchangeable.

Briefly, the functions of the stop codons are:

The UGA stop codon specifies that the ribosome reader is to release the emerging protein and disassemble. It is used to specify the end of the code for the last, or only, protein in the mRNA. It does not specify any alteration to the mRNA's 3' end. It is used in prokaryotic and viral genomes.

The UAA stop codon specifies that the ribosome reader is to release the emerging protein and then continue reading the mRNA's code and look for another start codon. UAA is used in mRNAs in all three domains which contain code for multiple proteins in sequential order. It is used to specify the end of each protein's code, except the last.

The UAG stop codon specifies that the ribosome reader is to release the emerging protein and disassemble. The ribosome reader is also to cause a portion of the Poly(A) tail attached to the mRNA is to be removed. This codon is used in the human genome, and perhaps other genomes in eukaryotic cells, to specify the end of the code for the last, or only, protein in the mRNA.

Prokaryotic and eukaryotic cells use different means of controlling the lifespans of their mRNAs. In prokaryotic cells, a Poly(A) tail is attached to an mRNA to order its destruction. In eukaryotic cells, it is used to keep track of the number of times the mRNA has been read. The UGA stop codon does not specify any alteration to the mRNA's 3' end which is what is needed in prokaryotic cells. However, eukaryotic cells require that an action to the Poly(A) tail be specified which is what the UAG stop codon requires.

Discussion

The Genetic Code identifies the codons used by the ribosome readers to translate the RNA code in the mRNAs into proteins. It has been a point of interest as to why nature needs three stop codons, but only one start codon. In this study we begin to address that question. Our hypothesis is that nature would only have multiple stop codons if each had a different function.

As one attempts to understand the intent of different sequences of DNA and RNA code one is faced with trying to understand what the creator of the sequence had in mind. Further, when one attempts to create a sequence for a specific purpose, like an mRNA to produce a particular protein, one is also placing nucleotides into the sequence at precise locations to instruct the reader, as well as other molecules, to carry out specific functions in a defined order. Thus, in examining or creating a sequence the reader's response to each nucleotide or set of nucleotides must be precisely known; in examining the sequence to determine the reason it was used in a specific position, and in creating a sequence to ensure that the desired functions are carried out at each specific position. That is, each nucleotide or set of nucleotides in a sequence represents a command or set of commands to the reader and, in some situations, other molecules. With that in mind it is easy to see that sequences of nucleotides can be viewed as a machine language, base-4, digital computer program, or parts thereof, including subroutines.

Material

For this study we selected genes from genomes in all three domains: Prokaryotes cells, Eukaryotes cells and Viruses. To be sure we are clear on the stop codon usage, we take our data from the DNA portions of the genes and genomes to be analyzed. By doing this we can show the exact locations of the start and stop codons as they appear in the genes and genomes themselves. However, in doing the analysis, one must remember that in the 'U' in the RNA form of the Genetic Code is replaced by a 'T' in the DNA form[17].

For the Prokaryotes cells we used the E. coli genome. In this genome we selected the lactose operon in the NCBI GenBank, reference number J01636.1, which can be found at http://www.ncbi.nlm.nih.gov/nuccore/146575.

For the eukaryotes cells we used a random assortment of genes from the homo sapiens genome in the NCBI database[18].

For viruses we used the HIV genome we cited in Volume III of the series Changing the Global Approach to Medicine, NCBI K03455.1, which can be found at http://www.ncbi.nlm.nih.gov/nuccore/k03455.1.

Analyses[19]

1. Lactose Operon

The lactose operon genes are translated in two parts: LacI is translated alone while LacZ, LacY and LacA are translated as a sequential group. We start our analyses by extracting the information shown in Figure 53 for the four genes of the operon from the DNA portion of the lactose operon data in GenBank reference j01636.1. Section A contains the

[17] Both the DNA and RNA forms are given where it would seem to be helpful.

[18] The specific reference for each gene selected is shown in the text.

[19] In this study the DNA is viewed as a base 4, machine language digital computer program. Genes are sbroutines. The mRNAs are transformed snippets of that code. The codons shown in the Genetic Code are viewed as commands for RNA ribosome, the biological complex that reads the mRNA code. That is, the Genetic Code is the operational code (opcode) for the mRNA processor. The readers of the DNA use a different processor or processors, which has or have a different opcode or set of opcodes.

information for the LacI gene and Section B the information for the three sequential genes. The small arrows and dots represent reader continuation. Dots without an arrow indicate code continuation which is not read. The numbers given are the DNA locations, in the GenBank reference, of the nucleotides to which the arrow points.

The code for the LacI gene starts at position 79[20] and ends at position 1161. Proceeding from the start codon in positions 79-81 one finds the first stop codon, the TGA (UGA), in positions 1159-61. That stop codon instructs the ribosome reader to end the emerging protein and to disassemble since there are no more proteins to be translated in this reading.

The code for the for the LacZ, LacY and LacA proteins is contained in positions 1284 to 6356. Proceeding from the start codon in positions 1284-86 one finds the first stop codon in positions 4356-58. However, it is not a TGA (UGA). That stop codon would cause the reader to disassemble which would prevent the remaining protein code from being translated. Here the TAA (UAA) stop codon is used. This stop codon instructs the ribosome reader to end the emerging protein and continue to the next start codon, which it finds in positions 4410-12, and which happens to be the start codon for the LacY protein.

The same is true at the end of the code for the translation of the LacY protein except the next start codon is for the LacA protein.

The same TAA (UAA) stop codon appears at the end of the LacA protein code. However, six codons later a TGA (UGA) stop codon is found which instructs the reader to disassemble. This arrangement is actually expected in an evolutionary environment where code is reused without change. For example, programmers often use a subroutine for a number of purposes rather than writing a number of subroutines. They put code in the calling routines to adjust the output of the subroutine to fit the specific purpose of the part of the program that is calling the subroutine. Here, Nature simply added an instruction for the reader to disassemble rather than change the last TAA (UAA) stop codon. In any event, it is clear that two different procedures are required and the two stop codons provide for those procedures. It is also clear that these two stop codons are not interchangeable.

---

[20] NCBI reference specifies lac repressor protein, LacI, uses a GTG start codon.

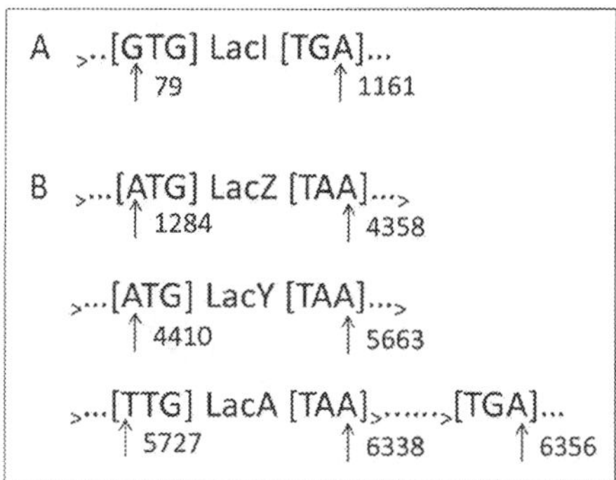

Figure 53
Layout of Lactose Operon Genes.

2. Homo Sapiens

The genes investigated in the Homo sapiens' genome are shown in Figure 54. They were not selected for any specific reason, except that they seem to be unrelated. It is noted that all three of the genes are monocistronic in that their mRNAs each produce a single protein. This is not to exclude polycistronic genes which occur in eukaryotic cells, will be dealt with later, but to concentrate on a new stop codon requirement which has been brought about by the emergence of the nucleus in the cell.

Figure 54 shows the start and stop codons for the genes presented in this section. It also shows the locations[21] of those start and stop codons as found in their DNA[22,23,24]. It is noted that each of the genes starts with the normal start codon. On the other hand they don't end with either of the stop codons shown in Figure 53, but end with the third stop codon TAG (UAG)[25]. Let us examine why.

---

[21] Using the locations specified by the Coding Sequence (CDS) where available.

[22] INS (Insulin): from NCBI sequence NC_000011.10 at http://www.ncbi.nlm.nih.gov/nuccore/nc_000011.10

[23] OCA2 (Eye Color): from NCBI sequence NM_000275.2 at http://www.ncbi.nlm.nih.gov/nuccore/NM_000275.2

[24] CYGB (Cytoglobin aka HGB): from NCBI sequence NC_000017.11 at http://www.ncbi.nlm.nih.gov/nuccore/nc_000017.11

[25] The stop codon in the NCBI reference is a TAA at locations 2625-27. The next codon at 2628-30 is the TAG stop codon. This is the same code reuse observation discussed with the

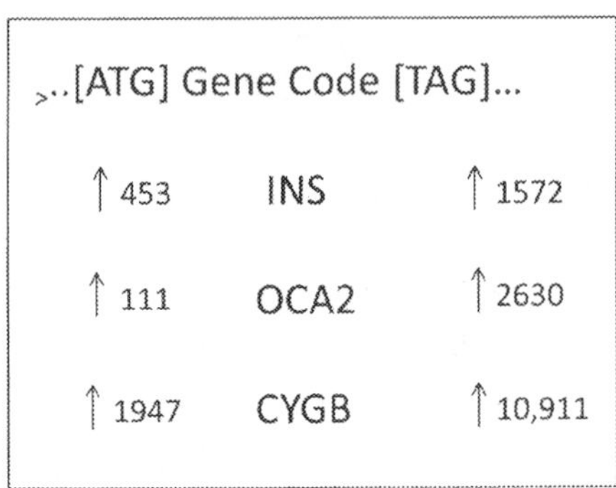

Figure 54
Examples of Homo Sapiens Genes.

In prokaryotic cells there is a close relationship between the reading of the gene's code in the DNA and the translation of the code in the resulting mRNA which produces the protein. They are done together in the cell's cytoplasm. As eukaryotic cells emerged with their DNAs, as well as the operations done on them, in the nucleus, and their mRNA translations done separately in the cytoplasm, Nature added a Poly(A) tail to the mRNAs to provide an indication of wear out, i.e., the number of times the mRNA has been read. To facilitate this, Nature added a means to reduce the number of <u>adenine</u> acids in the tail each time the mRNA is read (Beelman, Tourriere). To help prevent an mRNA from being used past its projected useful life, Nature also add poly(A) ribonuclease (PARN) to initiate destruction of an mRNA when its Poly(A) tail reaches a specified minimum length.

But what can provide the signal to shorten the tail? The stop codon that ends the reading of the code for the last protein in the mRNA is an obvious choice. That lets out the TSS (USS) codon. The TGA (UGA) codon has potential, but would need to be modified to add the signal. Such a modification might have been deemed to cause confusion or harm in the case of mRNAs which don't use Poly(A) tails in this manner. In any event, it seems that Nature gave this task to the stop codon TAG (UAG). That is, the TAG (UAG) stop codon instructs the reader to end the emerging

---

lactose operon above.

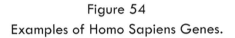

protein, provide a signal to remove a specific number of adenine acids from the mRNA's Poly(A) tail, and to disassemble.

This is not to claim that eukaryotic cells do not use the TGA stop codon as they do[26]. How the eukaryotic cells keep track of the usage of the mRNAs which utilize the TGA stop codons is beyond the scope of this report.

3. HIV

When one looks at the gene map of the HIV genome like the one shown in the Landmarks of the HIV-1 Genome, HXB2 strain[27], shown here in Figure 55, one gets the feeling that Nature just jumbled the genes together into a genome. The fact that some genes overlap others and some have parts at distant locations gives rise to the feeling that showing a consistent use of stop codons might be very difficult in this case. However, that is not true. In fact, it turns out to be very interesting.

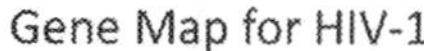

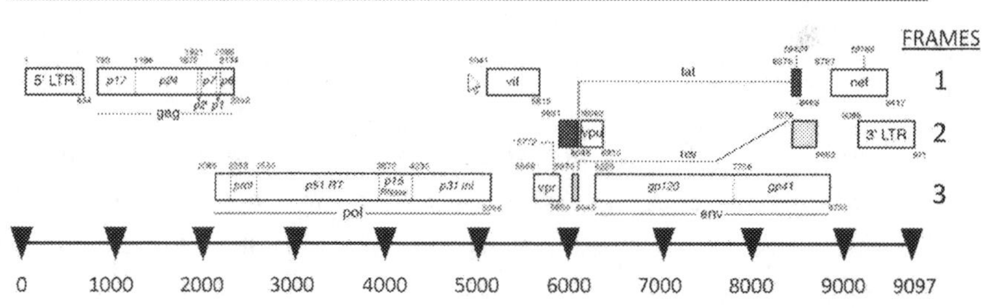

Figure 55
Gene Map for HIV-1 HXB2 Strain.

Identifying the mRNAs in the HXB2 Strain of HIV-1, which describes the seven mRNAs the T-Helper cells use to produce the HIV-1 proteins in the HXB2 strain, we extract the information shown in Figures 56 and 57.

---

[26] See, for example, the Homo Sapiens ACTN3 gene at NCBI reference sequence NM_001104.

[27] Landmarks of the HIV-1 genome, HXB2 strain which can be found at http://www.hiv.lanl.gov/content/sequence/HIV/MAP/landmark.html

Figure 56 shows that all seven of the mRNA start with the 'g' in position 456 and end with the 'a' in position 9719. That is, they all have the same initial set of code and the same tail. All but the first mRNA undergo significant splicing. For mRNAs two through seven, the initial set of code ends at the 'g' nucleotide in position 743. The code spliced out varies with the protein to be translated. Tat and Rev undergo additional splicing. The translation of Nef follows that of Env in mRNA 7.

```
1a g------------ Gag Group ------------------------------------------------a
1b g-------------------------------- Pol Group ------------------------------a

2  g--------g   Spliced Out      --------------- Vif -------------------------a

3  g--------g   Spliced Out        --------------- Vpr -----------------------a

4  g--------g   Spliced Out          --------------- Tat 1 ------- Tat2 ------a

5  g--------g   Spliced Out             ------------- Rev1 ------- Rev2 ------a

6  g--------g   Spliced Out               --------------- Vpu ---------------a

7  g--------g   Spliced Out                 --------------- Env -------Nef----a
   ↑456  ↑743                |<  Various  >|                             9719↑
```

Figure 56

Overview of HIV-1 HXB2 mRNAs.

Figures 57 and 58 show the stop codons used to end the translation of each of the genes along with their locations. Also shown for the mRNAs that have undergone splicing are the locations where the code is reattached to enable translation of each protein along with its start codon and the location of the start codon.

Figure 57 shows the data for the first mRNA. There are two possibilities in the translation of the code in the first mRNA depending on the location at which the reading begins. One position resulting in the translation of the gag group of genes and the other in the translation of the pol group of genes. As indicated in the figure, there are no stop codons internal to the gag complex of genes. This is also true of the pol group.

The gag group ends with a TAA (UAA) stop codon at 2292 with a TAG (UAG) following one codon later. This is the same code reuse observation discussed with the lactose operon above.

The translation of the pol group ends in a TAG (UAG) codon at 5096.

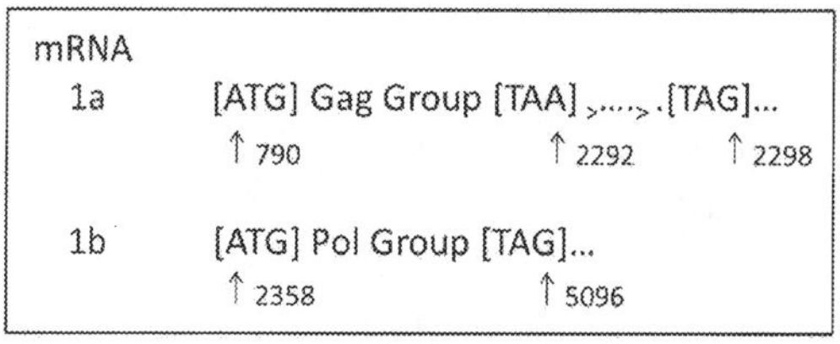

mRNA
1a [ATG] Gag Group [TAA] >....> .[TAG]...
↑ 790 ↑ 2292 ↑ 2298

1b [ATG] Pol Group [TAG]...
↑ 2358 ↑ 5096

Figure 57
Data for mRNA 1.

Figure 58 shows the data for mRNAs two through six. These mRNAs each contain code for a single protein as indicated. They all end with the UAG (TAG) stop codon. Tat and Rev are both further spliced as shown.

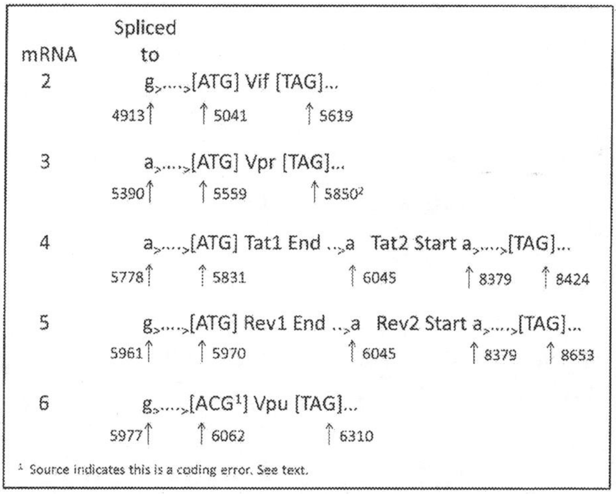

mRNA / Spliced to

2 g>....>[ATG] Vif [TAG]...
4913↑ ↑ 5041 ↑ 5619

3 a>....>[ATG] Vpr [TAG]...
5390↑ ↑ 5559 ↑ 5850[2]

4 a>....>[ATG] Tat1 End ..>a Tat2 Start a>....>[TAG]...
5778↑ ↑ 5831 ↑ 6045 ↑ 8379 ↑ 8424

5 g>....>[ATG] Rev1 End ..>a Rev2 Start a>....>[TAG]...
5961↑ ↑ 5970 ↑ 6045 ↑ 8379 ↑ 8653

6 g>....>[ACG[1]] Vpu [TAG]...
5977↑ ↑ 6062 ↑ 6310

[1] Source indicates this is a coding error. See text.

Figure 58
Data for mRNAs 2 through 6.

Figure 59 shows the processing of the Env and Nef proteins. What is interesting here is that the Env code ends with a TAA (UAA) stop codon at 8795 which, according to our observations above, instructs the reader to end the emerging protein and continue to the next start codon. The next start codon is located two nucleotides later at 8797. It is the start codon for the Nef protein. The code for the Nef protein ends with a TGA stop codon at 9417.

Why a TGA stop codon? A better question might be - Why does Nature bother to use TAG stop codons in a virus that is probably going the kill the host cell before the mRNAs wear out? Both questions are beyond the scope of this effort.

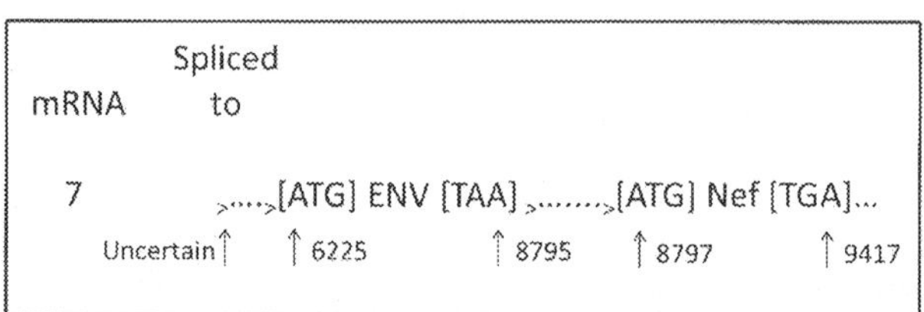

Figure 59
Data for mRNA 7.

Observations and Rational

Although admittedly the size of our data set is as yet small, it contains some interesting points. Let's look at them.

Observation 1: The TAA stop codon.

Rational: The TAA command has two parts. It directs the processor to end the current protein and read on to the next Start codon. It appears in all three domains.

Observation 2: While a stop codon is needed to direct the processor to disassemble after ending the last protein in the mRNA, there exist two additional stop codons.

Rational 2: This is a two-part rational:

1. There is another task that the processor needs to do in eukaryotic cells. The mRNA is a template and it has a predicted lifetime. That is, as the mRNA is read there needs to be an accounting of its use so that it is not used beyond its predicted lifetime which might results in the production of error filled proteins. Nature

is well aware of this lifetime. The question is 'How does Nature ensure that the mRNAs are not used beyond their lifetimes? 'There are two ways to do this, one based on time and a second based on actual usage.

The literature does not contain information on a time-stamp being placed on mRNAs when they are created, but it does provide information on a potential usage strategy. That is, when mRNAs are created in eukaryotic cells, a Poly-A tail (Tourriere) is attached to its 3' end. Poyaderation places a sequence of 250 adenine nucleic acids (As) at a location at the 3' end (Wahle). These acids are removed by a deadenylation process do to some signal (Hoshino). As the mRNA is used the Poly(A) tail is shortened. When the tail becomes shorter than a specific length, it becomes a signal that specifies that the mRNA must be destroyed.

What provides the signal telling the deadenylation process to trim the mRNA's tail? The only entity that knows a reading of the mRNA has been made is the ribosome reader. Thus, it seems that the stop command used in the eukaryotic cells, the TAG (UAG), provides that signal. That is, when a TAG codon is reached by the ribosome reader, the codon is interpreted by the reader to provide, in addition to instructions to end the protein and disassemble, a third instruction. This third instruction is to provide a signal to a specific molecule, or set of molecules, to reduce the mRNA's Poly(A) tail by one or more As. This also appears to be a necessary step in the cellular command and control process.

2. In prokaryotic cells the Poly(A) tail is attached to mRNAs for a different reason. It is a signal to destroy the mRNA. Thus, while the TGA stop codon might be made to work in eukaryotic type of cells, it seems more appropriate to use a different codon to prevent having to always check to ensure that the instructions are still appropriate every time changes are made to the DNA code. Thus, the use of the stop codon TAG.

Other Observations

The material for this study was specifically selected from three different entities with nothing in common, but the fact that all have DNA and molecules derived from them, and that all use the same nucleic and amino acids. It is striking that all entities operate the same at least as far as the currently available data permitted the study to go. Additional results, for or against the hypothesis, will be provided as new data becomes available.

The TAA followed by the TGA or TAG seems consistent with reusing code - inserting code from an outside source without change. In this case, not changing code that works, but putting a hard stop after the code to force the ribosome reader to disassemble.

It is interesting to look at the problem from two different ends: from an observer's point of view and from a needs point of view. An observer discovers three stop codons and sees three operations. Nature, looking at the requirements, sees three sets of functions and creates three stop codons.

References

Beelman, C., et al., Degradation of mRNA in eukaryotes, Cell, 4-21-1995.

Hoshino, S., et al., the Eukaryotic Polypepide Chain Releasing Factor (eRF3/GSPT) Carrying the Translation termination Signal to the 3'-Poly(A) Tail of mRNA. Direct Association of eRF3/GSPT With POLYADENYLATE-Binding Protein, J Bio Chem, 274, 16677-16680, 1999.

Tourriere, H., et al., mRNA degradation machines in eukaryotic cells, Biochimie, 2002.

Wahle, E., Poly(A) Tail Length control Is Caused by Termination of Processive Synthesis, Journal of Biological Chemistry, 1995.

APPENDIX THREE

PROTEIN BUILDING INSTRUCTIONS EMBEDDED IN THE AMINO ACID CODON CODE

Introduction

One of the most intriguing mysteries of molecular biology is the fact that there exist sixty-four codons used to identify twenty amino acids, and the three STOP codons. Given there are 20 differing recognized amino acids, a cursory view of the subject would suggest there should be only 23 differing codons with twenty codons coding for the 20 amino acids and three STOP codons. Therefore, 41 of the 64 codons should be nonfunctional. Nature tends to contrive systems that conserve energy requirements to produce the most efficient processes. Redundancy tends to occur only when there is a clear advantage to survivability of the life form that has been created. The most efficient approach to labeling the amino acids would have been to assign only one codon to identify one specific amino acid. Such an approach would have created the most precise means of identifying to the cell machinery the code to generate proteins by stringing together amino acid molecules. Excluding the three STOP codons, there are 61 differing codons that are used to identify the 21 amino acids. There exist three STOP codons due to each STOP codon represents a different STOP function when read by the ribosomes.

The key point in deciphering the reason behind why 64 codon codes exist rather than 23 codon codes directs attention to how the amino acid molecules are attached to a fledgling protein. The purpose of the codon code may be in identifying the spatial position of the amino acid as the amino acid is bonded to the protein molecule's amino acid chain.

Observation of how proteins are created as three-dimensional objects, that the functionality of many proteins is dependent of the spatial orientation of the amino acids comprising the protein. Many protein-protein interactions function as a lock-and-key mechanism. Lock-and-key protein interactions refer to one protein inserting a specific portion of the molecule into the binding site of a second protein. The inserting of a portion of one protein molecule into another protein molecule acts to (1) bond the two proteins together or (2) in the case of receptors or enzymes, causes a physical action or a chemical reaction to take place. The specifics of the three-dimensional design of a protein act to either create a successful protein that is able to properly participate in a lock-and-key process. The successful design of a protein is dependent upon the amino acids being positions in space.

The basic equation of an amino acid is HN2-CHR-COOH. When one amino acid is attached to another amino acid position of the side chain (R) of the amino acids dictates the functional position of the amino acid. Some of the amino acids reach out their side chain (R) to bond to either other nucleotides in a separate protein molecule or to a nucleotide comprising a segment of DNA or an RNA. With respect to molecular architecture, both the type and position of an amino acid's side chain can influence bending and folding parameters of a protein's structure, in both positive and negative ways.

In Table 15 the Amino Acid are listed using IUPAC notation, with the name of each of the twenty-one amino acids in the left column. The three-letter abbreviation and the one letter abbreviation for the amino acids are listed in the adjacent columns. In the right most column of Table 15 are listed the DNA Nucleotide Codes as described by convention. Note, T (thymine) can be swapped out for U (uracil) when discussing the actual construct of an mRNA molecule.

The column listing the DNA Nucleotide Codes demonstrates: (1) three amino acids have six different codons, (2) five amino acids have four different codons, (3) one amino acid has three different codons, (4) nine amino acids have two different codons and two amino acids have one differing codon. Given the sixty-four possible combinations all amino acid codons described above are represented by a different three letter combination of nucleotides. The only codon that is used twice is the unique situation where the codon 'ATG' represents both the amino acid molecule 'methionine' but 'ATG' also represents the 'START' codon for purposes of transcription.

Review of the right most column of Table 15 demonstrates that other than the three amino acids of Arginine, Leucine and Serine which have six codons, the codons of the remaining amino acids have two of the three nucleotides are the same.

Further study of the codons shows that the three amino acids which have six different codons and the five amino acids which have four different codons contain a series of four codons where two of the nucleotides are the same and in each of the four one nucleotide represents either an A, C, G or T.

Regarding the nine amino acids that have two different codons review of the codons demonstrate that two letters are the first to nucleotides are the same for the amino acid the third nucleotide is either an 'A' or a 'G' or the third nucleotide is either an 'C' or a 'T'.

Amino Acid	Three Letter Abbreviation	One Letter Abbreviation	DNA Nucleotide Codes
Alanine	Ala	A	GC**A** GC**C** GC**G** GC**T**
Arginine	Arg	R	CG**A** CG**C** CG**G** CG**T** AGA, AGG
Asparagine	Asn	N	AA**C** AA**T**
Aspartic acid	Asp	D	GA**C** GA**T**
Cysteine	Cys	C	TG**C** TG**T**

Glutamine	Gln	Q	CA**A** CA**G**
Glutamic acid	Glu	E	GA**A** GA**G**
Glycine	Gly	G	GG**A** GG**C** GG**G** GG**T**
Histidine	His	H	CA**C** CA**T**
Isoleucine	Ile	I	AT**A** AT**C** AT**T**
Leucine	Leu	L	CT**A** CT**C** CT**G** CT**T** TTA, TTG
Lysine	Lys	K	AA**A** AA**G**
Methionine	Met	M	ATG
Phenylalanine	Phe	F	TT**C** TT**T**
Proline	Pro	P	CC**A** CC**C** CC**G** CC**T**
Serine	Ser	S	TC**A** TC**C** TC**G** TC**T** AGT, AGC
Threonine	Thr	T	AC**A** AC**T** AC**C** AC**G**
Tryptophan	Typ	W	TGG
Tyrosine	Tyr	Y	TA**C** TA**T**

Valine	Val	V	GT**A** GT**C** GT**G** GT**T**
START	---	---	ATG
STOP	---	---	TAA, TGA, TAG

Table 15

Amino Acid table using IUPAC notation.

If randomness was the basis of the design criteria, as suggested by the concept of Evolution, then there should be no order to the arrangement of the triplicate coding assignments to the amino acids. The fact that there is a consistent order, suggests reason and intent for the assignments of the triplicate codon codes to the twenty amino acids.

From a molecular design perspective, the four differing 'third' nucleotides in the codon code might dictate position of the side chain of the amino acid as the amino acid is attached to the protein's amino acid chain. A circle is 360 degrees in circumference. In essence an amino acid being attached to an amino acid chain can be attached to that amino acid chain with its side chain positioned anywhere in the 360 circumference about the axis of the protein molecule being built. Where an amino acid has assigned at least four codon codes, the codon codes have four differing nucleotides (the third nucleotide), the existence of these four codes may divide the circumference of a circle into four 90-degree quadrants surrounding the axis of the molecule. Such a coding system would dictate how proteins would be configured in relation to the position of the side chains of the amino acids comprising their structures. Position of an amino acid side chain would influence folding of the overall molecule and/or bonding capacity of the finished molecule. Where the codon code has only two assigned codons for an amino acid, the two codon codes may divide the circumference of the circle into 180 degrees about the axis of the molecule; that is binding the amino acid with its associated side chain R in one of two choices such as either the side chain is positioned right-handed or left-handed or the position of the side chain is positioned either top or bottom in relation to the axis of the molecule being constructed.

The amino acids with three, four and six codon codes assigned to them, are amino acids that have the smaller side chains. The smaller side chains are most likely amendable to positioning in quadrants around the circumference of the axis of the molecule. The amino acids with large side chains, most likely contain side chains of such a size that the end of the side chain moves so freely in space that it is only necessary to distinguish the position of the side chain in a range of a 180-degree sweep about the axis of the molecule. If such a format is true, this is a clever coding system to dictate the internal architecture of protein molecules.

As illustrated in Figure 60, some form of code must exist to set the R-side chain alignment of the amino acid being added to the existing chain in relation to the amino acids that are already present comprising the protein under construction.

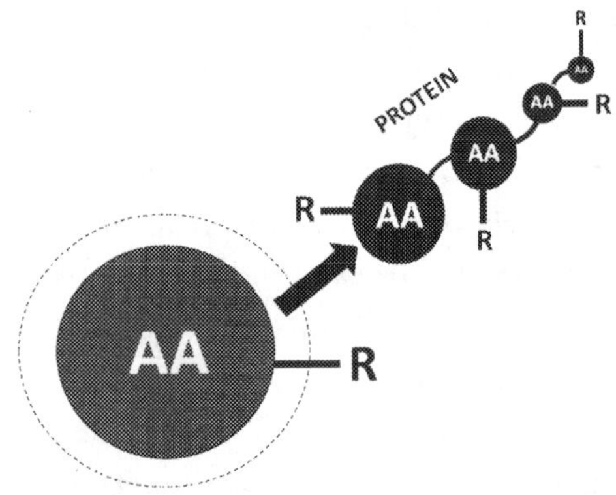

Figure 60
Amino acid to being added to a protein chain.

As seen in Figure 61, one of the nucleotides comprising the codon code may act as a means of defining the orientation of the R-side chain of the amino acid being attached as the amino acid is bound to the protein under construction.

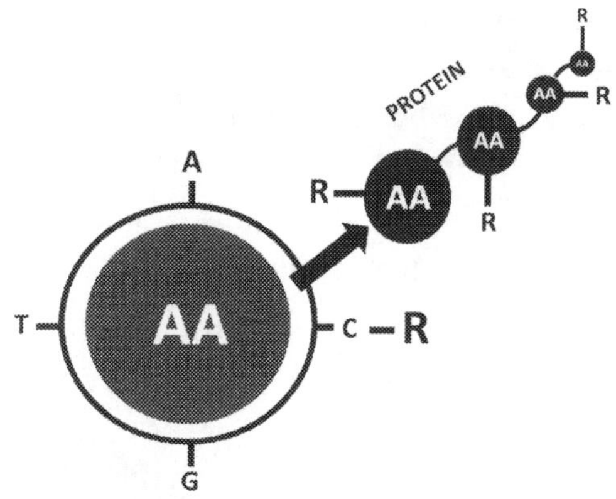

Figure 61
Codon code used to assign orientation of the R-side chain of an amino acid.

As illustrated in Figure 62, the amino acids in one of the three codons may be assigned distinct degrees of orientation so that the R-side chain of an amino acid being added to a protein under construction will be oriented properly in relation to the amino acids already comprising the protein. Such precise orientation of the R-side chain of an amino acid facilitates folding of the protein and exposes potential bonding sites of the protein.

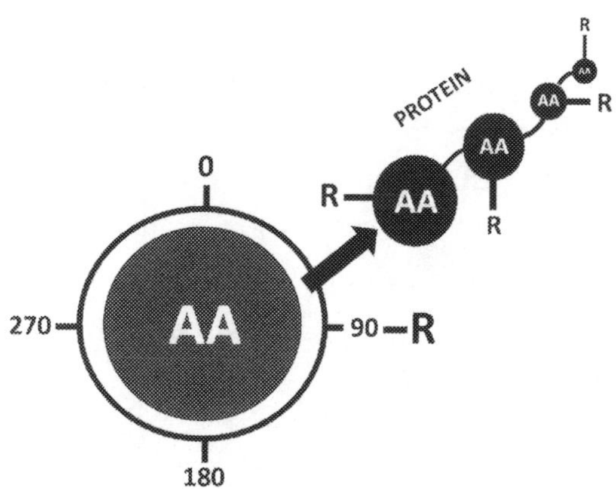

Figure 62
Distinct degrees of orientation assigned to a nucleic acid in the codon code.

Below, Figure 63, shows the four possible attachments at 0, 90, 180, and 270 degrees, marked as A, C, G, and T respectfully. This correlates with the four versions of the codon code associated with the amino acid alanine. Likely the third letter of the three letter codon code indicates to the ribosome which angle in relation to the primary axis of the protein to mount the R side chain of the alanine amino acid.

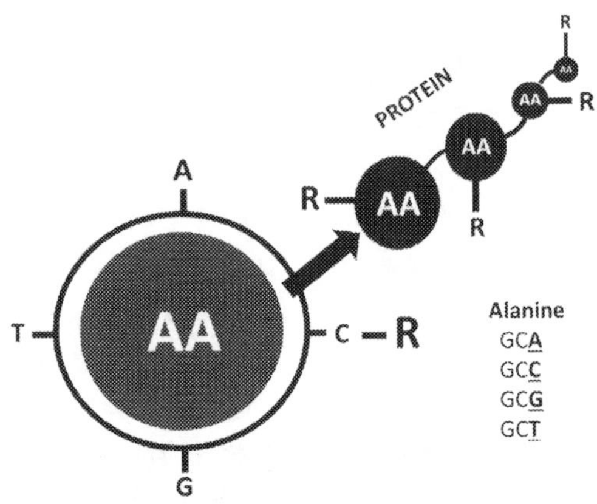

Figure 63
Distinct degrees of orientation assigned to a nucleic acid in the codon code.

The design secrets of creating the bends and folds in the special three-dimensional structure of a protein may be as simple as deciphering the intent of the amino acid codon code. The codon code may act in the dual function of identifying both which amino acid to add to a protein chain as well as the spatial orientation the amino acid should have in relation to the primary axis of the protein as the amino acid is added to the protein molecule.

APPENDIX FOUR

NCBI TRANSCRIPTION FACTOR IIIA MRNA AS OF 16 JUNE 2020

Introduction

As technology progresses, the understanding of the DNA and RNA continue to widen in scope. As of June 16, 2020, the mRNA for Transcription Factor IIIA (GTF3A) taxon:9606 is presented below. The information was obtained from the following website: https://www.ncbi.nlm.nih.gov/nuccore/1519315333.

Would like to celebrate and honor the hard work and dedication of the many researchers whose efforts made accessing this information on the NCBI website possible, so that the study and understanding of human genetics could advance toward a cure for a variety of challenging diseases.

Homo sapiens general transcription factor IIIA (GTF3A), mRNA

```
NCBI Reference Sequence: NM _002097.3

FASTA Graphics
Go to:

LOCUS         NM _002097 1443 bp mRNA linear PRI 16-JUN-2020
DEFINITION    Homo sapiens general transcription factor IIIA
              (GTF3A), mRNA.
ACCESSION     NM _002097 XM _001715623 XM _001716951 XM _001717641
VERSION       NM _002097.3
KEYWORDS      RefSeq; RefSeq Select.
```

```
SOURCE      Homo sapiens (human)
  ORGANISM  Homo sapiens
            Eukaryota; Metazoa; Chordata; Craniata; Vertebrata;
            Euteleostomi; Mammalia; Eutheria; Euarchontoglires;
            Primates; Haplorrhini; Catarrhini; Hominidae; Homo.
REFERENCE   1 (bases 1 to 1443)
AUTHORS     Sloan KE, Bohnsack MT and Watkins NJ.
TITLE       The 5S RNP couples p53 homeostasis to ribosome
            biogenesis and nucleolar stress
JOURNAL     Cell Rep 5 (1), 237-247 (2013)
PUBMED      24120868
REFERENCE   2 (bases 1 to 1443)
AUTHORS     Speliotes EK, Willer CJ, Berndt SI, Monda KL,
            Thorleifsson G, Jackson AU, Lango Allen H, Lindgren
            CM, Luan J, Magi R, Randall JC, Vedantam S, Winkler
            TW, Qi L, Workalemahu T, Heid IM, Steinthorsdottir
            V, Stringham HM, Weedon MN, Wheeler E, Wood AR,
            Ferreira T, Weyant RJ, Segre AV, Estrada K, Liang
            L, Nemesh J, Park JH, Gustafsson S, Kilpelainen TO,
            Yang J, Bouatia-Naji N, Esko T, Feitosa MF, Kutalik
            Z, Mangino M, Raychaudhuri S, Scherag A, Smith AV,
            Welch R, Zhao JH, Aben KK, Absher DM, Amin N, Dixon
            AL, Fisher E, Glazer NL, Goddard ME, Heard-Costa
            NL, Hoesel V, Hottenga JJ, Johansson A, Johnson
            T, Ketkar S, Lamina C, Li S, Moffatt MF, Myers RH,
            Narisu N, Perry JR, Peters MJ, Preuss M, Ripatti
            S, Rivadeneira F, Sandholt C, Scott LJ, Timpson NJ,
            Tyrer JP, van Wingerden S, Watanabe RM, White CC,
            Wiklund F, Barlassina C, Chasman DI, Cooper MN,
            Jansson JO, Lawrence RW, Pellikka N, Prokopenko I,
            Shi J, Thiering E, Alavere H, Alibrandi MT, Almgren
            P, Arnold AM, Aspelund T, Atwood LD, Balkau B,
            Balmforth AJ, Bennett AJ, Ben-Shlomo Y, Bergman RN,
            Bergmann S, Biebermann H, Blakemore AI, Boes T,
            Bonnycastle LL, Bornstein SR, Brown MJ, Buchanan TA,
            Busonero F, Campbell H, Cappuccio FP, Cavalcanti-
            Proenca C, Chen YD, Chen CM, Chines PS, Clarke R,
            Coin L, Connell J, Day IN, den Heijer M, Duan J,
            Ebrahim S, Elliott P, Elosua R, Eiriksdottir G, Erdos
            MR, Eriksson JG, Facheris MF, Felix SB, Fischer-
            Posovszky P, Folsom AR, Friedrich N, Freimer NB, Fu
            M, Gaget S, Gejman PV, Geus EJ, Gieger C, Gjesing AP,
            Goel A, Goyette P, Grallert H, Grassler J, Greenawalt
            DM, Groves CJ, Gudnason V, Guiducci C, Hartikainen
            AL, Hassanali N, Hall AS, Havulinna AS, Hayward C,
            Heath AC, Hengstenberg C, Hicks AA, Hinney A, Hofman
            A, Homuth G, Hui J, Igl W, Iribarren C, Isomaa B,
            Jacobs KB, Jarick I, Jewell E, John U, Jorgensen
            T, Jousilahti P, Jula A, Kaakinen M, Kajantie E,
            Kaplan LM, Kathiresan S, Kettunen J, Kinnunen L,
            Knowles JW, Kolcic I, Konig IR, Koskinen S, Kovacs P,
            Kuusisto J, Kraft P, Kvaloy K, Laitinen J, Lantieri
            O, Lanzani C, Launer LJ, Lecoeur C, Lehtimaki T,
```

Lettre G, Liu J, Lokki ML, Lorentzon M, Luben RN, Ludwig B, Manunta P, Marek D, Marre M, Martin NG, McArdle WL, McCarthy A, McKnight B, Meitinger T, Melander O, Meyre D, Midthjell K, Montgomery GW, Morken MA, Morris AP, Mulic R, Ngwa JS, Nelis M, Neville MJ, Nyholt DR, O'Donnell CJ, O'Rahilly S, Ong KK, Oostra B, Pare G, Parker AN, Perola M, Pichler I, Pietilainen KH, Platou CG, Polasek O, Pouta A, Rafelt S, Raitakari O, Rayner NW, Ridderstrale M, Rief W, Ruokonen A, Robertson NR, Rzehak P, Salomaa V, Sanders AR, Sandhu MS, Sanna S, Saramies J, Savolainen MJ, Scherag S, Schipf S, Schreiber S, Schunkert H, Silander K, Sinisalo J, Siscovick DS, Smit JH, Soranzo N, Sovio U, Stephens J, Surakka I, Swift AJ, Tammesoo ML, Tardif JC, Teder-Laving M, Teslovich TM, Thompson JR, Thomson B, Tonjes A, Tuomi T, van Meurs JB, van Ommen GJ, Vatin V, Viikari J, Visvikis-Siest S, Vitart V, Vogel CI, Voight BF, Waite LL, Wallaschofski H, Walters GB, Widen E, Wiegand S, Wild SH, Willemsen G, Witte DR, Witteman JC, Xu J, Zhang Q, Zgaga L, Ziegler A, Zitting P, Beilby JP, Farooqi IS, Hebebrand J, Huikuri HV, James AL, Kahonen M, Levinson DF, Macciardi F, Nieminen MS, Ohlsson C, Palmer LJ, Ridker PM, Stumvoll M, Beckmann JS, Boeing H, Boerwinkle E, Boomsma DI, Caulfield MJ, Chanock SJ, Collins FS, Cupples LA, Smith GD, Erdmann J, Froguel P, Gronberg H, Gyllensten U, Hall P, Hansen T, Harris TB, Hattersley AT, Hayes RB, Heinrich J, Hu FB, Hveem K, Illig T, Jarvelin MR, Kaprio J, Karpe F, Khaw KT, Kiemeney LA, Krude H, Laakso M, Lawlor DA, Metspalu A, Munroe PB, Ouwehand WH, Pedersen O, Penninx BW, Peters A, Pramstaller PP, Quertermous T, Reinehr T, Rissanen A, Rudan I, Samani NJ, Schwarz PE, Shuldiner AR, Spector TD, Tuomilehto J, Uda M, Uitterlinden A, Valle TT, Wabitsch M, Waeber G, Wareham NJ, Watkins H, Wilson JF, Wright AF, Zillikens MC, Chatterjee N, McCarroll SA, Purcell S, Schadt EE, Visscher PM, Assimes TL, Borecki IB, Deloukas P, Fox CS, Groop LC, Haritunians T, Hunter DJ, Kaplan RC, Mohlke KL, O'Connell JR, Peltonen L, Schlessinger D, Strachan DP, van Duijn CM, Wichmann HE, Frayling TM, Thorsteinsdottir U, Abecasis GR, Barroso I, Boehnke M, Stefansson K, North KE, McCarthy MI, Hirschhorn JN, Ingelsson E and Loos RJ.

CONSRTM MAGIC; Procardis Consortium
TITLE Association analyses of 249,796 individuals reveal 18 new loci associated with body mass index
JOURNAL Nat. Genet. 42 (11), 937-948 (2010)
PUBMED 20935630
REFERENCE 3 (bases 1 to 1443)

AUTHORS Wu C, Ma MH, Brown KR, Geisler M, Li L, Tzeng E, Jia CY, Jurisica I and Li SS.

TITLE Systematic identification of SH3 domain-mediated human protein-protein interactions by peptide array target screening

JOURNAL Proteomics 7 (11), 1775-1785 (2007)

PUBMED 17474147

REFERENCE 4 (bases 1 to 1443)

AUTHORS Weser S, Riemann J, Seifart KH and Meissner W.

TITLE Assembly and isolation of intermediate steps of transcription complexes formed on the human 5S rRNA gene

JOURNAL Nucleic Acids Res. 31 (9), 2408-2416 (2003)

PUBMED 12711686

REFERENCE 5 (bases 1 to 1443)

AUTHORS Hanas JS, Hocker JR, Cheng YG, Lerner MR, Brackett DJ, Lightfoot SA, Hanas RJ, Madhusudhan KT and Moreland RJ.

TITLE cDNA cloning, DNA binding, and evolution of mammalian Transcription factor IIIA

JOURNAL Gene 282 (1-2), 43-52 (2002)

PUBMED 11814676

REFERENCE 6 (bases 1 to 1443)

AUTHORS Fridell RA, Fischer U, Luhrmann R, Meyer BE, Meinkoth JL, Malim MH and Cullen BR.

TITLE Amphibian transcription factor IIIA proteins contain a sequence element functionally equivalent to the nuclear export signal of human immunodeficiency virus type 1 Rev

JOURNAL Proc. Natl. Acad. Sci. U.S.A. 93 (7), 2936-2940 (1996)

PUBMED 8610146

REFERENCE 7 (bases 1 to 1443)

AUTHORS Drew PD, Nagle JW, Canning RD, Ozato K, Biddison WE and Becker KG.

TITLE Cloning and expression analysis of a human cDNA homologous to Xenopus TFIIIA

JOURNAL Gene 159 (2), 215-218 (1995)

PUBMED 7622052

REFERENCE 8 (bases 1 to 1443)

AUTHORS Arakawa H, Nagase H, Hayashi N, Ogawa M, Nagata M, Fujiwara T, Takahashi E, Shin S and Nakamura Y.

TITLE Molecular cloning, characterization, and chromosomal mapping of a novel human gene (GTF3A) that is highly homologous to Xenopus transcription factor IIIA

JOURNAL Cytogenet. Cell Genet. 70 (3-4), 235-238 (1995)

PUBMED 7789179

REFERENCE 9 (bases 1 to 1443)

AUTHORS Moorefield B and Roeder RG.

TITLE Purification and characterization of human transcription factor IIIA

JOURNAL J. Biol. Chem. 269 (33), 20857-20865 (1994)

PUBMED 8063702

REFERENCE 10 (bases 1 to 1443)

AUTHORS Seifart KH, Wang L, Waldschmidt R, Jahn D and Wingender E.

TITLE Purification of human transcription factor IIIA and its Interaction with a chemically synthesized gene encoding human 5 S rRNA

JOURNAL J. Biol. Chem. 264 (3), 1702-1709 (1989)

PUBMED 2912980

COMMENT REVIEWED REFSEQ: This record has been curated by NCBI staff. The reference sequence was derived from D32257.1, BP254755.1, U20272.1, AW627732.1 and AL137059.20.
On Nov 23, 2018 this sequence version replaced NM_002097.2.

Summary: The product of this gene is a zinc finger protein with nine Cis[2]-His[2] zinc finger domains. It functions as an RNA polymerase III transcription factor to induce transcription of the 5S rRNA genes. The protein binds to a 50 bp internal promoter in the 5S genes called the internal control region (ICR), and nucleates formation of a stable preinitiation complex. This complex recruits the TFIIIC and TFIIIB transcription factors and RNA polymerase III to form the complete transcription complex. The protein is thought to be translated using a non-AUG Translation initiation site in mammals based on sequence analysis, protein homology, and the size of the purified protein. [provided by RefSeq, Jul 2008].

Publication Note: This RefSeq record includes a subset of the publications that are available for this gene. Please see the Gene record to access additional publications.

```
##Evidence-Data-START##
Transcript exon combination :: SRR3476690.289034.1,
                               SRR3476690.656735.1
                               [ECO:0000332]
RNAseq introns              :: single sample
                               supports all introns
                               SAMEA1965299,
                               SAMEA1966682
                               [ECO:0000348]
##Evidence-Data-END##

##RefSeq-Attributes-START##
non-AUG initiation codon :: inferred from conservation
RefSeq Select criteria   :: based on single protein-
                            coding transcript
##RefSeq-Attributes-END##
COMPLETENESS: full length.
```

PRIMARY

REFSEQ_SPAN	PRIMARY_IDENTIFIER	PRIMARY_SPAN	COMP
1-53	D32257.1	76-128	
54-125	BP254755.1	110-181	
126-1298	U20272.1	1-1173	
1299-1329	AW627732.1	2-32	c
1330-1443	AL137059.20	102072-102185	c

```
FEATURES             Location/Qualifiers
     source          1..1443
                     /organism="Homo sapiens"
                     /mol _type="mRNA"
                     /db _xref="taxon:9606"
                     /chromosome="13"
                     /map="13q12.2"
     gene            1..1443
                     /gene="GTF3A"
                     /gene _synonym="AP2; TFIIIA"
                     /note="general transcription factor IIIA"
                     /db _xref="GeneID:2971"
                     /db _xref="HGNC:HGNC:4662"
                     /db _xref="MIM:600860"
     exon            1..320
                     /gene="GTF3A"
                     /gene _synonym="AP2; TFIIIA"
                     /inference="alignment:Splign:2.1.0"
     CDS             120..1217
                     /gene="GTF3A"
                     /gene _synonym="AP2; TFIIIA"
                     /note="non-AUG (CUG) translation initiation
                     codon"
                     /codon _start=1
                     /product="transcription factor IIIA"
                     /protein _id="NP  002088.2"
                     /db _xref="CCDS:CCDS45019.1"
                     /db _xref="GeneID:2971"
                     /db _xref="HGNC:HGNC:4662"
                     /db _xref="MIM:600860"
/translation="MDPPAVVAESVSSLTIADAFIAAGESSAPTPPRPALPRRFICSF
PDCSANYSKAWKLDAHLCKHTGERPFVCDYEGCGKAFIRDYHLSRHILTHTGEKPFVC
AANGCDQKFNTKSNLKKHFERKHENQQKQYICSFEDCKKTFKKHQQLKIHQCQHTNEP
LFKCTQEGCGKHFASPSKLKRHAKAHEGYVCQKGCSFVAKTWTELLKHVRETHKEEIL
CEVCRKTFKRKDYLKQHMKTHAPERDVCRCPREGCGRTYTTVFNLQSHILSFHEESRP
FVCEHAGCGKTFAMKQSLTRHAVVHDPDKKKMKLKVKKSREKRSLASHLSGYIPPKRK
QGQGLSLCQNGESPNCVEDKMLSTVAVLTLG"
     misc  feature   243..311
                     /gene="GTF3A"
                     /gene _synonym="AP2; TFIIIA"
                     /note="Region: zinc finger"
     misc  feature   333..401
                     /gene="GTF3A"
                     /gene _synonym="AP2; TFIIIA"
                     /note="Region: zinc finger"
     misc  feature   423..494
                     /gene="GTF3A"
                     /gene _synonym="AP2; TFIIIA"
                     /note="Region: zinc finger"
     misc  feature   519..587
                     /gene="GTF3A"
                     /gene _synonym="AP2; TFIIIA"
                     /note="Region: zinc finger"
     misc  feature   609..677
                     /gene="GTF3A"
                     /gene _synonym="AP2; TFIIIA"
                     /note="Region: zinc finger"
     misc  feature   690..758
```

```
                     /gene="GTF3A"
                     /gene _synonym="AP2; TFIIIA"
                     /note="Region: zinc finger"
     misc feature    774..836
                     /gene="GTF3A"
                     /gene _synonym="AP2; TFIIIA"
                     /note="Region: zinc finger"
     misc feature    861..932
                     /gene="GTF3A"
                     /gene _synonym="AP2; TFIIIA"
                     /note="Region: zinc finger"
     misc feature    954..1022
                     /gene="GTF3A"
                     /gene _synonym="AP2; TFIIIA"
                     /note="Region: zinc finger"
     exon            321..421
                     /gene="GTF3A"
                     /gene _synonym="AP2; TFIIIA"
                     /inference="alignment:Splign:2.1.0"
     exon            422..518
                     /gene="GTF3A"
                     /gene _synonym="AP2; TFIIIA"
                     /inference="alignment:Splign:2.1.0"
     exon            519..607
                     /gene="GTF3A"
                     /gene _synonym="AP2; TFIIIA"
                     /inference="alignment:Splign:2.1.0"
     exon            608..681
                     /gene="GTF3A"
                     /gene _synonym="AP2; TFIIIA"
                     /inference="alignment:Splign:2.1.0"
     exon            682..762
                     /gene="GTF3A"
                     /gene _synonym="AP2; TFIIIA"
                     /inference="alignment:Splign:2.1.0"
     exon            763..992
                     /gene="GTF3A"
                     /gene _synonym="AP2; TFIIIA"
                     /inference="alignment:Splign:2.1.0"
     exon            993..1052
                     /gene="GTF3A"
                     /gene _synonym="AP2; TFIIIA"
                     /inference="alignment:Splign:2.1.0"
     exon            1053..1443
                     /gene="GTF3A"
                     /gene _synonym="AP2; TFIIIA"
                     /inference="alignment:Splign:2.1.0"

ORIGIN

        1 aagtgtgccg gcgtcgcgcg aaggttcagc agggagccgt gggccgggcg cgccggttcc
       61 cggcacgtgt ctcggcacgt ggcagcgcgc ctggccctgg gcttggaggc gccggcgccc
      121 tggatccgcc ggccgtggtc gccgagtcgg tgtcgtcctt gaccatcgcc gacgcgttca
      181 ttgcagccgg cgagagctca gctccgaccc cgccgcgccc cgcgcttccc aggaggttca
      241 tctgctcctt ccctgactgc agcgccaatt acagcaaagc ctggaagctt gacgcgcacc
      301 tgtgcaagca cacgggggag agaccatttg tttgtgacta tgaagggtgt ggcaaggcct
      361 tcatcaggga ctaccatctg agccgccaca ttctgactca cacaggagaa aagccgtttg
      421 tttgtgcagc caatggctgt gatcaaaaat tcaacacaaa atcaaacttg aagaaacatt
      481 ttgaacgcaa acatgaaaat caacaaaaac aatatatatg cagttttgaa gactgtaaga
```

541 agacctttaa gaaacatcag cagctgaaaa tccatcagtg ccagcatacc aatgaacctc
601 tattcaagtg tacccaggaa ggatgtggga aacactttgc atcacccagc aagctgaaac
661 gacatgccaa ggcccacgag ggctatgtat gtcaaaaagg atgttccttt gtggcaaaaa
721 catggacgga acttctgaaa catgtgagag aaacccataa agaggaaata ctatgtgaag
781 tatgccggaa aacatttaaa cgcaaagatt accttaagca acacatgaaa actcatgccc
841 cagaaaggga tgtatgtcgc tgtccaagag aaggctgtgg aagaacctat acaactgtgt
901 ttaatctcca aagccatatc ctctccttcc atgaggaaag ccgccctttt gtgtgtgaac
961 atgctggctg tggcaaaaca tttgcaatga aacaaagtct cactaggcat gctgttgtac
1021 atgatcctga caagaagaaa atgaagctca aagtcaaaaa atctcgtgaa aaacggagtt
1081 tggcctctca tctcagtgga tatatccctc ccaaaaggaa acaagggcaa ggcttatctt
1141 tgtgtcaaaa cggagagtca cccaactgtg tggaagacaa gatgctctcg acagttgcag
1201 tacttaccct tggctaagaa ctgcactgct ttgtttaaag gactgcagac caaggagcga
1261 gctttctctc agagcatgct tttctttatt aaaattactg atgcagaaca tttgattcct
1321 tatcatttcc atggtctttg ttcaaagtgt ctctttcctg ggtctcttga gtttctttat
1381 atgccttctc ctcattttg ctgaaagcac gaagaacaca cattaaagct tttcctcctt
1441 gaa

SUMMARY OF DEVELOPMENT OF A CURE TO COMBAT COVID-19:

1. Unique RNA target: Uracil tail of the negative-sense COVID-19 genome.

2. Molecule to bind to RNA: Transcription Factor IIIA.

3. Bonding algorithm for amino acids to nucleotides: Lysine (K) binds to uracil (u).

4. Modification to bonding molecule to create a hunter-killer protein: Modifications made to TFIIIA.

5. Package hunter-killer protein: mRNA to deliver modified TFIIIA protein.

6. Delivery system: nanomicelles to deliver therapeutic mRNA to lung cells.

PARTING THOUGHT

'Humans are the only known lifeform,

capable of altering the universe...

we need to wield such power wisely.'

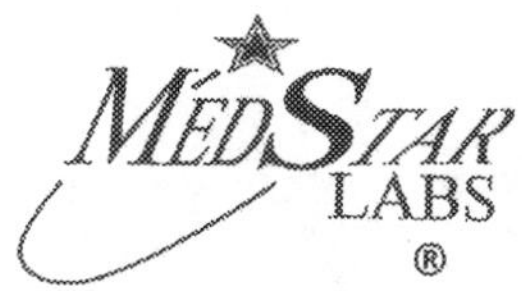

FINAL SPECULATION

Root cause analysis suggests

the Earth was seeded by a pod,

having traversed vast distance of deep space,

encapsulated in a magnetic bubble,

this precious galactic vehicle carrying

the Prime Genome genetic code and

an atmosphere activating catalyst,...

It is highly likely we are not alone

in the universe and our cousins are scattered amongst the stars.

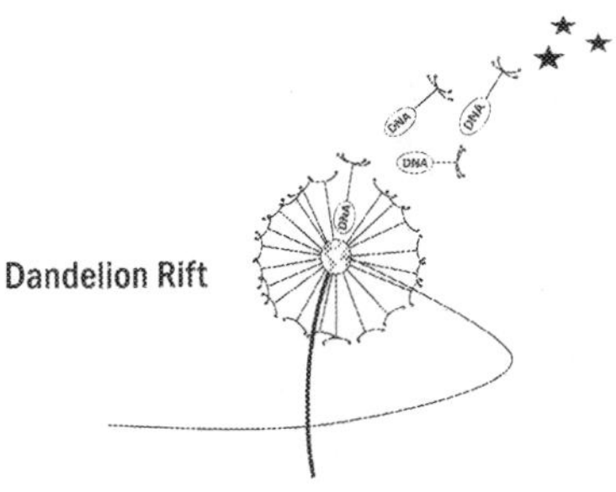

Printed in the United States
By Bookmasters